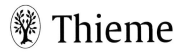

Essentials of Septorhinoplasty

Philosophy—Approaches—Techniques

Hans Behrbohm, M.D.
Professor
Department of Otorhinolaryngology
Neck and Facial Plastic Surgery
Park-Klinik Weissensee, Academic Teaching Hospital
of the Humboldt University, Charité,
Berlin, Germany

M. Eugene Tardy, Jr., M.D., FACS
Professor of Clinical Otolaryngology
Head and Neck Surgery
Division of Facial Plastic and Reconstructive Surgery
University of Illinois Medical Center at Chicago
Chicago, Illinois, USA

With contributions by:
H. Behrbohm, R.B. Capone, M. Goldstein, M. Hamilton, T. Hildebrandt, D. Jaeger, O. Kaschke, D.W. Kim, G. Mlynski,
I. Papel, S.S. Park, S. Perkins, W. Pirsig, W. Seidner, M.E. Tardy, Jr., R. Thomas, D.M. Toriumi

626 illustrations

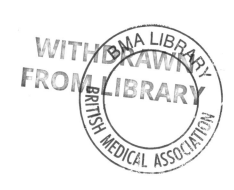

Thieme
Stuttgart · New York

Library of Congress Cataloging-in-Publication Data
is available from the publisher

Translators:
Terry C. Telger, Fort Worth, USA
Carola Wark, Cologne, Germany

Illustrator:
Robert J. Brown, Chicago, USA

Important note: Medicine is an ever-changing science undergoing continual development. Research and clinical experience are continually expanding our knowledge, in particular our knowledge of proper treatment and drug therapy. Insofar as this book mentions any dosage or application, readers may rest assured that the authors, editors, and publishers have made every effort to ensure that such references are in accordance with **the state of knowledge at the time of production of the book.**

Nevertheless, this does not involve, imply, or express any guarantee or responsibility on the part of the publishers in respect to any dosage instructions and forms of applications stated in the book. **Every user is requested to examine carefully** the manufacturers' leaflets accompanying each drug and to check, if necessary in consultation with a physician or specialist, whether the dosage schedules mentioned therein or the contraindications stated by the manufacturers differ from the statements made in the present book. Such examination is particularly important with drugs that are either rarely used or have been newly released on the market. Every dosage schedule or every form of application used is entirely at the user's own risk and responsibility. The authors and publishers request every user to report to the publishers any discrepancies or inaccuracies noticed.

Some of the product names, patents, and registered designs referred to in this book are in fact registered trademarks or proprietary names even though specific reference to this fact is not always made in the text. Therefore, the appearance of a name without designation as proprietary is not to be construed as a representation by the publisher that it is in the public domain.

© 2004 Georg Thieme Verlag,
Rüdigerstrasse 14, 70469 Stuttgart, Germany
http://www.thieme.de
Thieme New York, 333 Seventh Avenue,
New York, NY 10001 USA
http://www.thieme.com

Cover design: Martina Berge, Erbach
Typesetting by primustype Hurler GmbH, Notzingen
Printed in Germany by Druckhaus Götz, Ludwigsburg
ISBN 3-13-131911-9 (GTV)
ISBN 1-58890-208-0 (TNY)

1 2 3 4 5

Preface

Surgical refinements in rhinoplasty presage a bright future for this century-old procedure. Advances in the *science* dedicated to this procedure increasingly embellish the traditional *art* of rhinoplasty. The body of work contained in this volume, envisioned by Professor Hans Behrbohm, blends in a unique manner the inevitable intertwining of the two.

Similarly, the surgical link between aesthetic rhinoplasty and functional endoscopic sinus surgery is not well established. Patients regularly present with a combination of sinus disorders and structural nasal deformity. There is a paucity of guidelines in the medical literature on when and how to combine these two operations safely and efficiently. As far as possible the dedicated student will gain special insight into this surgical interrelationship as a consequence of the combined experience of the contributing German and American authors to this volume.

A resounding improvement in rhinoplasty outcomes in the past two decades has resulted from a profound emphasis on and understanding of detailed and specific *preoperative analysis*. Diagnostic nuances never considered in the early training of experienced surgeons now comprise a routine part of the analytic evaluation of the preoperative patient. Reliable avenues for honing these diagnostic skills can be realized by the dedicated learner: in-depth postgraduate courses, fresh cadaver dissection, the ready availability of videotaped surgery performed by master surgeons, as well as the emergence of a plethora of textbooks devoted to the subject. These opportunities expedite the learning process and provide knowledge previously available only through surgical trial and error. I am convinced, after 35 years of experience in rhinoplasty, that there does exist a universe of surgical principles that, when unveiled, respected, and embraced, can lead the rhinoplasty surgeon to predictable and favorable outcomes.

Rhinoplasty remains unique in that the preoperative planning of each procedure may be enacted with great accuracy by establishing the exact anatomy through inspection and evaluation. With precise analysis, few surprises should be encountered during the actual procedure. Yet every single rhinoplasty is a planned but uncharted adventure, in which similar but often different techniques are required to accomplish the desired outcome. As important as personal technical skill and knowledge is the surgeon's acquired ability to image the ultimate intended outcome, by blending the patient's request with what is realistically achievable given the anatomy encountered. An individual concept of what constitutes the "ideal aesthetic norm" must be developed, and then modified, to suit each patient's facial features and aesthetic needs. Thus, rhinoplasty surgeons must be flexible, nimble, and innovative, possessing knowledge of many diverse approaches and surgical techniques to successfully manage the myriad anatomic variations encountered.

That said, rhinoplasty continues to spawn far too many postoperative complications. As the dynamics of the interrelated maneuvers required in nasal surgery become more clear and surgical training improves worldwide, the number and magnitude of untoward outcomes should decline. A current factor of concern is the increasing employment of the open approach to rhinoplasty by less experienced surgeons, who apply this approach early on in the earnest hope that more extensive exposure of the entire nasal anatomy will allow enhanced surgical control of the healing process. This philosophy can too often pose an inviting snare. There is little doubt that properly employed, open rhinoplasty, *when indicated*, allows structural reorientation and rebuilding of the nasal framework in an often elegant fashion. Clearly, however, greater surgical exposure alone does not in itself translate into a better result. Failure to properly understand and execute sophisticated rhinoplasty refinement is not overcome by an open exposure. More difficult surgical revisions are thus being witnessed. A plea is made for all surgeons passionate about rhinoplasty to master the refinements of *both* endonasal and external rhinoplasty, and to *select the preferred approach based on the anatomy encountered,* not on false bias, for a particular operation.

This volume provides a unique insight into the personal philosophies and surgical techniques of rhinoplasty experts from both Germany and the United States. Hans Behrbohm has assembled colleagues with unique perspectives and experience, and on behalf of the American authors gratitude is offered for the opportunity to share philosophies with distinguished colleagues about a unique operation. The artful and distinctive illustrations of the renowned artist Robert Brown bring these philosophies to life in an exciting manner.

Finally, to Stephan Konnry and his colleagues at Thieme International, a salute is due for the dedication, organizational skills, and editorial expertise that shepherded this textbook throughout its developmental process.

Chicago, Summer 2003   *M. Eugene Tardy, Jr.*

Preface

The publication of this book coincides with a very special anniversary. Exactly 100 years ago, the first functional–aesthetic rhinoplasty was performed by Jacques Joseph in Berlin. One year later he published his technique for the removal of nasal humps with a simultaneous straightening of the septum through an intranasal approach.

My occupation with the diseases and variations in form of the nose began approximately 80 years later while I was studying to become an ear, nose, and throat specialist at the Charité Hospital in Berlin. Later, as head of the Department of Rhinology, the inseparable interrelation between clinically relevant malfunctions of the nose and outer structural defects became more and more obvious.

Working from an almost exclusively function-oriented point of view, I found myself increasingly endeavoring to combine elements of aesthetic and reconstructive surgery into one concept, in order to accommodate the dual character of rhinoplasty.

I received the crucial impulses and ideas in this field from Professor M. Eugene Tardy, Jr. in Chicago. Besides surgical details, I was much influenced by his philosophy of precise anatomical analysis of an individual problem and its structure-preserving correction, taking into account individual characteristics of various tissues, while aiming for a natural and stable long-term result. M. Eugene Tardy, Jr. has decisively influenced the scientific standard and operating technique of surgery of the nose in the past decades.

The achievement of this mutual project, which resulted from an encounter in the summer of 2001 in Chicago, fills me with gratefulness and pride and creates a bond between the master and one of his pupils. This book condenses the treasure of experience of outstanding experts in the field of rhinoplasty, rhinology, and related fields, building a bridge of expertise across the Atlantic.

For me, the chance to put this book together was like my own personal American dream, a sophisticated project made possible by the spontaneous cooperation of the copublisher and the authors' valuable contributions. This book would not have been possible without them and I thank them most sincerely. For the excellent graphics in the entire book I would like to thank Mr Robert Brown (Chicago). I also thank the sponsors, without whom these graphic presentations would have been impossible, for supporting the project, especially Ms Sybill Storz (Karl Storz GmbH), Mr. Kramer (Aventis), and Ms Kutschera (Alcon).

I would like to extend a hearty thanks to the administration and hospital management of the Park-Klinik Weissensee and Schlosspark-Klinik, represented by Professor J Baumgarten, for the continual and extensive support of this project.

Thanks also at this time to Ms Kathi Ratz for her significant contribution to photo documentation and archive work.

Mr Stephan Konnry from Thieme International played a substantial part in realizing the project on schedule. He was always the motor and coordinator between the publishers, authors, and publishing company.

Finally, I would like to thank all patients who willingly provided permission for their photographs to be published.

Berlin, June 2003   Hans Behrbohm

Contributors' Addresses:

Hans Behrbohm, M.D.
Professor
Department of Otorhinolaryngology
Neck and Facial Plastic Surgery
Park-Klinik Weissensee,
Academic Teaching Hospital of the Humboldt University,
Charité, Berlin, Germany
behrbohm@park-klinik.com
Institute of medical development
and further education Berlin e.V.

Randolph B. Capone, M.D.
Department of Otolaryngology
Head and Neck Surgery
The John Hopkins University School of Medicine
Baltimore, Maryland, USA

Michael Goldstein, M.D.
Chairman
Department of Anesthesiology
Park-Klinik Weissensee,
Academic Teaching Hospital of the Humboldt University,
Berlin, Germany

Mark Hamilton, M.D.
Meridian Plastic Surgery Center
Indianapolis, Indiana, USA

Thomas Hildebrandt
Clinic for Rhinologic Surgery
Medical Center
Berlin, Germany

Dieter Jaeger
Potsdam, Germany

Oliver Kaschke, M.D.
Professor
Department of Otorhinolaryngology
Neck and Facial Plastic Surgery
Sankt Gertrauden-Krankenhaus,
Academic Teaching Hospital of the Humboldt University,
Berlin, Germany
Institute of medical development
and further education Berlin e.V.

David W. Kim, M.D.
Assistant Professor
Division of Facial Plastic and Reconstructive Surgery
Department of Otolaryngology
Head and Neck Surgery
University of California
San Francisco, California, USA

Gunter Mlynski, M.D.
Professor
Department of Otorhinolaryngology
Ernst-Moritz-Arndt-Universität Greifswald
Greifswald, Germany

Ira Papel, M.D.
Facial Plastic Surgicenter, Ltd.
Owings Mills, Maryland, USA

Stephen S. Park, M.D.
Department. of Otolaryngology
Charlottesville, Virginia
USA

Steve Perkins, M.D.
Meridian Plastic Surgery Center
Indianapolis, Indiana, USA

Wolfgang Pirsig, M.D.
Professor
Department of Otorhinolaryngology
Ulm University ENT Clinic
Ulm, Germany

Wolfram Seidner, M.D.
Professor
Chairman, Department of Phoniatrics and Pediatric Audiology
Medical Faculty, Humboldt University
Charité University Clinic
ENT Clinic
Berlin, Germany

M. Eugene Tardy, Jr., M.D., FACS
Professor of Clinical Otolaryngology
Head and Neck Surgery
Division of Facial Plastic and Reconstructive Surgery
University of Illinois Medical Center at Chicago
Chicago, Illinois, USA
GTardy@aol.com

Regan Thomas, M.D.
Chairman, Department of Otolaryngology
University of Illinois
Chicago, Illinois, USA

Dean Toriumi, M.D.
Deparment of Otolaryngology
Head and Neck Surgery
University of Illinois Medical Center at Chicago
Chicago, Illinois, USA

Contents

12 The Saddle Nose—Causes and Pathogenesis, Approaches and Operative Techniques, Principles of Tissue Replacement in the Nose 201

H. Behrbohm

13 Nasal Trauma 219

O. Kaschke

14 Postoperative Care and Management 233

O. Kaschke

Index 243

1 The Dual Character of Nasal Surgery

H. Behrbohm

Contents

Introduction

Young sailors in the International Optimist class trim their sails with the help of a tensioning pole called a sprit. The stronger the wind, the more tightly the sprit is set. The lower the tension on the sprit, the more the sail will billow open. This change in the shape of the sail is clearly reflected in the adjacent top triangles.

A similar mechanism is at work in the nose. The height and tension of the anterior septum significantly affect the aperture angle of the nasal valve and the tension and shape of the tip and supratip area.

The goal of any structure-conserving surgery of the nose, as in the sprit sail, is to change the shape of the internal and external nose by altering the tension and traction on specific structural elements (Fig. 1.**1**).

The nose performs a variety of functions. It is a respiratory and sensory organ and has a special esthetic importance as a central feature of the face. It is a reflex organ and adds resonance to phonation. The functional and esthetic aspects of the nose are inseparably linked in a morphological sense. It is our experience that functional and esthetic problems of the nose almost always coincide. Rhinosurgery aimed exclusively at improving function will very quickly reach its limits if it disregards external form. This is clearly illustrated by the "tension nose," deviated nose, and saddle nose.

Conversely, rhinosurgery that is done purely for esthetic goals forfeits valuable opportunities, as in cases where the impact of septal surgery on nasal tip esthetics is not utilized to modify tip definition, projection, and rotation (9, 46).

Goldman found that in more than 70% of his cases, the presence of septal deviation coexisted with a deformity of the external nose (31). Meyer performed a concomitant septoplasty in 80% of his primary and secondary rhinoplasties (80). Masing explained the importance of external nasal shape in respiratory function by noting the smaller cross-sectional areas of the external nose compared with the internal nose (79).

Farrior states that surgical correction of the external nose is often the prerequisite for normal, unobstructed nasal breathing (29). Our own experience confirms the results of Schulz-Coulon, (116), who addressed the question of whether rhinoplasty is a predominantly esthetic or functional procedure. When statistical analysis was applied based on patients' motivations for surgery and their satisfaction or dissatisfaction with the outcome, this question could not be answered in terms of a predominantly esthetic or functional operation. This led the author to agree with Haas that both terms should be discarded in favor of the more accurate term, *corrective rhinoplasty* (38, 116).

But the concept of functionality does not apply just to the improvement of nasal breathing. It includes the following aspects as well:

- Peripheral olfactory disturbances
- Recurrent and chronic sinusitis
- Middle ear ventilation problems
- Rhinogenic headache
- Poor vocal quality
- Nasal ventilation problems due to rhonchopathy

Functional–esthetic rhinoplasties are among the most demanding procedures in plastic facial surgery. In themselves, they pose a significant challenge to the rhinosurgeon. It is logistically and technically feasible to include the above indications without getting lost in too many details while still addressing the patient's desire to solve multiple problems in a single operation (131).

Surgeon should have all the techniques and approaches of rhinoplasty and endoscopic endonasal microsurgery in their repertoire. We caution against the current trend toward the exclusive use of the open approach, because the advantage of clear operative exposure is offset by a substantial increase in tissue trauma and subcutaneous scarring. Circumstances will dictate the best choice from among the available options: the *cartilage-splitting approach*, *delivery approach*, or *open approach* (Fig. 1.**2**).

The approach should be as effective as possible and as invasive as necessary. Minimizing surgical trauma is of key importance, as it is the best means that the surgeon has for influencing postoperative wound healing and scar formation. While surgeons can directly alter the size and position of cartilage and bone, they can influence wound healing, and ultimately the definitive outcome, only by working atraumatically in the appropriate favorable *surgical planes*, creating small and appropriate graft beds, and reducing bleeding by preserving the muscular and vascularized planes of the nose (Fig. 1.**3**).

Besides selecting the approach, surgeons can choose from among several techniques (incision, suturing, or grafting) to achieve the desired goal in various ways. Nevertheless, all techniques are rarely of equal suitability. The technique of choice will depend upon skin type, connective-tissue type, and factors such as the age of the patient and the resiliency of the cartilage.

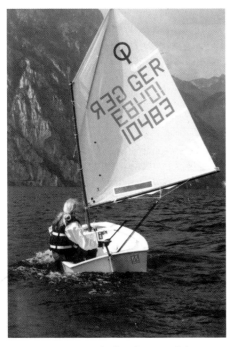

Fig. 1.**1** As in a sail, the shape and function of the nose can be influenced by altering (cartilage) tensions.

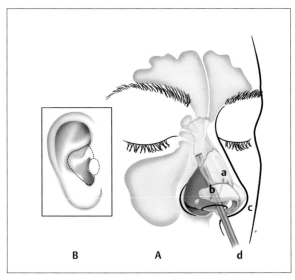

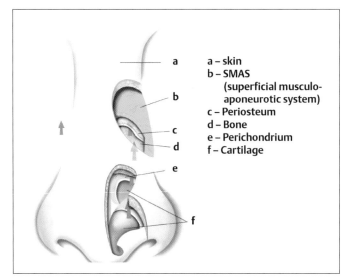

Fig. 1.**2 A**   All approaches to the nasal tip and nasal dorsum can be combined with the endoscopic endonasal approach to the internal nose and paranasal sinuses. (**a**) Intercartilaginous or transcartilaginous route. (**b**) Alar cartilage rim incision combined with intercartilaginous incision in the delivery approach. (**c**) Columellar incision, columellar rim incision, and alar cartilage rim incision in the open approach. (**d**) Endoscopic approach to the posterior septum and ethmoid—the gateway to the paranasal sinuses.

Fig. 1.**2 B**   "The external ear exists as a marvelous storehouse of skeletal spare parts for the nose" M. E. Tardy Jr. (130)

Fig. 1.**3**   The surgical plane in septorhinoplasty.

Historical Review

Origins of Plastic Nasal Surgery

The partial or complete loss of the nose causes severe disfigurement of the face. This kind of trauma injures not just the human body but also the mind. The destruction of the esthetic and psychological integrity of a personality is among the cruelest testimonials of bygone eras. Many ancient sculptures bear witness to this act in symbolic form (94, 110).

Cutting off the ears and nose as a form of punishment motivated the earliest attempts at reconstructive plastic surgery in India approximately 1500 years ago (41, 55, 110). The *Indian rhinoplasty* was performed with a midline forehead flap in a concept that resembles methods still in use today. This technique was described by Sushruta in approximately 600 BC. Galenus mentioned that the Egyptians performed nasal operations, but they kept their methods a secret (41).

Much later, around 1430, the Branca family (first the father, later the son) developed a procedure for reconstructing the nose with a flap from the upper arm.

Gaspare Tagliacozzi (1545–1599), writing in the first textbook on plastic surgery, described techniques for nasal reconstruction that he adopted from Branca and refined. Although that occurred about a century after the Brancas used the upper arm flap, Tagliacozzi is still considered the founder of *Italian rhinoplasty* (41, 55, 94, 124).

The human desire for the esthetic rehabilitation of traumatic or congenital disfigurement, with an opportunity for social reintegration, was definitely the original motivation for reconstructive rhinoplasty.

The age of corrective esthetic rhinoplasty was inaugurated by John Orlando Roe (1848–1915), an otorhinolaryngologist

from Rochester, New York. This surgeon corrected saddle nose deformities through an endonasal approach (112). In 1891, Roe also used intranasal approaches for dorsal hump removal (41, 79). Innovations in the functional aspects of rhinoplasty were later introduced by Mink, van Dishoek, Cottle, and others (20, 25, 89).

The Development of Plastic Surgery in Berlin and at the Charité Hospital from the 18th to 20th Centuries

Surgeons and rhinologists who practiced in Berlin from the 18th to 20th centuries greatly influenced the subsequent development of functional–esthetic rhinosurgery.

Carl Ferdinand von Graefe (1787–1840) became a full professor at the Institute of Clinical and Surgical Ophthalmology at the University in Berlin in 1810 when he was just 23 years old. He was a skilled surgeon who had a keen interest in plastic surgery of the face and jaws. He performed the first successful repair of a cleft palate in 1816. For autologous nasal reconstruction, he used both the Indian and Italian techniques and added his own refinements. He corrected deformities of the face, especially those involving the lips, eyelids, cheek, and nose (33, 114) (Fig. 1.**4**).

Johann Friedrich Dieffenbach (1792–1847) succeeded von Graefe, who kindled his enthusiasm for plastic facial surgery. Dieffenbach dedicated himself to refining the plastic surgical procedures of his day. He did pioneering work in such areas as cleft lip and palate repair, blepharoplasty, the surgical correction of strabismus, and tenotomy for the treatment of clubfoot. He promoted modern rhinoplasty by developing a dual flap technique that repaired both cutaneous and mucosal defects, thereby reducing the problem of flap shrinkage.

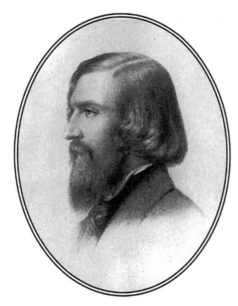

Fig. 1.**4** Carl Ferdinand von Graefe (1787–1840).

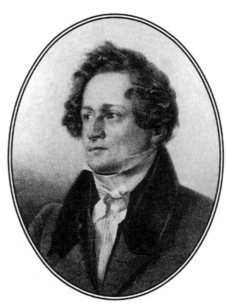

Fig. 1.**5** Johann Friedrich Dieffenbach (1792–1847).

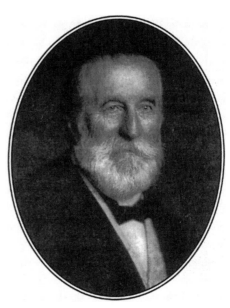

Fig. 1.**6** Ernst von Bergmann (1836–1907).

He became internationally known through his first strabismus operation and numerous monographs. Along with Guillaume Dupuytren of France, Ashley Cooper of England, and Nikolai Pirogow of Russia, Dieffenbach was among the greatest surgeons of his time and is considered the founder of plastic surgery (23, 24, 114) (Fig. 1.**5**).

The following episode helped to establish Dieffenbach's special reputation in 19th-century Berlin: A charming young woman who attended society balls in 1831 and 1832 attracted considerable attention by always hiding her face behind a golden mask. Elvira Tondeau's secret was that her face had been disfigured by deep ulcerative lesions of the nose, presumably a result of tuberculosis cutis luposa. Dieffenbach was able to reconstruct her nose in several sittings. One year later, Elvira entered into a much-publicized engagement. Dieffenbach's accomplishment was immortalized in a contemporary folk song which claimed that "…he makes the nose and ears like new" (114).

General anesthesia was developed in 1846, making painless surgery a reality. In 1878 Robert Koch published his paper "Studies on the etiology of wound infections." Joseph Lister (1827–1912) paved the way for germ-free operations. Berhard von Langenbeck (1810–1887) was Dieffenbach's successor at the Berlin Charité Hospital, specializing in plastic surgery.

Langenbeck's successor, Ernst von Bergmann (1836–1907), was one of the most influential surgeons of his time, introducing the principle of asepsis to surgery. His guiding rule was that everything that came into contact with the operative field and especially with the surgical wound had to be absolutely sterile (Fig. 1.**6**).

Jakob Lewin (Jacques) Joseph (1865–1934) was a pioneer of modern rhinoplasty. He studied medicine in Berlin, graduated in Leipzig in 1861, and opened a private practice in Berlin. Shortly thereafter he joined the Berlin University Orthopedic Hospital, headed by Julius Wolff, where he received extensive surgical training. In 1896 he was referred to the hospital for the correction of prominent ears (94).

In 1898, Joseph performed the first reduction rhinoplasty at his office, using an external approach. He also did pioneering work in several other areas, including the treatment of both morphological and functional abnormalities in one sitting, the use of intranasal approaches, and the establishment of esthetic surgery as a medical specialty.

It is "not vanity which is the driving motivation, but the feeling of being disfigured and, conversely, the aversion to disfigurement and its psychological consequences." Rhinoplasty "seeks to cure psychological depression by restoring a normal shape to the nose. Its social importance is beyond question, and it represents a significant branch of surgical psychotherapy."

In 1904, Joseph reported on the first operation in which the intranasal removal of a dorsal hump was combined with correction of the anterior septum (54). At that time intranasal operative techniques were considered "unsurgical" procedures that were handicapped by poor exposure and a high infection risk (Fig. 1.**7**).

From 1916 to 1921, Joseph was director of the Department of Facial Reconstruction at the Charité Ear and Nose Clinic in Berlin, headed by Passow (1859–1926) (42, 95). At that time he worked mainly in the plastic reconstructive surgery of extensive facial injuries that were sustained during World War I.

Owing to his great success, Passow received an honorary professorship in 1918. Later he started his own hospital and specialized in esthetic surgery with an emphasis on rhinoplasty and mammoplasty. His colleagues included Gustav Aufricht and Joseph Safian (93).

Jacques Joseph is considered the founder of modern rhinoplasty. Curiously, three professors named Joseph were working in Berlin at the same time. The nasal surgeon among them was popularly known as "Noseph" to distinguish him from his gastroenterologist and dermatologist colleagues.

Aufricht later traveled to America, published numerous works, and became a respected nasal surgeon in the United States. He died in New York in 1984.

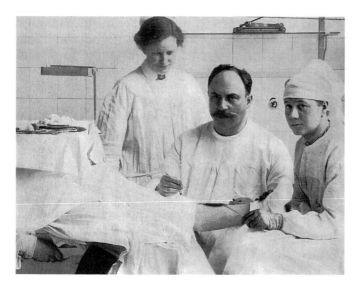

Fig. 1.**7**　Jacques Joseph (1865–1934) during an operation.

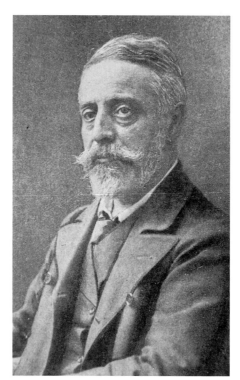

Fig. 1.**8**　Emil Zuckerkandl (1849–1921).

Joseph summarized his experience in an atlas and text-book with the lengthy title "*Rhinoplasty and Other Facial Plastic Surgery with an Appendix on Mammoplasty and Several Other Operations in the Area of External Plastic Surgery.*"

Joseph was buried in the Jewish Cemetery in Berlin-Weissensee, not far from our hospital. Unfortunately, his gravesite was destroyed by bombs during World War II. Joseph's wife, Leonore, emigrated to the United States, where she died at a grand old age, impoverished, in 1968.

History of Surgery of the "Internal Nose"

Diseases of the "internal nose" have their own history. The oldest documented record of medical treatment in which the patient and physician were named is that of the ancient Egyptian rhinologist Ni-Ankh Sekhmet, the physician to King Sahura, who presumably suffered from nasal polyps (15).

For centuries, efforts were made to improve the dreaded, bloody techniques for the operative treatment of nasal diseases, especially nasal polyps. New instruments, approaches, and techniques were constantly devised for that purpose. This brought no real improvement, however, because surgeons knew little about the actual location and origin of the diseases.

During the Renaissance, intense study was devoted to the anatomy of the skull, including the nose and paranasal sinuses (Leonardo da Vinci [1452], Versalius [1452], Highmore [1651]). Many new discoveries were made about the human skull. In the late 19th century, the anatomical studies of Zuckerkandl (1882), Onodi (1893), and Grünwald (1925) yielded precise information on the anatomy of the nose, facial bones, and para-nasal sinuses (21, 35, 44, 97, 134, 141) (Figs. 1.**8**, 1.**9**).

By first describing narrow anatomical passages in the ethmoid bone and middle meatus, Zuckerkandl (1882) promoted the development of new, endonasal operative procedures such

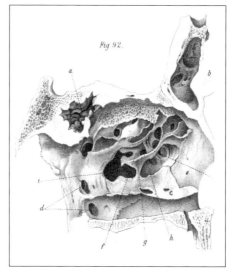

Fig. 1.**9**　Sectional view of the ethmoid labyrinth (from Zuckerkandl 141).

as ostial enlargement, maxillary sinus fenestration, and ethmoid infundibulotomy (39, 63, 118).

Gustav Killian, who became a professor in the Department of Otorhinolaryngology of the Charité Hospital in Berlin in 1921, already recognized the pathogenic significance of the anterior ethmoid cells. He introduced *median rhinoscopy* with a specially developed speculum for examining the middle meatus (Fig. 1.**10**).

Without optical aids, the endonasal operations were hazardous and were practiced by only a few pioneers (39). The fact that other operative methods were developed at the same time was another reason for the lack of popularity of endonasal operations. Mikulicz was the first surgeon, in 1887, to open the

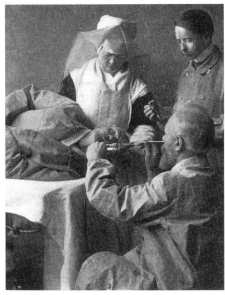

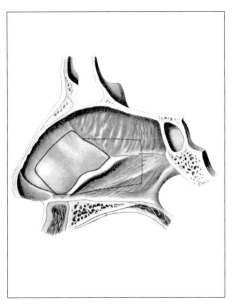

Fig. **1.10** Gustav Killian (1860–1921) during an endoscopic examination. Killian is the founder of suspension laryngoscopy and of bronchoscopy. He was nominated for the Nobel Prize for this work, but he died from the complications of appendix surgery before the prize could be awarded.

Fig. **1.11** Killian resection of the nasal septum.

maxillary sinus from the inferior meatus. Caldwell published his technique of maxillary sinus surgery in New York in 1893.

Boenninghaus modified the technique by transposing a mucosal flap into the maxillary sinus window. Luc published the same operative technique as Caldwell in Paris (18, 73, 88).

In 1867, Leinhardt described the first submucous resection of the nasal septum for correction of the anterior septum. Hartmann and Petersen expanded the method, also applying it to deviations of the posterior septum. The septum was approached through a horizontal and vertical incision of the mucosa on the deviated side. The major problem with this method and its refinements (e.g., 107) was the poor exposure caused by heavy mucosal bleeding. Rethi (123) helped to control this problem by the local administration of cocaine (40, 72, 78, 100, 107, 133).

Killian injected a cocaine–epinephrine solution beneath the two mucosal layers and elevated the mucosa from the cartilage on both sides, developing the technique of the *submucous resection* (62). This procedure involved a broad resection of the septal cartilage, leaving a dorsal and caudal strut in place for support. It also involved removing portions of the bony septum (i.e., the perpendicular plate of the ethmoid and vomer) that were believed to obstruct nasal airflow. Special emphasis was placed on gaining "sufficient working room to resect the bony septal wall" (12) (Fig. **1.11**).

The principle of the submucous resection was later abandoned because the overresection of cartilage from the anterior septum tended to cause unfavorable late sequelae. Destroying the supportive function of the septum between the rhinion (keystone area) and the anterior nasal spine often led to depression of the cartilaginous nasal dorsum and retraction of the columella, with the functional and esthetic problems of a saddle nose and hidden columella (20).

Corresponding mucosal lesions or poor vascularization of the scarred mucosal layers led to perforations. When the supportive function of the cartilaginous septum is withdrawn, there is a general tendency for the mucosa to become dry and atrophic. Although the septal layers are located near the midline and the nose appears broadened, the rhinitis sicca still causes a subjective feeling of nasal stuffiness. Another problem is the "septal flutter" that occurs during forced respiration and phonation.

In 1884, Sir Morrell MacKenzie founded the specialty of otorhinolaryngology when he published his first standard work on rhinology and laryngology (81). Rhinology began to be established as a separate field in the early 20th century. When the anatomical studies of Emil Zuckerkandl (141) supplied the first accurate information on the structural anatomy of the nose and paranasal sinuses in the late 19th century, interest also grew in using endoscopy to explore the complex spaces of the nose and its connections with the paranasal sinuses.

The first instruments used for this purpose were cystoscopes, because special endoscopes for the nose were not yet available. In 1901, A. Hirschmann first examined the maxillary sinus endoscopically through an enlarged dental alveolus, also examining the middle meatus (48).

Despite the progress made in optical examinations, these initial steps in nasal endoscopy did not lead at once to new approaches in diagnosis and treatment.

Substantial progress in these areas was not made until the postmortem studies of Walter Messerklinger (83,84) on mucous transport in the human nose and paranasal sinuses. Such studies are possible because the respiratory epithelium continues to show ciliary activity for up to 48 hours after death. Messerklinger discovered that secretions from the large paranasal sinuses are transported along specific pathways to the ostia and flow from there through narrow passages in the lateral nasal wall to the mucosa of the nose (83, 84).

The nose and sinuses constitute a physiological and morphological unit.

This principle seems obvious today, but before it was discovered, textbooks devoted separate chapters to diseases of the nose and diseases of the paranasal sinuses.

In recent years, the nasal mucous blanket has again attracted special interest because of its central role in the hypothesis of fungus-induced sinusitis. Fungal spores are trapped by the two layers of the mucous blanket. They penetrate the mucus and reach the epithelial surface, where they evoke an eosinophilic reaction. A mucosal inflammation is incited by major basic protein (MBP) and other cytokines, leading to polyposis (103).

On July 16, 1959, a patent for the "rod lens system" was filed by its inventor, the English physicist Harold Horace Hopkins. It attracted considerable attention when unveiled as a new optical system at the Photokina photo exposition in Cologne. Karl Storz recognized the innovative potential of the invention for medicine and signed a licensing contract with Hopkins in 1965. The Hopkins rod lens system employs special glass rods with optically finished ends that replace conventional lenses. This has distinct advantages over a conventional lens system: better resolution and contrast, a wider viewing angle, superb clarity and brilliance, and an extremely fine depiction of details over the entire visual field (11).

Messerklinger used the new endoscopes to examine the lateral nasal wall, where he observed both normal and abnormal mucosal findings. He discovered that recurrent and chronic sinusitis had a rhinogenic cause in the great majority of cases. This led him to develop an *endoscopic diagnostic strategy for the nose and paranasal sinuses* (85, 86, 87).

Endoscopy could reveal the often subtle signs of mucosal inflammation, septal deformities located in the deeper areas of the nose, as well as anatomical factors predisposing to sinusitis. The pathways for the spread of rhinogenic sinusitis could be traced by endoscopic visualization.

One challenge at this point was to make this optical pathway accessible for a new type of surgery. The endoscopic surgeon would be able to reach the pathogenic nidus of recurrent or chronic–hyperplastic sinusitis and, by restoring ventilation and drainage, create the conditions necessary for the hyperplastic epithelium of the functionally dependent sinuses (maxillary and frontal) to heal (120).

The operative techniques and indications for this type of surgery have been constantly expanding along with the development of increasingly fine instruments and new endoscopes (27, 60, 116, 137, 138).

Phylogenesis

Phylogenetically, the necessity of having a nose is based upon the transition from aquatic to terrestrial life. Originally all vertebrates breathed through gills, but this type of respiration was preserved only in lampreys (agnathians) and fish. Ectothermic amphibians marked the metamorphosis from gill-breathing to lung-breathing animals, with only a few water-dwelling forms continuing to breathe with gills. Amphibians have other mechanisms of respiration through their gland-studded outer skin and oral mucosa. Reptiles are obligate lung breathers that have become independent of aquatic life and have adapted to various environments. Some groups, like the sea turtles, have returned to life in the water. The development of choanae, which are the morphological prerequisite for nasal breathing, first appeared in primitive amphibians and later arose in all vertebrates.

This development is reflected in human ontogenesis. Through active growth, the epithelium of the nasal mucosa leads to the formation of the lateral nasal wall in the third month of fetal development. The rudiments of the nasal turbinates and paranasal sinuses also appear at this stage.

Over the course of evolution, the human nose has developed into a highly efficient aerodynamic body with specialized functions (4, 6, 92).

The Nose as a Respiratory Organ

Only nasal breathing is physiological in humans. Mouth breathing tends to dry out the lower respiratory tract, predisposing to various diseases (pharyngitis, laryngitis, bronchitis, bronchial hyperreactivity, asthma).

The nose has an immense regulatory capacity. Although the mucociliary apparatus is affected by the temperature and humidity of the inspired air and by the pH and osmolarity of the surrounding medium, air entering the nose is warmed to a relatively constant 31–34 °C in the epipharynx. This occurs largely independently of the external temperature (113). The nose also humidifies the inspired air to a relative humidity of 90–95 % (51).

Most warming and humidification takes place in the anterior part of the nose (59). Both functions are linked to the ability of the nose to undergo rapid changes in cross section.

The nasal mucosa is the "front line" of the human immune system. With each breath, it responds to and defends against a variety of antigens and allergens. The mechanisms of this response include nonspecific (e.g., interferon, protease inhibitors) and specific humoral reactions (immunoglobulins A, M, and G), as well as cellular reactions by macrophages, mast cells, and granulocytes. At the same time, entirely different reactions such as absorption and secretion can take place on the mucosa.

The phylogenic development of the upper and lower airways accounts for their functional interrelationship. The upper and lower airways form a functional unit. The mucosa, submucosa, and vascularity are similar in both regions. Also, the biochemical control mechanisms in the upper and lower airways have the same mediators. The mucosa of both the upper and lower airways responds to allergic and physical stimuli, chemical irritants, and inflammatory microbial irritants with cellular infiltration (mostly eosinophilic granulocytes), mucosal edema, and increased mucus production (104, 115).

The time required for a mucosal disease to "change levels" by spreading to the posterior wall of the pharynx, trachea, and bronchi varies in different individuals. The rhinologist should always keep in mind the principle of *one airway, one disease* (115) (Fig. 1.**12**).

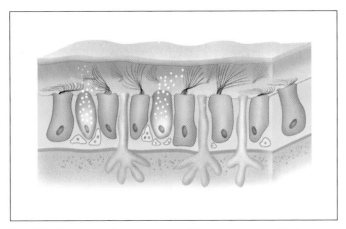

Fig. 1.**12** The mucociliary apparatus of the respiratory epithelium is an important defensive and regulatory mechanism of the nose. Goblet cells and seromucous glands secrete a substance onto the surface of the mucosa, forming a two-layer film. The beating cilia located in the deeper, less viscous mucous layer actively propel the superficial, more viscous layer toward the esophagus.

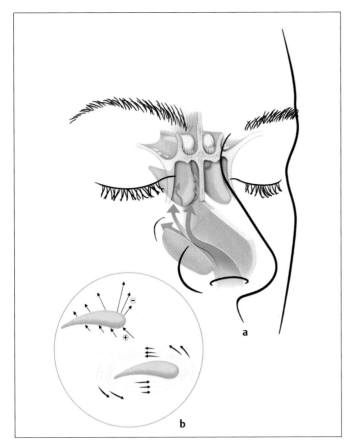

Fig. 1.**13 a** Intranasal airflow patterns during olfaction.
b and its share in sense of taste

The Nose as a Sensory Organ

The Olfactory Sense

The area of respiratory epithelium located in the human olfactory groove measures approximately 2 x 5 cm. This area is many times larger in numerous mammalian species. In the speechless world of animals, the olfactory sense is the most important means of communication next to vision. Humans have approximately 10 million olfactory cells. These are bipolar sensory cells with an elongated cell body and a short process, the dendrite, with numerous cilia extending into the nasal mucous blanket. At the opposite end of the cell is a long neural process, the axon. The olfactory cells are classified as primary sensory cells.

The axons pass through the basement membrane of the olfactory epithelium and join to form the *fila olfactoria*. These filaments pass through the *cribriform plate* to enter the *olfactory bulb* in the brain. There they synapse with the *dendritic tree* of the *mitral cells*. Approximately 1000 olfactory cells converge toward one mitral cell.

The processes of the approximately 60 000 mitral cells form the *olfactory tract*, which passes to the olfactory cortex, the primitive rhinencephalon. Information is relayed from there to the thalamus, hypothalamus, and amygdala. This intimate contact with the hypothalamus, which controls behavior patterns such as eating, drinking, sexual behavior, hormonal regulation, and the perception of emotions, probably explains why olfactory stimuli have rapid and direct access to the deepest centers of human emotion. Information is relayed from the thalamus to the neocortex, where the pathways terminate in old, nonspecific brain regions (75, 91). The human olfactory sense is less rooted in the conscious mind than seeing and hearing, for example.

Generally speaking, olfaction must still be considered the "neglected" sense. The analytical perception of visual and auditory stimuli is constantly being trained and reinforced, whereas the processing of odors is a more intuitive process (9, 10). Cortical representation in the phylogenically old brain areas of the limbic system establishes a close, essentially nonverbal link with affect, emotions, and distant memories. For example, the smell of freshly polished linoleum can bring back vivid memories of grade school simply because that is how the school used to smell. Often it is difficult to describe an odor in words, and the best we can do is compare the smell to something else or describe it as "flowery," "fruity," etc.

In the isthmic region of the *limen nasi*, the inspired air is slowed and separated into two streams. The main stream is directed over the nasal floor to the choana. A smaller stream is directed upward and sweeps over the dorsum of the inferior nasal turbinate. At this point the air is warmed and continues to move upward. On reaching the head of the middle turbinate, the "updraft" splits into a lateral stream that ventilates the paranasal sinuses and another stream that is directed medially upward. The alignment of the middle turbinate is crucial for ventilation of the olfactory groove. It has the shape of an airfoil suspected between three points of attachment. A negative pressure prevails on the medial or "lee" side of the turbinate, causing the inspired air to rise into the olfactory fossa. Gustatory olfaction is subject to the same basic flow patterns following convection of the flow around the body of the turbinate (see Fig. 1.**13**).

Respiratory hyposmia can result from obstruction or deficient aeration of the olfactory groove caused, for example, by septal deviation, polyps, or tumors. Deformities of the nasal turbinates (e.g., lateralization, atrophy, paradoxical curvature) can also lead to hyposmia (Fig. 1.**13**).

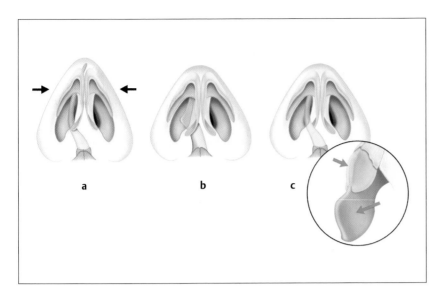

Fig. 1.**14**   The most common types of septal deviation. Explanation in text.

The Vomeronasal Organ

A. Butenandt, the Nobel Prize winner from Munich, coined the term *pheromones* for molecules that are produced by a species and evoke certain reactions in animals of the same species.

The vomeronasal organ (Jacobson's organ) is essential for the social and mating behavior of all mammals (102). Except for some higher primates, mammals mate only when the female is fertile. Information on the timing of ovulation is conveyed to males by means of pheromones.

Numerous observations and studies indicate that pheromones also convey signals in humans.

The vomeronasal organ consists of tiny, paired, blindly terminating canals located in the anterior nasal septum. Its morphology suggests that the vomeronasal organ is a functioning sensory epithelium. Further studies are needed to identify its central connections with the hypothalamus and elucidate its functional significance (52).

Prerequisites for the Concept of Functional–Esthetic Nasal Surgery

Several prerequisites have been essential in developing a common concept in rhinosurgery that places equal emphasis upon functional and esthetic demands.

Septal Surgery with Functional and Esthetic Goals

The *nasal septum* is the central connecting link between the internal and external nose. It supports the lateral cartilages and provides a secure attachment of the cartilaginous nose to the facial skeleton between the rhinion (keystone area) and the anterior nasal spine, premaxilla, vomer, and perpendicular plate of the ethmoid.

The successful correction of axial deformities of the nose is not possible without fully utilizing the capabilities of the submucous septoplasty.

Aufricht (2) said: "Where the septum goes, there goes the nose" (1). This is equally true for the reconstruction of saddle nose deformities, where a stable buildup of the septum is the key to a successful outcome.

While the nasal septum may be affected by numerous deformities, three patterns are most commonly encountered (Fig. 1.**14**):
a) The septum is too long in the basal-to-dorsal direction. This situation is common in the overprojected nose and functional tension nose with hyperplasia of the upper lateral cartilage or alar cartilage.
b) Phylogenically, the connection between the vomer and basal septal cartilage is a zone of "tectonic unrest." Originally it had the form of an articulation (92). Even slight growth or forward movement of the vomer, usually during puberty, leads to elevation of the cartilaginous nasal dorsum due to the wedged shape of the underlying vomer or to characteristic vomerine ridges that run obliquely upward.
c) The septum is too long in the craniocaudal direction. This situation is often seen in axial deformities and is associated with two sites of nasal airway obstruction. Subluxation is common (Fig. 1.**14**).

The external shape of the septum can be selectively modified in septal operations. Resections of the anterior septal margin can be helpful in shortening the nose and in establishing a symmetrical nasal tip with an equilateral rhomboid shape. An infratip triangle that is too long can be shortened. Also, the anterior septal margin can be beveled to rotate the tip upward and accentuate the *double break* in the nasal profile. Septal modification is an essential part of creating a subtle, esthetically pleasing *supratip break* in women (46).

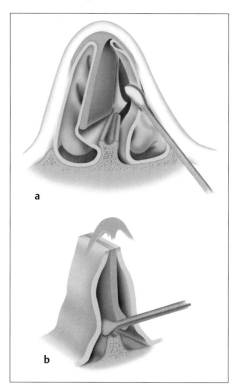

Fig. 1.**15** Submucous septoplasty. Principles: mobilisation, reorientation and fixation.
a) The mucoperichondrium remains adherent to the septal cartilage on the right side (Cottle technique), swinging door
b) Sometimes it is useful to mobilize the entire septal cartilage

Principles of Submucous Septoplasty

Cottle (1948) introduced his cartilage-conserving operation as an alternative to the Killian septal resection (see p. 6). The Cottle operation attempts to preserve the supporting function of the septal cartilage and the physiological function of the nasal mucosa. After the anterior margin of the septum has been exposed, the mucoperichondrium is undermined to create a superior tunnel on the left side and an inferior tunnel on both sides. The mucosa remains adherent to the septal cartilage on the right side. This provides good septal mobility. The classic Cottle operation has been continually modified over the years. One modification is the *swinging door* technique in which the septal cartilage is detached just anterior to the perpendicular plate to increase the mobility of the cartilage during the operation (Fig. 1.**15 a**). The mucoperichondrium is left in place. Also, small strips or wedges can be excised from the cartilage to eliminate redundant material that would create undesired stresses. The cartilage can also be scored or cross-hatched to modify its bending properties.

In our experience a large percentage of septal deviations can be managed with this technique. For greater, sharp-edged deviations that are combined with axial deformities, the mucosa can be completely elevated from the septal cartilage to form two superior and inferior tunnels in preparation for an extracorporeal septoplasty (36). In this technique the cartilaginous and bony septum is completely removed, straightened, and reimplanted. A *compound graft* is made by suturing pieces of septal cartilage in a mosaiclike pattern to a sheet of polydioxanone suture material (PDS). This sheet gives

the composite implant the necessary mechanical stability until the material is absorbed (13, 36).

If the potential of the septoplasty is to be fully realized in terms of improving function and esthetics, this procedure must take the form of a technically demanding plastic operation. As Adamsen put it, "The only easy septum is the one which has no need to be done" (1) (Fig. 1.**15**).

The Pediatric Nasal Septum

Traditionally, the main argument against septal surgery in childhood has been the belief that the septal cartilage is an essential pillar for the primary growth of the midfacial region (58).

Today it is known that the septum, maxilla, and premaxilla develop independently of one another (90, 101). Strict criteria should be applied in selecting children for septal operations. Nevertheless, even small children can be successfully operated for traumatic deformities or malformations of the septum that cause significant nasal obstruction. Deformities of the antero-inferior septum are the most common problem (117). It is important that the surgery preserve the perichondrium, the growth zones (e.g., the caudal septum), the premaxilla, and the sutural junctions with the perpendicular plate and vomer (109).

The pediatric septum consists mainly of the quadrilateral plate; the vomer and perpendicular plate are relatively small. This calls for an atraumatic, chondroplastic mode of surgery. Pieces of cartilage that are removed should be straightened and reimplanted. Even after surgical trauma, the septal cartilage still has considerable regenerative capacity (101).

The Nasal Valve

As early as 1882, Zuckerkandl described the nasal valve as follows: "The fold of the upper lateral cartilage and the wall of the nasal septum form a space leading into the nasal cavity that is much narrower than the external naris." Mink called this area the *nasal valve* because of its dynamic function in regulating the cross-sectional area of the nasal airway (89, 141). The resistance to nasal airflow is to a large degree determined by the nasal valve (25).

Over the years, numerous operations have been described for widening the nasal valve and preventing alar collapse (18, 32, 47, 108, 127, 135).

A history of obstructed nasal breathing plus visual inspection of the external and internal nose (preferably with an endoscope) will direct attention to the underlying problem and suggest the best technique for widening or stabilizing the nasal valve.

A positive *Cottle maneuver* indicates a problem with the nasal valve: When the ala is pulled laterally upward, the nasal valve opens and breathing improves (Fig. 1.**16**).

Principles of Nasal Valve Surgery

1. A morphologically tight nasal valve can restrict nasal breathing even when there is no obvious collapse of the lateral nasal wall during forced inspiration. The nasal valve width and tightness and their changes during respiration

are readily assessed by endoscopic examination. A tight nasal valve is a common finding in the tension nose and is an indication for *spreader grafts*. When placed on the extramucous plane between the upper lateral cartilages and the dorsal septal cartilage, these grafts provide effective widening of the nasal valve (127).

2. If forced inspiration leads to aspiration and collapse of the alar or upper lateral cartilage, this signifies deficient stability and resiliency of these cartilages. This is most often caused by a rhinoplasty in which too much material has been resected from the lateral alar cartilage or from the anterior margins of the upper lateral cartilages. Treatment consists of reinforcing the lateral nasal wall in the area of the nasal valve with autologous cartilage implants from the septal or auricular cartilage. These implants should be fitted into suitable, slightly narrow recipient beds to preserve their natural curvature and reinforce the alar convexity. The implants can be placed in a horizontal or vertical alignment. They are braced against the piriform aperture and attached with sutures or fibrin glue (32, 130).

3. If extensive scar-tissue bands are found in the area of the nasal valve, they can be resected and the wound epithelialized with split-thickness or thin full-thickness skin grafts.

4. In cases with combined cartilage and skin loss, tissue must be added to this region in order to open up the valve. An auricular composite graft is excellent for this purpose. R. Goode said: "Replace what is missing with like material."

5. Curling of the caudal end of the upper lateral cartilage may cause restriction of the nasal valve. This can be corrected by carefully shortening the anterior cartilage margin. Also, a long caudal lateral cartilage that is overlapped by the alar cartilage is functionally unfavorable and should be shortened.

Detailed information on operative techniques is presented in the sections below.

Physiological Limits of Nasal Breathing

Our experience in the treatment of speed skaters at the Olympic Center in Berlin has demonstrated an interesting phenomenon. Good nasal breathing is particularly important in this sport, where very cold, dry air is forcibly inspired in short, deep breaths taken through the mouth or through the nose and mouth combined. Twelve top athletes who had septal deviation, turbinate hyperplasia, inflammatory ethmoid changes, or an anatomical variant (concha bullosa, paradoxical curve of the middle turbinate, pneumatized agger nasi) underwent a septoplasty that usually included an endoscopic ethmoidectomy or turbinate reduction. But even patients who showed very good postoperative nasal breathing by rhinomanometry reverted to oronasal breathing during exercise. The reason is a physiological collapse of the nasal valve that occurs with extreme inspiration to protect the lower airways and lungs from unconditioned air that is too cold or too hot. Activation of the sympathoadrenergic system in response to physical exercise leads to a decongestion of the nasal mucosa. This results in increased airflow through the nose and a lowering of nasal resistance, accompanied by an acceleration of mucociliary secretion (4). Nevertheless, the resistance to open mouth breathing is still less than the resistance to nasal breathing. The athletes adopt a

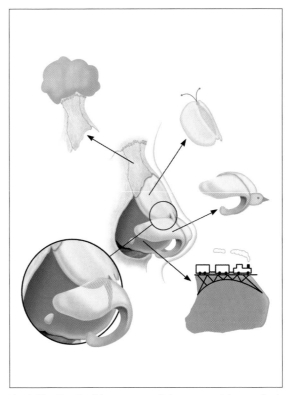

Fig. 1.**16**   The flexible structure of the nose and the nasal valve. The flexibility of the nose increases in the craniocaudal direction. The bony portion is completely rigid, and the flexible cartilaginous portion begins at the rhinion. The distal caudal lateral cartilages are mobile, similar to the wings of a butterfly. This flexibility is supported by the upper alar cartilages, which perform an important supporting function medially and distally along with the septum. This arrangement imparts a special functional elasticity to the nasal valve. The nasal skin shows an opposite pattern: It is thin and mobile over the bony nasal pyramid but is relatively thick and immobile over the nasal tip. Neither "internal" nor "external" nasal operations should needlessly traumatize this sensitive system of flexible and inflexible elements.

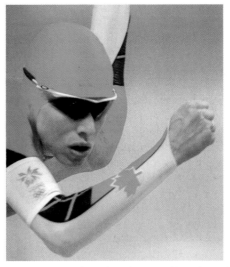

Fig. 1.**17**   Typical combined oronasal breathing, demonstrated by Olympic speed skating gold medallist Catriona Le May Doan.

combined oronasal mode of breathing that includes a degree of nasal breathing while regulating the airway resistance so that the work of respiration (pressure and volume) does not become too great (26, 28, 43, 79) (Fig. 1.**17**).

Atraumatic, Structure-Conserving Techniques of Septorhinoplasty

The description of new principles of rhinoplasty, especially by Tardy, has changed the fundamental character of this surgery (125, 126, 128, 130).

The key is a detailed analysis of the presenting anatomical problems, taking into account other fundamental factors such as skin type, connective-tissue type, and the age of the patient (129).

Surgical access is gained through adequate, usually intranasal approaches that are as minimally invasive as possible.

The surgery is structure-conserving and aimed at preserving and reorienting the cartilages. The strategies include circumscribed resections and the use of suture techniques to shape the nasal tip. Any unnecessary tissue trauma is avoided. The following measures are helpful in achieving these goals:

- Selective, local vasoconstriction is added to general anesthesia to minimize bleeding.
- Osteotomies are performed with micro-osteotomes that do not damage the periosteum or the overlying vascular and muscle plane. Traditional transverse osteotomies are avoided.
- Intranasal sutures or splints eliminate the need for laborious packing (106).
- By minimizing tissue trauma, intraoperative bleeding is reduced. A well-defined surgical concept based on an analysis of the specific morphological problem and of preoperative photographs helps to shorten the operating time. Less bleeding and shorter operating times are the prerequisites for expanding the range of indications for rhinosurgical operations that include endoscopic microsurgery.

An understanding of the tip-supporting mechanisms will protect against unnecessary destabilization of the nasal tip and dorsum during the operation. The *dynamics of rhinoplasty* refers to a system of surgically induced interactions to fine-adjust the position of the nasal tip. Dissection strictly in the favorable surgical planes can minimize unnecessary bleeding, edema, and subsequent scarring. The task of the surgeon is to lay the groundwork for a stable long-term result (96, 98, 105, 130).

Functional Aspects of Septorhinoplasty

Olfactory Disturbances

Disturbances of olfaction are the second most common leading symptom of nasal obstruction reported by our patients. Olfactory disturbances may be described as quantitative or qualitative. *Hyposmia* and *hyperosmia* signify a change in the olfactory threshold, while *anosmia* denotes an absence of the smell sensation. This may affect the perception of certain odors or of all smells. *Parosmia* refers to an altered perception of smells under certain physiological conditions, such as pregnancy. *Pseudosmia* refers to the misidentification of perceived smells, as in cacosmia. *Phantosmia* is an olfactory hallucina-

tion, or the perception of an odor with no stimulus present. In *agnosmia*, olfactory information is perceived but is not recognized. The most important distinction for the rhinosurgeon is between *respiratory* and *sensory hyposmia* (9, 10).

Basic Diagnostic Workup of Olfactory Disturbances and Paranasal Sinus Diseases

Olfactometry

Olfactometry should precede every surgical operation on the nose or paranasal sinuses. We use the butanol threshold test and the Cain odor identification test. The Kobal "Sniffin' Sticks" are also recommended (37, 65).

Computerized Rhinomanometry

Active anterior computerized rhinomanometry with a decongestion test can be used to differentiate between fixed stenoses, dynamic stenoses, and pseudostenoses.

In our practice, rhinomanometric measurements are an indispensable tool in selecting patients for septoplasty or septorhinoplasty (9).

Computed Tomography

Computed tomography (CT) in the coronal plane provides an excellent overview of the ethmoid region and paranasal sinuses. The marked individual variations in the degree of ethmoid pneumatization can be appreciated on CT scans. CT can also demonstrate pathological mucosal changes, the relative locations and special features of major structures like the optic nerve, the presence of Onody cells, the depth of the olfactory fossa, and the distance from the medial infundibular wall to the orbit. Thus, CT can provide both an inventory of pathological changes and a "roadmap" for endoscopic operations.

Endoscopic Examination of the Nose

Nasal endoscopy, with its ability to explore the internal nose, has become an essential tool for modern finding-oriented rhinological diagnosis and treatment. The endoscopist looks for signs of inflammatory mucosal disease such as abnormal mucous tracks, areas of mucosal edema, or mucosal polyps on the lateral nasal wall. Attention is also given to anatomical variants of pathogenic significance such as conchae bullosa or paradoxical middle turbinates.

Nasal endoscopy also permits the topographic evaluation of aerodynamic obstructions such as ridges or spurs on the posterior septum or perpendicular plate, nasal valve stenosis, and alar collapse.

Frequent Causes of Respiratory Hyposmia

- Large deviations of the nasal septum
- Septal deviation with compression or lateralization of the middle turbinate
- Prominent spurs and ridges
- Nasal and sinus polyps
- Papillomas
- Morphological variants of the middle turbinate (e.g., concha bullosa, large pneumatized labyrinth–turbinate complex)
- Synechiae
- Rhinitis sicca

Surgery in the Olfactory Groove

Surgical manipulations in the olfactory groove should be carried out with extreme care. Olfactory and respiratory epithelium are indistinguishable from each other.

To avoid a cerebrospinal fluid (CSF) leak caused by the avulsion of fila olfactoria, the surgeon should use only sharp, low-profile, 70–90° angled instruments that *cut through* the tissue. The middle turbinate should be displaced laterally during the dissection to afford maximum exposure.

The Storz minishaver has proved especially useful for operations in the olfactory groove. Floating tissue is aspirated into the window of the outer sheath and cut off cleanly with a rotating blade. The sheath protects the opposing mucosa from accidental injury.

Recurrent and Chronic Sinusitis

Significant deviation of the nasal septum, like that often found in axial deformities of the nose, is a predisposing factor for recurrent sinusitis.

The diagram in Figure 1.**18** illustrates the most important cellular structures and their variants that may have causal significance in recurrent sinusitis.

Endoscopic Surgery of the Paranasal Sinuses

Endoscopic surgery of the paranasal sinuses is a minimally invasive microsurgical operating technique. Dissection through a well-exposed field will cause minimal intraoperative bleeding. With some practice and good anatomical orientation, it is our experience that endoscopic microsurgery and septorhinoplasty can be effectively combined.

Algorithm for Simultaneous Septorhinoplasty and Endonasal Microsurgery

The recommended sequence of surgical steps is shown below, based on the example of a long, humped nose:
- Decongestion of the nasal mucosa with nose drops.
- Local anesthesia plus vasoconstriction of the external nose and septum.
- A pledget soaked with tetracaine and epinephrine is placed in each naris for 10 minutes for vasoconstriction.
- Infiltration of the lateral nasal wall under endoscopic control.
- Endoscopic microsurgery of the ethmoid and paranasal sinuses, including adjunctive measures. This presumes that a strong septal deviation is not obstructing the middle turbinate. The beginner can determine this by noting whether a 4-mm telescope can be easily positioned at the antrum of the middle meatus. If not, a submucous septoplasty should be performed first.
- A pledget is inserted into the ethmoid at the end of the ethmoid surgery.
- Submucous septoplasty is carried out, usually through a hemitransfixion or superior transfixion incision, paying attention to esthetic aspects such as:
  - Shortening the entire caudal or dorsocaudal edge to shorten the nose, reducing an infratip triangle that is too long, or tip rotation;
  - Resecting a narrow basal strip to relax a tight nasal valve;

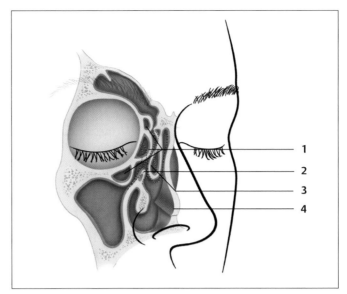

Fig. 1.**18**   Anatomical variants of the ethmoid that may contribute to the pathogenesis of recurrent sinusitis.
1. Cells of the medial orbital wall.
   - Large ethmoid bulla, often in contact with the middle turbinate
   - Orbital ethmoid cells near the maxillary sinus ostium
   - Frontal cells
2. Variants of the uncinate process
   - Shape: free-standing, varying curvature, length, and thickness
   - Insertion: lamina papyracea, anterior skull base
   - Pneumatization
3. Middle turbinate
   - Pneumatization: head, neck, attachment
   - Curvature: paradoxical
4. Septum
   - Deviation: anterior, posterior, high, low
   - Ridge: vomer, traumatic
   - Prominent premaxilla
   - Septal tubercle
5. Agger nasi
   - Pneumatization
6. Combination of several variants

- Removing or shortening the nasal spine if there are signs of vestibular tension or an obtuse nasolabial angle. The soft tissues of the nasolabial angle are augmented as required.
- The nasal tip and dorsum are accessed through a non-delivery or delivery approach or an open approach. In the splitting approach, the transcartilaginous or intercartilaginous incision is combined with a hemitransfixion or transfixion incision. The intracartilaginous incision may also be combined with these incisions (e.g., for a delivery approach).
- The nasal tip is corrected, according to the anatomical situation.
- The cartilaginous hump is removed first, then the bony hump.
- Medial oblique and lateral curved osteotomy.

Principles of Endonasal Microsurgery

A detailed endoscopic evaluation is an essential prelude to microsurgery of the lateral nasal wall and paranasal sinuses. The endoscopic and imaging findings provide the basis for designing an individualized concept for operative treatment. The

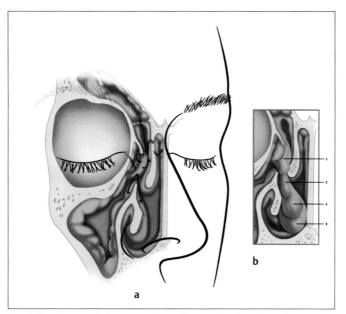

Fig. 1.**19**   Phases of the generation of a nasal polyp from the anterior ethmoid:
- Mucosa inflammation, edema
- Subsidence of the growing polyp
- Obstruction of the middle meatus, the anterior ethmoid and compression of the polyp tissue
- Complete nasal obstruction

value of this endoscopic–microsurgical concept is that it provides the means for detecting and eliminating the often subtle causes of recurrent or chronic inflammatory diseases of the maxillary, frontal, and sphenoid sinuses. The mucosal pathology begins in the anterior ethmoid and spreads from there in a centrifugal pattern. Foci of mucosal edema in the tight spaces of the lateral nasal wall hamper mucous drainage from the frontal and maxillary sinuses, causing infected secretions to dam back. If the mucosal disease persists, the edematous foci become organized. This leads to disturbances of the mucociliary apparatus such as restricted ciliary beating and rheological mucus changes. These are followed by morphological mucosal changes such as an altered ratio of ciliated cells to goblet cells, loss of cilia, and mucous transformation of the seromucous glands (Fig. 1.**19**).

This sets up a vicious circle that should be interrupted as soon as possible to halt the spread of inflammation to the entire ethmoid labyrinth and to the frontal, maxillary, and sphenoid sinuses. The goal of mucosa-conserving surgery is to create the conditions necessary for morphological and functional reparative processes to occur in the epithelium.

The metabolic products of eosinophilic granulocytes are toxic to the epithelium and play a central role in the pathogenesis of chronic hyperplastic rhinosinusitis. A mixed-cell inflammation is perpetuated by immune mechanisms, in most cases by T-lymphocyte activated eosinophilic granulocytes.

Against the backdrop of these immune responses, eosinophil-associated "rhinosinubronchopathy"—especially the triad of analgesic intolerance, bronchial asthma, and sinonasal polyps—should be viewed as a separate disease entity (115).

Surgery in these cases is only one component of a treatment concept consisting of finding-oriented endoscopic aftercare and topical medical treatment, with systemic therapy added in selected cases.

Indications

Based on our experience in 920 simultaneous septorhinoplasties with endoscopic microsurgery of the paranasal sinuses, we can recommend the following indications:

> **Indications**
> - Recurrent ethmoid and maxillary sinusitis
> - Recurrent ethmoid and frontal sinusitis
> - Chronic hyperplastic sinusitis with circumscribed mucosal changes
> - Cysts of the maxillary and sphenoid sinus
> - Postinflammatory or postoperative synechiae

Contraindications

As a general rule, any complications of inflammatory diseases, tumors, and suppurative inflammations should be excluded prior to the simultaneous operative treatment of extensive pansinusitis.

Revision procedures (e.g., of the ethmoid or frontal sinus) for mucoceles or obliterative scarring of the frontal recess should be performed separately. One should never compromise the functional or esthetic outcome in order to achieve a one-stage operation.

> **Contraindications**
> - Chronic hyperplastic pansinusitis
> - Acute exacerbation of chronic or recurrent sinusitis
> - All types of complication (orbital, central, vascular)
> - Tumors
> - Revisions

Complications

The complication of endoscopic endonasal microsurgery can be classified as *orbital*, *central*, or *vascular*.

Orbital Complications

The most frequent orbital complication is injury to the lamina papyracea, resulting in a hematoma of the upper or lower eyelid. If the periorbita is injured, orbital fat will herniate into the ethmoid cells. The ocular compression test described by Stankiewicz can be used to assess the magnitude of the injury (123). It is important for the surgeon to detect any orbital injuries at once so that the use of sharp and cutting instruments can be avoided. If an orbital perforation is suspected, the eye should be opened to check for concomitant movement of the globe. Lesions ≥ 0.4 cm^2 should be repaired with fascia or perichondrium, while smaller lesions can be covered with mucosa. Injury to the anterior ethmoid artery can lead to the formation of a intrabulbar or retrobulbar hematoma. In severe cases the associated effect on intraorbital pressure can lead to blindness. The best first aid in these cases is to compress the orbital contents with external pressure on the closed eyelid. If this does not stop the hemorrhage, the pressure can be relieved by a lateral canthotomy or endonasal incision of the periorbita.

The bony canal of the optic nerve forms a typical prominence in the lateral wall of the sphenoid sinus. It may also encroach upon the posterior ethmoid, especially in the presence of Onody cells. This is the area in which most optic nerve injuries occur. Pupillary response should be checked during the operation. Direct or indirect injuries are manifested by a reflex mydriasis. Injuries to the orbit always require specific or empirical antibiotic therapy as an adjunct (30, 50, 56).

Intracranial Complications

CSF leak is the most common intracranial complication. Particular danger sites are located in the cribriform plate and anterior skull base at the level of the canal of the anterior ethmoid artery. The skull base is very thin in that area, and the surgeon approaches it directly after opening the anterior ethmoid. The surgeon should be alert for any leakage of the colorless fluid.

Small defects can be covered with free grafts of nasal or turbinate mucosa. Lesions of the bony skull base larger than 4 mm should be repaired with autologous fascia lata harvested from the thigh. Fibrin glue is excellent for attaching the graft. The fascia should be supported for one week with antibiotic-impregnated packing. Coverage with an antibiotic agent that will enter the subarachnoid space is also required.

Vascular Complications

The most serious vascular complication is injury to the carotid artery in the lateral wall of the sphenoid sinus. The surgeon should take every precaution to avoid this disaster. This includes the use of coronal CT scans and high-performance endoscopes with a wide-angle view that will encompass peripheral surgical landmarks.

Even when opening the sphenoid sinus, the surgeon should proceed very carefully while noting key landmarks such as the attachment of the middle turbinate, the choana, the sphenoethmoid recess, and the posterior ethmoid artery. When dissecting in the ethmoid labyrinth, the surgeon should always work in a medial and caudal direction. The sphenoid sinus is not always the last posterior ethmoid cell, and the latter may project past the sinus. The posterior ethmoid cell may even be larger than the sphenoid sinus itself. The sphenopalatine artery runs level with the floor of the sphenoid sinus and may bleed profusely when injured. This vessel is easy to locate, however, and can be coagulated with a bipolar cautery even through the mucosa.

The anterior and posterior ethmoid arteries may or may not traverse a bony canal in the anterior skull base. The vessels are easily identified and can be coagulated. There is a danger of vessel retraction into the orbit (120, 138).

Endoscopic Surgery of the Paranasal Sinuses

Based on our own experience, we can recommend the following procedures in cases where septorhinoplasty is to be combined with endoscopic paranasal sinus surgery.

Surgery of the Anterior Ethmoid

Infundibulotomy

The goal of this procedure is to join the ethmoid infundibulum with the nasal cavity. The first step is to cut around and remove

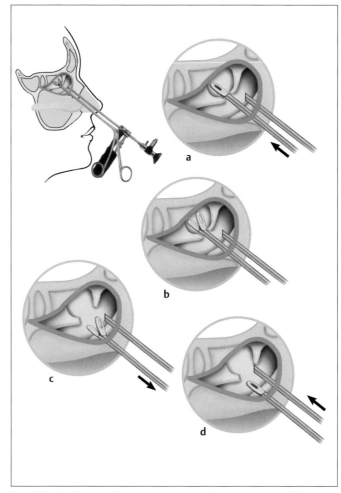

Fig. 1.**20**   Endoscopic dissection technique in microsurgery of the paranasal sinuses, shown here for removal of the ethmoid bulla. (**a**) The anterior wall of the ethmoid bulla is bluntly perforated. (**b**) A Blakesley nasal forceps is inserted through the perforated bony plate and opened. (**c**) The opened instrument is withdrawn. (**d**) Endoscopic surgery of the opened cell: bone and mucosa are removed.

the uncinate process, which basically forms the medial wall of the infundibulum. After removing the medial wall, the surgeon can inspect the ostium of the maxillary sinus, which opens anteroinferiorly. The intraoperative endoscopic findings will determine whether it is necessary to remove additional cells during the infundibulotomy—especially the ethmoid bulla, which bounds the infundibulum dorsally. In all cases at least an exploratory opening should be made in the anterior wall so that the endoscope can be passed into the bulla.

This procedure is indicated for recurrent maxilloethmoid sinusitis with circumscribed changes in the ethmoid epithelium.

Anterior Ethmoidectomy

Removal of the anterior ethmoid cells creates a uniform cavity through which the frontal and maxillary sinuses communicate with the nose. Care is taken to obtain a clean, complete excavation of the cells. Not infrequently, walled-off residual cells create a nidus for recurrent inflammation (139).

The resection cavity is bounded dorsally by the basal lamina of the middle turbinate with its hyperbolic line of insertion on the lamina papyracea (Fig. 1.**20**).

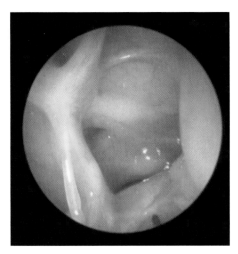

Fig. 1.**21**   View into the sphenoid sinus with the 4-mm 0° endoscope (Karl Storz, Tuttlingen), showing the typical contour of the bony optic-nerve canal.

Supraturbinate Fenestration of the Maxillary Sinus

Supraturbinate fenestration of the maxillary sinus is done to improve mucus drainage and ventilation in patients with diffuse hyperplastic maxillary sinusitis. It also affords access for intracavitary maxillary surgery.

After infundibulotomy is completed, the maxillary ostium can be located by viewing laterally with the 30° oblique scope. The ostium is extended anteriorly with back-biting forceps, taking care to preserve the epithelium of the dorsal circumference to avoid a circular wound with a strong tendency to restenose.

Diffuse hyperplastic ("cobblestone") mucosa is left to heal by reparative processes. Cysts and polyps can be removed through a 9- to 12-mm window under vision using the 70° scope. Maxillary sinus cysts smaller than 1.5 cm that are not causing complaints do not need to be removed (6).

Larger cysts should be removed as they disrupt the mucociliary apparatus of the maxillary sinus, leading to secondary functional disturbances of the nasal mucosa. The cysts can be harpooned with a thin, pointed plastic tube carried on the end of a small Killian probe. The contents are then aspirated and the cyst follicle pulled forward into the nose. The follicle can be grasped low with a Kuhn-Bolger or Stammberger-type giraffe forceps and resected without damaging the parietal mucosa.

Endoscopic Frontal Sinus Surgery in the Context of Functional–Esthetic Nasal Surgery

Recurrent bouts of sinusitis are an indication for enlarging the frontal recess. A useful landmark for locating the frontal recess is the bony canal of the anterior ethmoid artery, which runs just dorsal to the recess. The frontal recess is bounded anteriorly by the agger nasi, which may be pneumatized. It should be noted that the frontal recess runs obliquely downward and backward at about a 120° angle to the infraorbitomeatal line. A 45° scope should be used to locate the region anterior to the bony canal of the ethmoid artery at the anterior skull base. The recess can be enlarged in the dorsoventral direction with a fine hook or with Kuhn-Bolger curettes. This dissection technique is also recommended when cranial ethmoid cells obstruct the frontal recess. Freeing the recess of these cells has been described as "uncapping the egg" (122).

It is essential to preserve the posterior circumference of the mucosa, for otherwise the recess is bound to become occluded by adhesions. If this is not possible, specially designed silicone stents (Rains drains) can be placed to provide temporary drainage and promote stable epithelialization. The drains are left in place for four to six weeks. They are very soft, are well tolerated by the patient, and are easy to remove.

Surgery of the Posterior Ethmoid and Sphenoid Sinus

The posterior ethmoid is entered by perforating the basal lamina of the middle turbinate. It is broader than the anterior ethmoid due to the funnel shape of the orbit. The number of cells is variable. The dissection proceeds in an inferomedial direction to reach the anterior wall of the sphenoid sinus. The optic nerve may be encountered at the lateral wall of the posterior ethmoid, and most optic nerve injuries occur at that location.

The sphenoid sinus may be entered by the transethmoid or transnasal route. The landmark for the transethmoid route is the canal of the posterior ethmoid artery, which runs a few millimeters in front of the anterior wall. Posterior ethmoid cells may extend past the level of the sphenoid sinus. We call them *Onody cells* when they have a pyramidal shape with a posteriorly directed apex and a prominent optic nerve canal.

The sphenoid sinus is the most caudally located posterior cavity and is not always the largest cell. The apex of the choana provides a good landmark for perforating the anterior wall of the sphenoid sinus. The wall is opened about 1 cm cranial to that point, preferably using a blunt instrument. If the anterior wall is exceptionally thick and difficult to perforate, it can be carefully thinned with a diamond bur until the sinus lumen is visible behind the thinned wall. If anatomical constraints limit access, the ethmoid part of the anterior sinus wall can be joined with the nasal part by removing the posterior portion of the middle turbinate. The intranasal route is always preferable for the beginner. It involves enlarging the ostium of the sphenoid sinus in the sphenoethmoid recess (Fig. 1.**21**).

Adjunctive Intranasal Measures

Adjunctive measures are endoscopic endonasal procedures in the nasal cavity and nasopharynx that are intended to:
- Improve nasal breathing;
- Correct rhinogenic ventilation problems in the maxillary, frontal, and sphenoid sinuses and in the middle ear;
- Decompress the middle meatus.

Adjunctive Septoplasty

Circumscribed ridges or spurs can be removed by a minimally invasive endoscopic technique. The selective removal of spurs or ridges from the septal cartilage or perpendicular plate is performed through dorsally based "trapdoor flaps."

The mucoperichondrium is undermined by selective subperichondral injection. The flap is outlined with a No. 15 blade and raised with a Freer elevator. The cartilage ventral to the deformity is divided with the Freer elevator, separated from the contralateral mucoperichondrium, and excised with nasal scissors.

The removed fragment can be straightened with cartilage-crushing forceps and reimplanted. The replaced mucosal flap is secured with several drops of fibrin glue (Fig. 1.**22**).

Treatment of the Middle Turbinate

The middle turbinate is the principal landmark for endoscopic microsurgery of the paranasal sinuses. The medial lamina separates the cribriform plate from the ethmoid roof, which is formed by the frontal bone. The middle turbinate should be preserved whenever possible because it bears olfactory epithelium and has an aerodynamic function in ventilating the frontal and maxillary sinuses and the olfactory groove.

Most Common Procedures on the Middle Turbinate

Splitting a Pneumatized Middle Turbinate

The middle turbinate is part of the ethmoid bone, and all potions of the turbinate (head, neck) may be pneumatized. The pneumatized middle turbinate behaves like a separate paranasal sinus. It is susceptible to concha bullosa sinusitis and can cause complications, usually headaches. A concha bullosa, or heavily pneumatized head of the middle turbinate, can obstruct the middle meatus of the nose. It is cleanly and completely split from before backward, continuing the split to the insertion of the pterygoid process, and removed.

Any bleeding from the sphenopalatine artery during this procedure can be quickly brought under control by submucous bipolar coagulation of the vessel.

Swinging Flap

If the middle turbinate is unstable and hypermobile due to pressure atrophy, it should be shortened. The mucosa is dissected from the bone, the bone is shortened with the nasal scissors, and the mucosa is swung over the bone in a medial to lateral direction (138).

"Trimming"

Trimming is a nautical term for opening a sail to a smooth, unfurled position by adjusting the tension on various lines. The middle turbinate is an aerodynamic body, and its treatment requires attention to aerodynamic principles. It should always be "trimmed" in a tension-free position within the nasal airstream (see the chapter on Olfaction).

Even an atraumatic ethmoid operation will lead to scarring and atrophy of the ethmoid bone with lateralization of the middle turbinate.

Every postoperative patient should receive a follow-up endoscopic examination, and the middle turbinate should be trimmed as required. If the turbinate has a tendency to deviate laterally, the following options exist:

- The turbinate attachment is fractured and the turbinate splinted with a Kennedy-type Merocel pack.
- The middle turbinate has three zones of attachment that keep it stable and properly aligned within the nose:
  - Anterior skull base—frontal bone
  - Lamina papyracea—ethmoid bone
  - Pterygoid process—sphenoid bone

The lateral attachment on the lamina papyracea can be weakened to medialize the turbinate and counteract the tendency toward lateral retraction due to scarring. For additional mobilization, the posterior part can be incised with curved shank scissors.

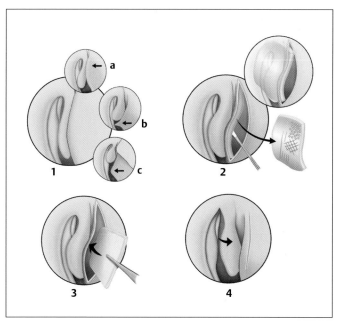

Fig. 1.**22** Procedure for the adjunctive endoscopic correction of a deviated septum.
a) high deviation, **b** vomer spur, **c** vomer ridge
1. Obstruction of the middle meatus by a high septal deviation
2. Removal of the deviated posterior septum, external straightening by cross hatching, morselization or incomplete cartilage incisions
3. Reimplantation of the cartilage
4. Straightening septum with decompression of the middle turbinate

Initial medialization of the turbinate can be accomplished by making a corresponding small incision in the septal mucosa and medial turbinate mucosa to produce a synechia, which is later divided after wound healing is complete (60).

Treatment of the Inferior Turbinate

Deviation of the septum and hyperplasia of the inferior turbinates are closely interrelated conditions. Deviations that narrow one side and broaden the opposite side lead to a compensatory hyperplasia of the inferior turbinate on the broader side.

The inferior turbinate was long considered off limits in rhinosurgery. Surgical manipulations of the inferior turbinate were performed only with great caution, if at all. Today that philosophy has been reversed, and the inferior turbinate is the target of various resections and laser procedures. This is not without its hazards, because the inferior turbinate functions as the thermostat of the nose. Once destroyed, its function cannot truly be replaced.

The results are irreparable functional deficits due to inadequate warming and humidification of the inspired air, olfactory disturbances, and mucosal atrophy combined with a feeling of nasal stuffiness in a broad nose.

It is our experience that inferior turbinate hyperplasia is often caused by a mucosal inflammation that spreads centrifugally from the ethmoid. After this region has been cleared of disease, the turbinate hyperplasia tends to resolve in the majority of patients.

There should be little hesitation in removing the hyperplastic ends of the inferior turbinate. They can significantly compromise nasal breathing and eustachian tube function,

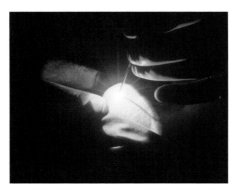

Fig. 1.**23**   Photocoagulation of the facial skin with an Nd:YAG laser in non-touch technique.

especially when they extend through the choana into the nasopharynx. In a subperiosteal turbinectomy, shrinkage of the submucous tissue is achieved by partial resection of the turbinate bone (132).

The inferior turbinate can be moved to a more lateral position by fracturing its muscular attachment (70).

A turbinate strip excision should be done sparingly, removing excess tissue at the lower margin of the inferior turbinate with *one* sharp cut. The bone should be left covered, as there is a danger that vessels may retract into the bone and cause serious bleeding.

Photocoagulation of the inferior turbinate is also mentioned as a special form of laser treatment. Different types of laser differ in their wavelength, absorption properties, penetration depth, and mode of operation. This accounts for their different effects in surgical procedures. Noncontact laser use does not ablate epithelial tissue but causes obliterative scarring of the erectile muscle tissue by inducing a vasculitis in the submucous venous plexus. The scarring leads to shrinkage of the affected turbinate. The advantages are that this is a noncontact, largely painless treatment option that causes minimal damage to the mucosa. The laser surgeon must watch for the desired tissue effect, which is recognized by the whitish discoloration ("spotting") of the mucosal surface.

We can offer the following general recommendations for laser treatment parameters based on our experience in more than 1000 cases: Nd:YAG laser, 10–15 watts, 0.2–0.3 seconds, distance of 2–4 mm from distal fiber end to tissue surface with a 600-µ fiber (5) (Fig. 1.**23**).

Tympanic Ventilation Problems

"The rhinologist must share in the responsibility for the ear." (Wigand, 139)

Abnormalities of eustachian tube ventilation have considerable importance in the pathogenesis of chronic middle ear diseases. The middle ear spaces are ventilated through the eustachian tube. The tube, which is lined with respiratory epithelium, contributes to the ventilation, clearance, and protection of the middle ear.

Eustachian tube function is an important criterion in selecting patients for ablative and tympanoplastic operations and in making a prognosis (70).

Pathophysiologically, the middle ear behaves like a paranasal sinus that is independent of the nose. The following questions should be considered:

- Is it feasible to correct nasal and septal deviations and turbinate hyperplasia as part of a septorhinoplasty in patients with middle ear ventilation problems?
- Should the nasal operation be done prior to tympanoplasty or middle ear surgery?
- By what interval should the nasal surgery precede otosurgery?

Koch (1977) found that rhinoplastic procedures could improve and normalize negative middle ear pressures in patients who had coexisting nasal obstruction (66). Deron (1993) showed that the surgical correction of septal deformities on both the deviated and nondeviated sides helps to normalize eustachian tube function (22). Numerous authors have affirmed the value of septoplasty in patients with eustachian tube dysfunction (3, 34, 53, 82).

This contrasts with the view that, while bilateral nasal obstruction affects middle ear pressure, a unilateral obstruction does not (3, 14).

While Holmquist (49) stated that every septal deviation should be corrected prior to tympanoplasty, Maier et al. (76) could not confirm this rule. Eustachian tube dysfunction is not demonstrable in every patient with chronic middle ear disease. Koch found that one third of patients with adhesive processes had no eustachian tube dysfunction (67, 68). The location of the septal deviation also affects tubal function. Gray distinguished between anterior, posterior, and combined septal deviations. He felt that only the combined forms were important in the pathogenesis of eustachian tube dysfunction (34).

We can offer the following recommendation based on personal experience: Besides otomicroscopy, all patients with signs of inflammatory ear disease or impaired tympanic ventilation should undergo pure-tone audiometry and also tympanometry, with the assessment of passive opening in cases with dry perforations.

The endoscopic examination starts with the nasal vestibule and proceeds across the limen nasi to the nasal cavity and the inferior and middle turbinates, using the 0° wide-angle endoscope. The 30° or 45° scope is then used to examine the sphenoethmoid recess, the choanae, and the epipharynx with the pharyngeal orifice of the eustachian tube. The opening mechanism of the eustachian tube can be evaluated during the act of swallowing.

Particular attention is given to any hyperplasia of the posterior tips of the inferior turbinates. The inferior turbinates have the same sagittal orientation as the pharyngeal orifice of the eustachian tube, and hyperplastic tips can obstruct the tubal orifice. Viscous mucus from the posterior ethmoid often flows over the pharyngeal orifice of the tube. A relative negative pressure in the middle ear can aspirate the mucus into the eustachian tube, leading to an acute exacerbation of chronic otitis media.

Deformities of the nasal septum are assessed endoscopically. If vomerine ridges are present, the endoscope must be advanced strictly over the nasal floor to reach the epipharynx. In children and adolescents, the endoscopist should watch for adenoids or their remnants and for scars.

If signs of inflammatory paranasal sinus disease are noted, coronal CT should be performed. The aerodynamic relevance of axial deformities of the septum and nose or of nasal valve stenosis in a tension nose can be interpreted by comparing the re-

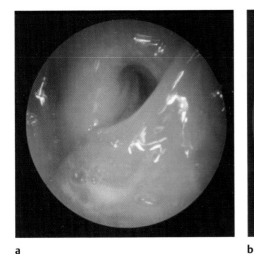 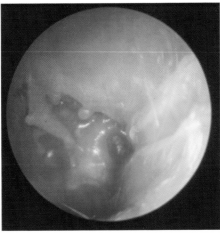

a **b**

Fig. 1.**24** Infected mucus tracks over the pharyngeal orifice of the eustachian tube, with an adhesive process on the left side.

sults of computerized rhinometry before and after a decongestion test with the tympanogram, taking into account the findings of nasal inspection and nasal endoscopy.

If rhinomanometry shows deficient nasal breathing parameters in conjunction with impaired eustachian tube function, surgical correction of the septum should be performed in patients with a deviated nose, saddle nose, or functional tension nose. The sparing reduction of hyperplastic inferior turbinates should be added in selected cases. If signs of inflammatory ethmoid and paranasal sinus disease are observed, an anterior ethmoidectomy may be indicated, depending on the findings.

Cellular structures such as pneumatized middle turbinates and large ethmoid bullae in contact with the middle turbinate are also treated (Figs. 1.**24 a, b**).

Rhinosurgical operations and tympanoplasties should not be carried out in one sitting. Postoperative mucosal swelling, intranasal packs or splints, and retained secretions in the nose or paranasal sinuses can lead to significant impairment of eustachian tube function following the surgery (66, 70, 76).

The nasal operation should precede the ear operation. It is prudent to wait until would healing is complete and postoperative swelling has subsided. An interval of four to six days to several weeks is recommended between the operations (66, 76).

Rhinogenic Headache

The differential diagnosis of unexplained headache is a frequent task for the rhinosurgeon, because rhinological patients often present with this complaint. A detailed endoscopic examination and imaging workup will often reveal findings in the nasal septum and lateral nasal wall that could account for potentially severe rhinogenic headaches.

The principal causes of rhinogenic headache are vasomotor processes, organic vascular lesions, vertebral pathology, psychoautonomic states, and toxic agents. Other potential causes are intracranial masses or inflammations, impaired CSF circulation, ophthalmological processes, and dental diseases.

Sinogenic and rhinogenic headaches are usually caused by direct irritation of the mucosa. This may occur between closely adjacent epithelial surfaces, for example. Mechanical irritation of the receptors in the nasal mucosa is transmitted via afferent nerve fibers to the cerebral cortex as pain. Also, neuropeptides such as substance P can induce vasodilation, secretion, and plasma extravasation. Mucosal edema develops via an axonal reflex, triggering a sensation of pain (16, 121).

The *trigger point* for this type of pain may be a sharp spur on a vomerine ridge that extends dorsally upward and comes into contact with the inferior turbinate or lateral nasal wall.

Sinogenic pain is caused by abnormalities of sinus ventilation and drainage that induce mucosal inflammation. Normally there is a constant equalization of pressures between the nose and paranasal sinuses. Valve mechanisms and incomplete pressure equalization can lead to barosinusitis. Local inflammatory processes lead to edema and the secretion of inflammatory mediators, causing a localized irritation of nerve endings in the mucosa. In this way, local mucosal inflammation can generate pain.

Essentially all pneumatized cells in the facial skeleton can incite this kind of pain. Previously operated paranasal sinuses that contain isolated residual cells can be a refractory source of misdiagnosed pain.

The quality of a rhinogenic headache depends on the underlying cause. Sinus inflammation is characterized by a dull, nagging, position-dependent headache that is associated with a feeling of pressure over the affected sinus.

The pain of acute sinusitis is more intense and is projected to adjacent regions (maxillary sinusitis to the forehead, sphenoid sinusitis to the parietal or occipital region). Typically the pain is aggravated by bending the head forward, coughing, straining, and blowing the nose.

Headache is a late symptom of tumors of the nose and paranasal sinuses. Usually the dominant features are unilateral nasal obstruction, bloody discharge, and impaired ventilation of the middle ear or peripheral sinuses.

Adenoid cystic carcinoma grows along nerve fibers and is associated with pain. A neoplasm that reaches the dura mater will produce intense, unremitting pain.

Mucoceles, which almost always occur in surgical or posttraumatic cavities, lead to pressure erosion of the adjacent bone. Typically the pain subsides when the mucocele can expand by eroding through the lamina papyracea or orbital roof toward the globe.

Facial Neuralgias

Trigeminal Nerve

It is difficult to evaluate facial neuralgias because they are seldom associated with objective organic findings. Idiopathic trigeminal neuralgia is marked by paroxysms of intense, stabbing pain on one side of the face (*tic douloureux*). The attacks may involve one or more branches of the trigeminal nerve and may be accompanied by hypoesthesia, facial redness, or lacrimation. Clonic spasms of the masticatory muscles may also occur during attacks.

Constant pain of varying intensity in the area supplied by the trigeminal nerve, sometimes with deficit symptoms and often combined with sensitivity to weather changes, should raise suspicion of symptomatic trigeminal neuralgia. It may be precipitated by inflammatory or neoplastic diseases of the paranasal sinuses, dental diseases, or infectious diseases (usually viral, such as herpes zoster) (16).

Nasociliary Nerve

Severe, unilateral, paroxysmal pain that is maximal at the medial canthus of the eye, epiphora with marked conjunctival injection, and edematous swelling of the ipsilateral nasal mucosa are features of nasociliary neuralgia (Charlin neuralgia). The pain typically radiates into the orbit, and many patients initially consult an ophthalmologist.

Pterygopalatine Ganglion

Unilateral, aching nocturnal pain centered in the lower half of the face ("lower half headache") combined with variable rhinorrhea and sneezing attacks may be symptomatic of pterygopalatine ganglion neuralgia (Sluder neuralgia). It is caused by tumors and inflammations of the nose, sinuses, orbit, or pterygopalatine fossa.

Post-Caldwell–Luc Syndrome

Inflammatory exacerbations of a previously operated maxillary sinus, scar traction on the infraorbital nerve, severe maxillary deformity, or scar-related infiltrates and abscesses can cause an aching or stabbing pain of variable and sometimes agonizing intensity. Anesthetic blockades can furnish clues to the nasal or sinogenic origin of the head and facial pain. If the pain is relieved by local mucosal anesthesia or conduction anesthesia of a trigeminal nerve branch and recurs after the anesthesia subsides, this confirms the origin of the pain.

Nasal Surgery and Sleep-Disordered Breathing

W. Pirsig

"Neither the site of obstruction during apnea nor the site of generation of snoring is in the nose." This statement by Hoffstein et al. (145) may give comfort to those who, despite successful nasal surgery in their patients with sleep-disordered breathing (SDB), have seen little or no reduction of snoring and apneic events, or perhaps even an exacerbation of these symptoms, in the sleep laboratory. A complete or incomplete obstruction of the nasal airways during sleep generally lessens the quality of sleep due to an increased amount of waking during the night and subsequent daytime tiredness.

The importance of obstructed nasal breathing in the pathogenesis of SDB, especially in primary snoring and obstructive sleep apnea (OSA), is still poorly understood, however. The dominant factor is increased nasal resistance, which leads to a greater reduction of intraluminal pressure during inspiration in the unstable pharyngeal segment and in the lower airways. If the inspiratory pressure falls below the critical closing pressure of the pharynx, the results are collapse of the pharyngeal airway and obstructive apnea. Nasal resistance is influenced by numerous factors such as climate, physical activity, and position. It is lower in the upright than supine position, and it is lower in healthy persons than in patients with OSA. Nasal resistance is approximately equal during sleep and waking. It is increased by nasal allergies and intranasal packing, leading to a greater risk of OSA. Some congenital midfacial and nasal malformations such as choanal atresia, Crouzon disease, Apert disease, and Treacher–Collins syndrome can contribute significantly to OSA by causing obstruction of nasal breathing. Another influence on nasal resistance was discovered by Kawano et al. (146) and Welinder et al. (153). Both groups found a significant decrease in nasal resistance following uvulopalatopharyngoplasty. While several investigators found no correlation between nasal resistance and the apnea–hypopnea index (AHI), Lofaso et al. (148) found in 541 nonselected snorers that nasal resistance in the waking state was an independent risk factor for OSA and added 21.3% to the AHI variance. Besides increased nasal resistance, the transition from nasal breathing to unstable mouth breathing during sleep also appears to have a role in SDB. While the nasal resistance is greater than the oropharyngeal resistance during waking, this relationship is reversed during sleep (149).

Results of Nasal Surgery

No long-term follow-ups have been done on the efficacy of nasal surgery in the treatment of SDB, and relatively few studies (most not comparable) meet the Class I and II criteria for evidence-based medicine. Several groups of authors have presented data on the subjective effects of nasal surgery on primary snoring based on questionnaires. Overall, 150 patients surveyed at one to two years' follow-up reported that the nasal surgery reduced or eliminated their snoring in 40–50% of cases.

There are several case reports in which OSA was cured by nasal surgery alone. By contrast, Simmons et al. (152) described cases in 1977 that had no significant reduction in the postoperative apnea index (AI) despite marked subjective improvement in some patients. As of 2000, only nine studies in a total of 130 patients had presented data on the severity of OSA before and after surgery (150). The follow-up periods ranged up to 44 months. Except for the oldest study by Rubin et al. (150), which described a significant postoperative reduction of AI from 37.8 to 26.7 in nine patients, none of the other investigators reported a significant reduction in the severity of OSA. Four studies even reported an increase in the AHI or AI in 58 out of 130 patients. While on average none of the studies found a polysomnographically measurable reduction of OSA after septoplasty, 12 out of 14 patients did feel less tired during the day and showed improvement in the quality of their sleep (147). Thus, a successful nasal operation alone cannot cure OSA in any given case based on the criteria of Sher et al. (151), which require at least a 50% decrease in AHI and a reduction to values less than 20. When the raw data for 57 patients were evaluated by the Sher criteria, an overall success rate of 18% was calculated for the results of nasal surgery in OSA patients.

Verse et al. (152) recently conducted a prospective study on the effect of nasal surgery in 26 patients with primary snoring (n = 7) or with OSA (n = 19) and reexamined them by polysomnography after an average period of 12.7 months. The body-mass index (BMI) was unchanged. The nasal resistance without decongestion was significantly lower at follow-up. The score in the Epworth Sleepiness Scale and the arousal index showed significant declines after surgery, but the AHI was not changed. Four patients even showed a greater severity of OSA at follow-up than before the surgery, despite unrestricted nasal breathing. Only three out of the 19 patients (15.8%) with OSA could be considered cured based on the success criteria described by Sher et al. (151).

Only a few studies report on the pressure-lowering effect of rhinosurgical procedures in OSA patients on continuous positive airway pressure (CPAP) therapy. In a prospective study of 50 adults with OSA, Friedman et al. (144) performed a submucous septal operation and reexamined 22 of the patients by polysomnography six weeks after the surgery. The average BMI was unchanged. Forty-nine patients reported a postoperative improvement of nasal breathing. Snoring was reduced in 14 of the patients (28%) and was eliminated in three (6%). Daytime activity increased in 78% of the patients even though the mean AHI increased from 31.6 to 39.5 after the surgery. In 22 patients, a postoperative decrease of 2.5 mbar was measured in the nCPAP therapy. In a retrospective study, Bierman (142) compared 35 men with severe OSA who had no nasal surgery with 35 men with severe OSA who had been successfully treated by a septoturbinoplasty before their nCPAP therapy. After three years, the mean necessary nCPAP mask pressure was significantly lower (by 1.5 mbar) than in the control group while the average daily use was 0.8 hours longer.

In older patients with moderately severe or severe OSA who require temporary intranasal packing because of nasal surgery or epistaxis, the AHI may increase to a potentially life-threatening level. This led Dorn et al. (143) to investigate the benefit of oral CPAP therapy in five nCPAP-dependent OSA patients who were wearing intranasal packs following nasal surgery. This therapy prevented the otherwise frequent packing-related abnormal respiratory events during sleep and achieved a permanent, average nCPAP pressure reduction of 3.2 mbar.

Practical Recommendations

There is evidence that two groups exist with regard to the effect of nasal surgery on sleep-related breathing disorders. In the long term, nasal surgery can achieve a desirable reduction of snoring and a marked improvement of OSA symptoms in only a small percentage of patients. In the majority of cases, surgery to reduce nasal airway resistance will relieve obstructed nasal breathing and improve the quality of sleep and life, but it will not eliminate the symptoms of OSA and will even aggravate them in some cases. Patients must be informed of this possibility and that success cannot be predicted in an individual case due to a lack of predictors. Nasal surgery can achieve success in up to 50% of primary snorers, but this rate is only 15–25% in OSA patients. Nasal surgery will reduce the nCPAP pressure in OSA patients with moderate to severe ob-

struction of nasal breathing, resulting in higher compliance for ventilation therapy.

Rhinophonia

W. Seidner

Judging the nasal component of the sound of the voice during diagnostic and therapeutic measures in the area of the nose and paranasal sinuses is not a conventional procedure. In functional diagnostics, only aerodynamic measurements have become routine. Spectral analysis, especially sonograms measurements of vibration or are less frequently measured. It is most important to perceive and document peculiarities in the sound of the voice, as these may be decisive in determining whether surgery is indicated.

The term nasality is mostly used to indicate a normal phenomenon, i.e., a nasal component of the voice sound, which is esthetically satisfying and which contributes to the carrying range of the voice. The latter is often a deliberate aim of artistic voice training. The extent of nasality in speaking, however, also depends on factors such as dialectal influences, models, and speech habits.

The term nasalization, on the other hand, describes changes in the sound of the voice that are characterized by a too prominent or too faint nasal component, changes, which often even sound unesthetic and which suggest a pathological organic or functional condition. There are two main varieties: An open form (sounding exaggeratedly open) and a closed form (sounding blocked). The open variety sounds flat, shifted backward, sometimes sharp, "irritating," and thus esthetically unsatisfactory. The closed variety sounds dull and also shifted backward; the inherent nasality of the phonemes [n], [m], and [ng] is missing. "Nancy needs new nighties" thus becomes "Dadcy deeds dew dighties," with a shift in the zone of articulation. It seems strange that there appears to be no discrimination between the two varieties in everyday usage. A combined variety can also occur.

If the changes mainly relate to the sound of the voice, the term rhinophonia with the subvarieties hyperrhinophonia (rhinophonia aperta), hyporhinophonia (rhinophonia clausa), or rhinophonia mixta is used. Sometimes pathological conditions such as hypernasality and hyponasality are distinguished from the normal condition of nasality. If, on the other hand, the changes mainly relate to impairment of articulation or changes in the pronunciation of phonemes, including consonants, they are designated by the term rhinolalia with the subgroups rhinolalia clausa, rhinolalia aperta or rhinolalia mixta (158, 159).

The diagnosis is mainly based on the perceptional assessment of spontaneous speech, the enouncing of certain sequences of words or reading of a text. In hyperrhinophonia or hyporhinophonia the roughness, breathiness, hoarseness (RBH) scale, often used for the assessment of hoarseness, can be used. The scale has the following degrees: 0 = nil, 1 = mild, 2 = moderate, 3 = severe. Voice recordings are a reliable method for documenting abnormalities and are absolutely necessary for precise follow-up checks on the course of therapy, and also, and above all, for apparative sound analyses. Descriptions of specific samples of nasalization will not be given here since these are mostly used for judging the function of the velum.

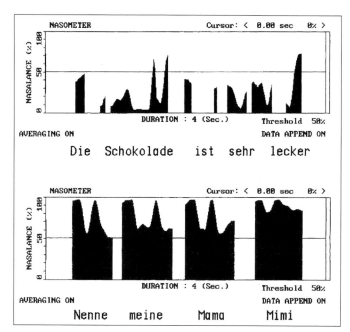

Fig. 1.**25** Nasalance illustration on the monitor (Müller et al.). Low nasalance (above), pronounced nasalance by means of well-formed nasal sounds (below)

It is always necessary to identify the underlying causes of rhinophonia and rhinolalia. The open varieties may be due to functional or organic disorders, mostly malformation or paralysis, or may result from surgery. Within the framework of this publication it is more important to focus on the closed forms, which may also be due to functional disorders, though this occurs extremely rarely. In most cases they are caused by organic changes of various kinds, which also impair breathing through the nose and thus affect the normal nasal component of the voice. Hyporhinophonia, even if barely perceptible, that persists for a longer period of time always calls for a thorough inspection of the nasopharynx and main nasal cavities.

In therapeutic measures, especially surgical ones, which may entail the risk of hyperrhinophonia, it should be noted that open nasalization is more conspicuous and sounds more unpleasant than the closed variety. As demands on oral communication skills are higher than ever today, this esthetic sound component should not be underrated.

Objectivization of nasality and its pathological varieties is made possible by means of a so-called nasometer, in which two microphones, separated by a plate, measure the oral and nasal sound energies. The acoustic passage of the nose is then described in terms of nasalance, i.e., the amount of nasal sound energy as a percentage of the total sound energy (155–157, see also Fig. 1.**25**).

Singers in the occidental tradition of artistic singing always aim at an optimum of sound quality of the voice and their term for this is "focus." This does not only relate to an acoustic category, which also comprises nasality, but also a physical one, as, while using his/her voice, the singer senses vibrations in the areas of nose, forehead, cheeks, and palate and uses this phenomenon for deliberate control of the voice ("singing into the mask").

According to our own experience (154), endoscopic surgery on the nose and the paranasal sinuses of patients in voice-intensive professions can have major consequences for

their voices. Apart from the improvement in voice quality and clearer vibrational sensations in the areas of forehead and cheek, a decrease in voice fatigue, a reduction of the compulsion to clear one's throat, and the ability to sustain high notes for a longer time were reported. Acoustic rhinometry showed a distinct postoperative increase in the volume of the nasal cavities, significant results of which were a wider range of higher tones as well as a higher sound pressure level in calling out.

These results should not be taken to suggest that specialists should be generous in providing indications for surgery on the area of the nose, as the hope of achieving major improvements in the sound of the voice by plastic septum surgery in students of singing or professional singers, which was widespread some decades ago, did not materialize. This does not mean, however, that the judgement of the voice sound and its potential alteration by therapeutic measures are unimportant. It should always be recognized that clearer vibrational sensations can be very useful, especially for professional singers.

In summary, we can say that the quality of the voice sound should always be considered in all diagnostic and therapeutic measures in the area of the nose and paranasal sinuses, the miminum requirement being the perceptional assessment of hyporhinophonia or hyperrhinophonia (hyponasality or hypernasality), which should be performed as soon as possible, as the procedure is quick and reliable. Nasalance measurements, on the other hand, though requiring a greater effort, have the advantage of objectivizing the measurement of the acoustic passage of the nose.

Esthetic Aspects of Septorhinoplasty

The nose is, quite literally, a prominent facial feature. It critically determines the facial appearance. Its symmetry, proportionality, and contours determine whether the facial features are perceived as harmonious. An impression of disharmony arises when the nose is perceived as too broad, too long, or too large. Patients tend to consult a rhinoplastic surgeon when they become aware of this disharmony and desire a change. Generally the physician will have developed a feel for these matters but will still try to apply objective criteria by measuring angles, proportions, or projections. It is less important in plastic facial surgery to form a single esthetically pleasing feature than to match the various features to one another in an harmonious, esthetically pleasing way. Moreover, there is an acknowledged hierarchy of facial features, starting with the eyes. The eyes can speak, and the nose should be subordinated to them with a certain understatement. For this purpose, a gently curved imaginary line is drawn from the medial point of the eyebrow to the pronasale (greatest anterior projection of the nasal tip).

Rhinoplastic surgeons should be a careful and patient listener as well as a keen observer and anatomical analyst. They should understand what is troubling the rhinoplasty candidate about his/her own face or nose.

The face is the most important means of communication, even without words. It is considered a mirror of the human psyche and conveys much about the personality.

Lavater correlated the shape of the nose with several basic human temperaments, relating a large, convex nose to a choleric or sanguine temperament (Fig. 1.**26**).

When combined with a prominent chin, this feature is generally associated with an active, aggressive type of personality (111).

Without belaboring this point, we may observe that the effect of physiognomy on human beings does follow certain principles. The nose is a personality trait and, as such, has been an object of studies in anthropology and constitutional research. Ziegelmayer could find no specific modes of inheritance for morphological variants and individual features of the human nose (140) (Fig. 1.**27a, b**).

The French caricaturist Honoré Daumier (1808–1879) used his brilliant talent to stereotype character traits by exaggerating certain physiognomic features.

Symmetry is an important criterion, but it is not synonymous with beauty. No face is exactly the same on both sides. Facial asymmetries are common and are combined with subtle axial deformities of the nose.

Whenever the physiognomy of a human being is altered, a reasonable *esthetic indication* should exist. Physicians should act responsibly and dissuade patients from changing their face in a desire to mimic current trends or idols. Surgeons should also be wary about altering ethnic characteristics.

As a general rule, the individual features of a human being should be respected and preserved. We have found that the great majority of our own patients have the same desire. As a general goal, we would recommend a somewhat large nose with a high dorsum and esthetic proportions. Type-altering operations or the desire for a "perfect nose" also have their justification if the current appearance of the nose is distressful to the patient. But physicians are obliged in these cases to use their "sixth sense" in distinguishing the reasonable desire for a morphological change from a psychopathological condition such as body dysmorphic disorder (see below).

"While knowledge of the anatomy, physiology, and surgery of the nose is a sine qua non, the artistic creative power is the most important factor in the success of the operation" (Aufricht, 2).

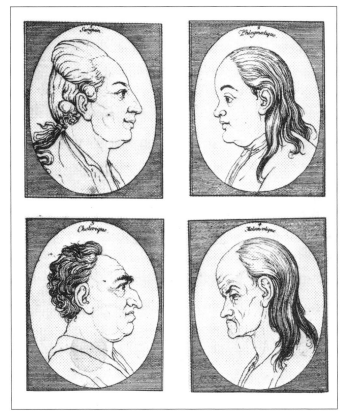

Fig. 1.**26**   Temperaments are reflected in facial features (69).

Fig. 1.**27**   The nose as an inherited character trait? Mother (**a**) and daughter (**b**).

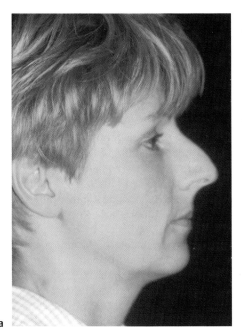

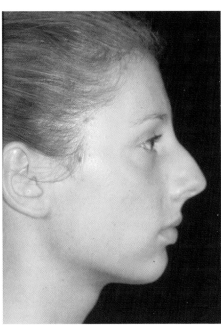

a

b

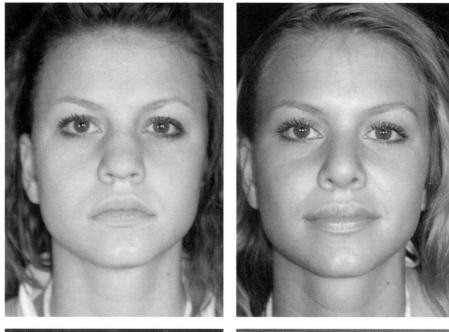

a

b

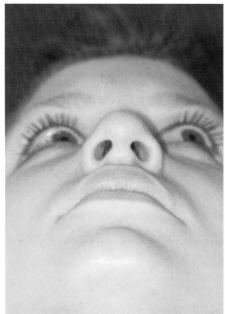

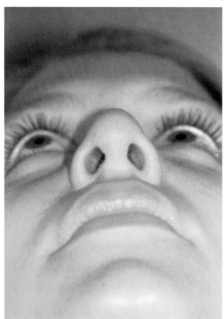

c

d

Fig. 1.**28 c** Note the broad, elliptical nares. Nasal breathing is obstructed by *ballooning* with inferior turbinate hyperplasia.
d Appearance after correction of vestibular stenosis.

Selecting an Approach for Septo-rhinoplasty

Various approaches are used to gain access to the nasal tip and dorsum in functional–esthetic surgery. The selection of a particular approach is based on a clinical analysis of the specific problem. Taking into consideration the patient's age and his/her skin type and connective-tissue type, the surgeon mentally composes a plan for the operative procedure.

Moderately thick nasal skin is favorable for rhinoplasty. Thick skin is more prone to scarring and postoperative problems such as pollybeak deformity. When dealing with thick skin, the surgeon should avoid removing too much cartilage in an effort to form a delicate tip. Thick skin and thin cartilage are a particularly unfavorable combination.

On the other hand, thicker skin will cover small irregularities in the nasal dorsum and allows for all techniques of nasal tip surgery, i.e., *incision, graft,* and *suture techniques.*

Thin skin is less susceptible to postoperative problems but requires a high degree of precision, since all contour imperfections and irregularities can be seen. Superficial contour-defining grafts cannot be used in the tip area. As a general rule, the tip should always be left slightly broader than is ideal, as it will tend to become narrower as the patient ages and the overlying skin–subcutaneous tissue complex shrinks (Figs. **1.28 a–d,** **1.29 a–d**).

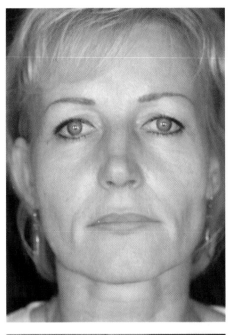

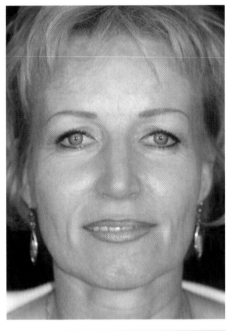

a

b

Fig. 1.**29 a**   Middle-aged woman with thin skin and thick cartilage tissue. A prominent, over-projected tip is combined with a saddle depression in the supratip area. The nose requires reduction and augmentation with septal cartilage.
b   Appearance three years after surgery (endonasal approach, double suture technique).

Fig. 1.**29 c, d**   Profile views before and after the operation.

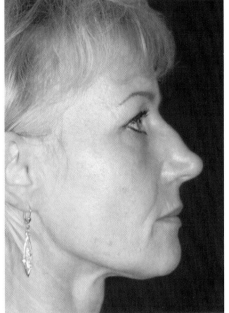

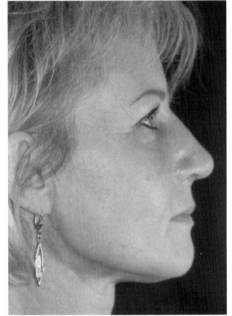

c

d

Endonasal Approaches

Endonasal approaches offer the advantage of an exacting and less invasive operation. By dissecting in the surgical plane, the operator can avoid injuring vessels of the superficial musculoaponeurotic system (SMAS). Undermining is done only over the cartilaginous and bony nasal dorsum and is used to develop precise pockets for deep or superficial graft placement. Suture fixation is unnecessary in most cases.

There is minimal tissue trauma in these approaches, and scar formation is limited to circumscribed areas. As a result, postoperative healing is rapid and uncomplicated. External scars and postoperative asymmetries due to scar contraction are avoided.

Cartilage-Splitting Approach

The cartilage-splitting approach is very well suited for reducing the volume of the upper alar cartilages to correct a bulbous nasal tip. The approach is suitable for correcting tip asymmetries only in exceptional cases. It is best for cases with a symmetrical, nonbifid tip that does not have a broad, obtuse dome (angle).

While the cartilage-splitting approach provides good access to the upper alar cartilages, the shape of the lower alar cartilages cannot be altered through this approach. The intracartilaginous incision typically runs cranial to the *tip-defining point*, which should be marked beforehand.

Narrowing of the supratip area and cranial rotation of the tip can be supported by beveling the anterosuperior septal

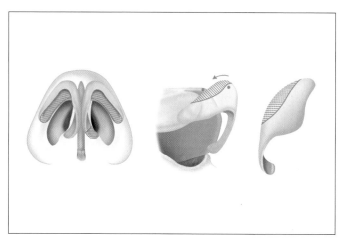

Fig. 1.**30** Principle of the cartilage-splitting approach.

margin. Cranial tip rotation is produced by scar contraction occurring between the caudal margin of the upper lateral cartilage and the intact alar cartilage. It depends on the extent of volume reduction of the upper alar cartilage.

The tip projection is unchanged when the tip-defining points are preserved. Owing to the low invasiveness of the cartilage-splitting approach and the minimal bleeding, endonasal operative steps can be performed concurrently with this approach (Figs. 1.**30**, 1.**31 a–f**, 1.**32 a–g**).

Delivery Approach

The delivery approach is an elegant endonasal technique that gives experienced surgeons a variety of options for correcting the nasal tip.

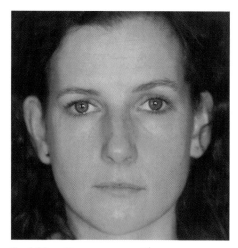

Fig. 1.**31 a** Young woman with an overprojected nose. The tip appears bulbous in relation to the thin, ridgelike bony and cartilaginous dorsum. She had a history of recurrent frontal sinusitis, predominantly on the right side, and severe obstruction of nasal breathing.

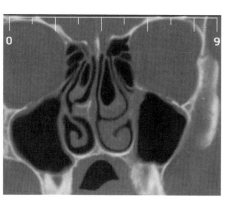

Fig. 1.**31 b** Coronal CT shows severe septal deviation with a spur on the right side, concha bullosa on both sides, and a long, narrow ethmoid infundibulum on each side. Mucosal swelling is noted in the left infundibulum and on the left middle turbinate.

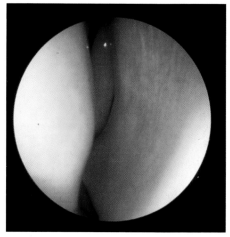

Fig. 1.**31 c** View into the middle meatus with the 0° endoscope (Karl Storz, Tuttlingen). There is severe obstruction of the middle meatus by a spurlike projection on the right vomerine ridge.

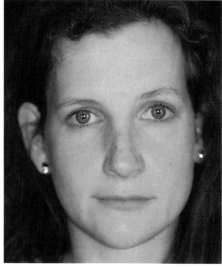

Fig. 1.**31 d** Appearance three years after cranial volume reduction of the alar cartilages. Spreader grafts were used to produce a gently curved eyebrow–tip line.

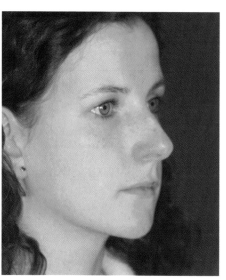

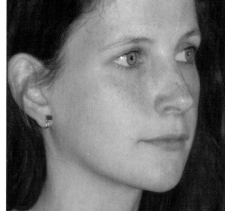

Fig. 1.**31 e, f** Half profile views before and after the operation.

e, f

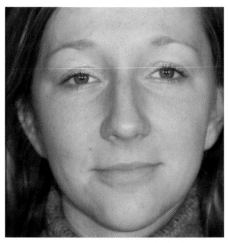

Fig. 1.**32a** Young woman with slight facial asymmetry, a somewhat broad supratip area, and unequal curvatures of the eyebrow-tip lines. The tip defining points are close together, and there is fullness of the upper lateral alar cartilages. The patient had a history of chronic, bilateral ethmoid and maxillary sinusitis, and frontal headaches.

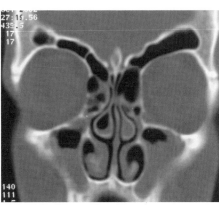

Fig. 1.**32b** Coronal CT scan of the paranasal sinuses shows mucosal swelling in relatively large ethmoid bullae on both sides, bilateral concha bullosa with inflammatory mucosal changes on the left side (concha bullosa sinusitis), and mucosal swelling in both maxillary sinuses.

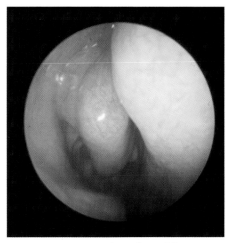

Fig. 1.**32c** View into the right middle meatus with the 0° endoscope: mucosal edema.

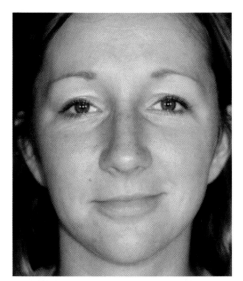

Fig. 1.**32d** Appearance three years after surgery.

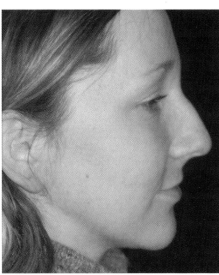

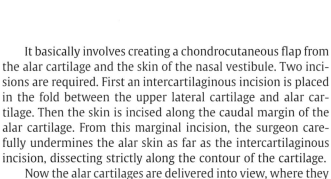

e, f

Fig. 1.**32e, f** Profile views before and after the operation. Slight cranial tip rotation has been achieved by cranial volume reduction of the alar cartilages (*complete strip*).

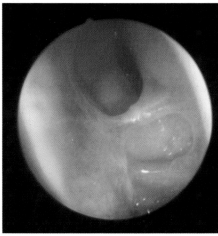

Fig. 1.**32g** View into the enlarged right frontal recess.

It basically involves creating a chondrocutaneous flap from the alar cartilage and the skin of the nasal vestibule. Two incisions are required. First an intercartilaginous incision is placed in the fold between the upper lateral cartilage and alar cartilage. Then the skin is incised along the caudal margin of the alar cartilage. From this marginal incision, the surgeon carefully undermines the alar skin as far as the intercartilaginous incision, dissecting strictly along the contour of the cartilage.

Now the alar cartilages are delivered into view, where they can be modified under direct vision with the benefit of side-to-side comparison. Wedges or strips can be resected from the cartilages for volume reduction, cartilage tension can be modified by scoring or cross-hatching, the cartilages can be augmented with autologous graft material, and intradomal or interdomal suture techniques can be applied.

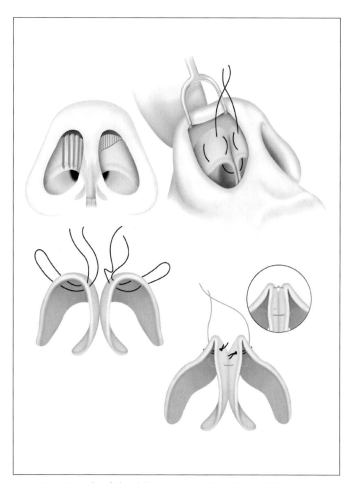

Fig. 1.**33**   Principle of the delivery approach, and possibilities.

This approach is suitable for asymmetrical and bifid tips. The tip projection can be assessed and modified. Cranial tip rotation can also be induced.

The *dome suture technique* is particularly suitable for patients with a broad or bifid nasal tip, thin skin, and scant subcutaneous fat and connective tissue. The alar cartilages themselves should be stable and resilient (99, 124).

Interdomal sutures are used to narrow the domes. Transdomal sutures are effective for approximating the tip-defining points, usually after removal of the interdomal fat or connective tissue.

Based on personal experience, we can recommend 5–0 PDS for these tip suturing techniques. Following suture absorption, the tip shape remains permanently stable as a result of shrinkage and submucous scarring. The knots should always be placed on the inside between the domes and should not be subcutaneous on the cartilage surface.

The intercartilaginous incision can be combined with a transfixion, hemitransfixion, or high transfixion incision, or with an oral vestibular incision for midfacial degloving through a transfixion approach (Figs. 1.**33**, 1.**34a–f**, 1.**35a–h**).

Open Approach

The open approach for rhinoplasty provides maximum exposure of the alar cartilages with their medial and lateral crura, the domes, and the nasal dorsum.

The skin incision is stepped or zig-zagged at the midcolumellar level. The incision is carried around the contour of the medial crura, runs on the lateral columella about 2 mm behind the anterior side of the columella, and joins with marginal alar incisions. Then the skin of the midcolumella is undermined with small, sharp scissors above the medial crura of the

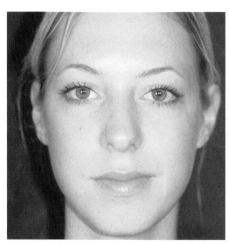

Fig. 1.**34a**   Young woman who had worked as a model and was emphatic in her desire to narrow the nasal tip. The tip-defining points are spaced widely apart. She had a history of recurrent maxillary sinusitis and difficulty with pressure equalization when flying.

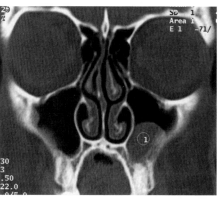

Fig. 1.**34b**   Coronal CT scan of the paranasal sinuses shows a high septal deviation toward the right side with compression of the middle turbinates. The ethmoid infundibula are extremely long and narrow on both sides. A cyst is present in the left maxillary sinus.

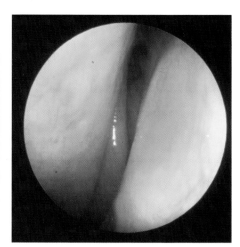

Fig. 1.**34c**   View into the right middle meatus with the 0° endoscope: high septal deviation.

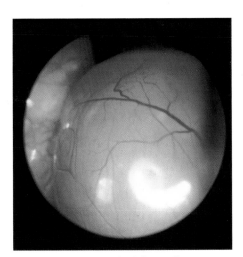

Fig. 1.**34 d** View into the left maxillary sinus with the 45° endoscope: large cyst.

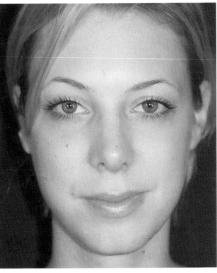

Fig. 1.**34 e** Appearance three years after surgery. The tip was narrowed through a delivery approach with cranial volume reduction of the lateral alar cartilages and the placement of intradomal and transdomal sutures.

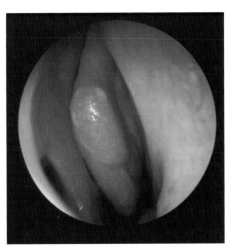

Fig. 1.**34 f** Postoperative view into the right middle meatus with the 0° endoscope. The middle turbinate and middle meatus are decompressed, and the middle turbinate has been medialized. Open supraturbinate window.

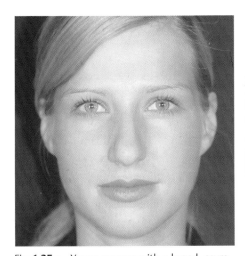

Fig. 1.**35 a** Young woman with a broad, asymmetrical tip and supratip area. She had severe nasal obstruction and a history of frontal headaches.

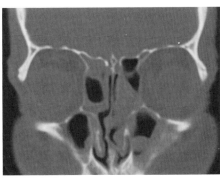

Fig. 1.**35 b** Coronal CT scan of the paranasal sinuses shows polypous mucosal swelling in the ethmoid cells, maxillary sinuses, and nasal cavity on both sides.

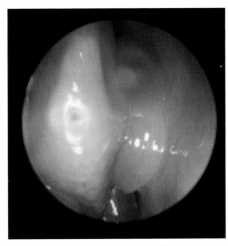

Fig. 1.**35 c** View into the left middle meatus with the 0° endoscope demonstrates severe obstruction by a mucosal polyp.

alar cartilages. Now the columellar flap is progressively developed. When the medial crura of the alar cartilages have been exposed, their medial surfaces provide a guide for dissecting in the cephalad direction. In this way the surgeon reaches the top of the domes and, after dividing the interdomal connective tissue, the lateral crura.

Later in the operation, the upper lateral cartilages and nasal valve can be exposed. They can be traced to the rhinion, or *keystone area*. The nasal bones and frontomaxillary process can also be directly visualized. While the dissection is supraperichondrial initially, it should be continued in the subpe-

riosteal plane at the level of the rhinion. This is done by carefully elevating the periosteum laterally from the midline with a sharp Freer or Joseph elevator (this produces a scratching sound).

The advantages of the open approach are the binocular, three-dimensional view of the operative site and the ability to dissect the structures bimanually and under vision with controlled hemostasis.

Larger grafts can be placed and secured with great precision (Figs. 1.**36**, 1.**37 a–e**, 1.**38 a–f**).

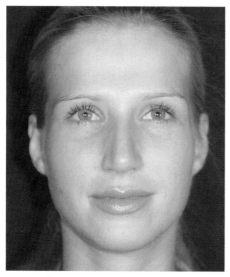
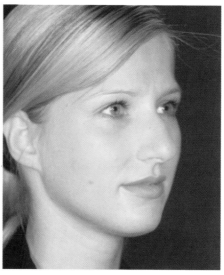
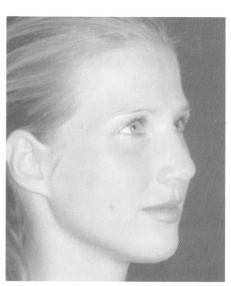

e, f

Fig. 1.**35 d**   Appearance three years after asymmetrical reduction of the lateral alar cartilages and a double suture technique.

Fig. 1.**35 e, f**   Half profile views before and after the operation.

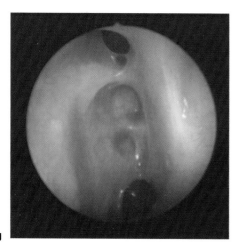
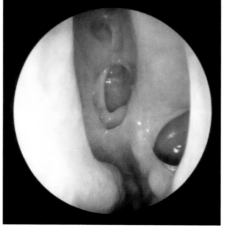

Fig. 1.**35 g**   View of the anterior skull base with the 30° endoscope three years after surgery, showing the frontal recess and the bony canal of the left anterior ethmoid artery. **h**   View into the excavated, well-epithelialized ethmoid with the 0° endoscope. Note the perforated basal lamina of the middle turbinate and the open supraturbinate window in the maxillary sinus.

g   h

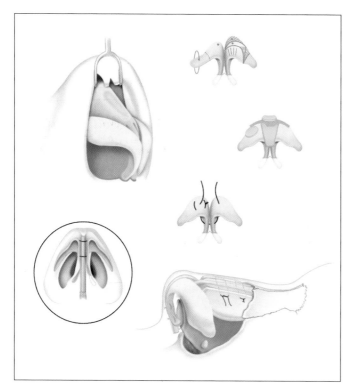

Fig. 1.**36**   Schematic diagram of the open approach and its possibilities.

Principal Graft Types

Autologous grafts should be used whenever possible. More detailed information on grafts and implants is presented in the section on the saddle nose (see p. 201 ff). Autologous grafts can be obtained from pieces of septal or alar cartilage (first choice), or auricular cartilage may be harvested from the conchal cavity or tragus (second choice). A distinction is made between deep grafts for replacing lost substance and superficial grafts for contouring the nose. Grafts can always be placed on one or both sides.

Surgical templates are available for harvesting the grafts and cutting them to size. "Carving" of the grafts is done on a small bench on the operating table.

Columella Strut

This graft is placed into a pocket between the basal medial crura of the alar cartilages over the anterior nasal spine and fixed between the medial crura with through-and-through sutures. It is used to control tip projection and provide tip support. It can correct for disparities in the height of the domes. Tip symmetry can be created by working upward from the base.

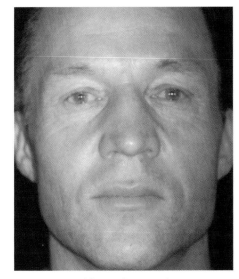

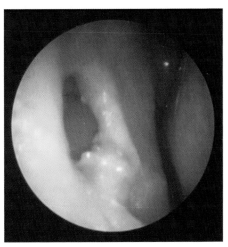

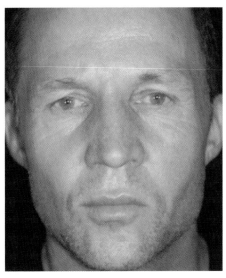

Fig. 1.**37 a** Middle-aged man with a posttraumatic saddle nose, severe nasal obstruction, a large septal perforation, and deviation of the septal remnant. The patient had worked as a professional boxer.

Fig. 1.**37 b** View of the anterior septum with the 0° endoscope demonstrates a large perforation.

Fig. 1.**37 c** Appearance four years after reconstruction of the septum with conchal cartilage and narrowing of the bony and cartilaginous nasal dorsum, which was also augmented.

Fig. 1.**37 d, e** Profile views before and after the operation.

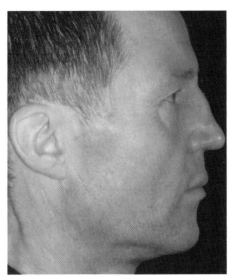

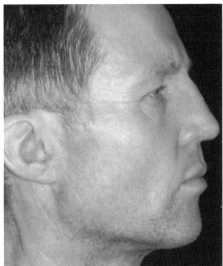

d

e

Tip Grafts

These can be placed on the domes as trapezoid-shaped grafts to contour the tip or improve its projection. They are fixed with 5–0 PDS.

Shield Grafts

Shield grafts can be placed to lengthen the nose, form a double break, or create a harmonious columella–lobule–tip junction. They can be combined with a columella strut to support the tip and dome contours.

Onlay Grafts

Onlay grafts are used on the nasal dorsum or lateral alar cartilages as *alar onlay grafts* to correct for loss of substance or contour the nose.

Camouflage

Peaked domes can be camouflaged by covering them with autologous tissue. This softens the tip contours and creates an harmonious junction with the facets. Tragal perichondrium and temporalis fascia have proved effective for this purpose.

Spreader Grafts

Spreader grafts are placed in the extramucous plane between the dorsal septal margin and the upper lateral cartilages. They are equally useful for both functional and esthetic goals. They may be placed after the removal of large humps, on a depressed nasal dorsum in a functional tension nose, or in a large nose with short nasal bones. They are equally useful for the correction of deviated noses.

Spreader grafts prevent the development of nasal valve stenosis and can create an harmonious eyebrow–tip line.

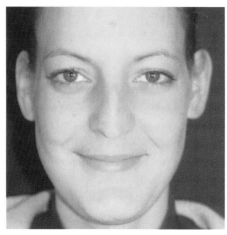

Fig. 1.**38 a**   Young woman with a broad, humped nose after trauma, an open roof, and an asymmetrical bifid tip with ptosis.

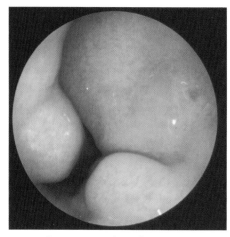

Fig. 1.**38 b**   View into the right anterior nose with the 0° endoscope shows a prominent pre-maxilla with severe midseptal deviation toward the right.

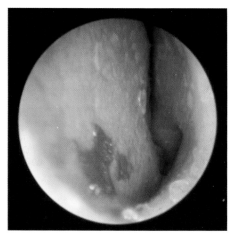

Fig. 1.**38 c**   View into the left anterior nose with the 0° endoscope shows marked deviation of the anterior septum toward the left side. There is rhinitis sicca with mucosal bleeding as a result of the deviation. Typical features of a *transverse septum*.

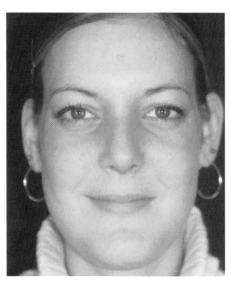

Fig. 1.**38 d**   Appearance three years after narrowing of the bony and cartilaginous nasal dorsum, construction of a symmetrical tip with alar onlay grafts, and camouflage with spreader grafts of tragal perichondrium.

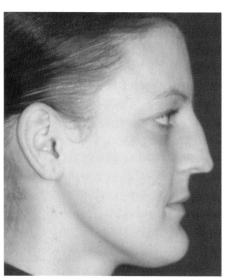

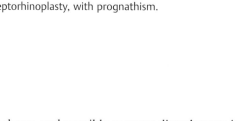

e, f

Fig. 1.**38 e, f**   Profile views before and after septorhinoplasty, with prognathism.

The open approach is a revelation for understanding the anatomy of the nose. It is common to discover fine curvatures and asymmetries (e.g., of the alar cartilages) that could not be appreciated preoperatively. The open approach does not help us to understand the dynamics of rhinoplasty, however, and the question must be asked whether this degree of exposure is necessary in any given case. The art of rhinoplasty includes the ability to choose an approach that is as invasive as necessary but as noninvasive as possible. In this regard, the open technique abandons the principle of conservatism in favor of a more aggressive approach. Large submucous wound areas lead to relatively extensive scarring. The results are prolonged wound healing, edema, and possible sensory disturbances in the tip area. Strict criteria should be applied, therefore, in selecting patients for this approach.

Indications

- Marked asymmetries of the nasal tip
- Revisions (usually after multiple previous operations)
- Septal perforations larger than 6 mm
- Severe axial deformities
- Cleft nasal deformities
- Pronounced saddle nose

References

1. Adamson P. Controversies in septorhinoplasty. One problem—one goal—one solution? Course in functional aesthetic septorhinoplasty, Ulm; June 2002.
2. Aufricht G. A few hints and surgical details in thinoplasty. *Laryngoscope.* 1943.
3. Becker W, Opitz HJ. Paukenergüsse bei Erwachsenen. *Z. Laryngol Rhinol Otol* 1977; 56:846–849.
4. Behrbohm H, Sydow K, Härtig W. Experimentelle Untersuchungen zur Physiologie der Nasennebenhöhlen. *HNO* 1991; 39:168–172.
5. Behrbohm H. Lasertherapie in der HNO-Heilkunde: Teil 1. *HNO-Nachr.* 2002; 2:26–28.
6. Behrbohm H, Kaschke O, Nawka T. *Endoskopische Diagnostik und Therapie in der HNO.* Stuttgart: Gustav Fischer: 1997.
7. Behrbohm H, Kaschke O. *Oto-Endoskopie–Otoskopie mit Endoskopen, Diag-nostik, Befundbewertung, Nachbehandlung nach Ohrchirurgie.* Tuttlingen: Endo-Press: 1999.
8. Behrbohm H, Hildebrandt T, Kaschke O, Jahnke,V. Funktionell-ästhetische Chirurgie der Nase Teil 1: Ziele, präoperative Diagnostik, Operationsplanung. *HNO akt.* 2000; 8:129–137.
9. Behrbohm H, Hildebrandt Th, Kaschke O. *Funktionell-ästhetische Chirurgie der Nase.* Tuttlingen: Endo-Press: 2001.
10. Behrbohm H, Kaschke O. Pathophysiologie, Differentialdiagnostik und Therapie von Störungen des Geruchsinns. *HNO akt.* 1999; 7:21–29.
11. Behrbohm H. Die endoskopische Untersuchung der Nase. Teil 1 und 2. *HNO akt.* 2000; 9:361–366, 409–414.
12. Bier A, Braun H, Kümmel H. *Chirurgische Operationslehre.* Leipzig: JA Barth: 1917.
13. Bönisch M, Mink A. Heilungsprozesse des Knorpels in Verbindung mit PDS-Folie. *HNO* 2000; 48:743–746.
14. Bonding P, Tos M. Middle ear pressure during brief pathological conditions of nose and throat. *Acta Otolaryngol.* 1981; 92:63–69.
15. Brain DJ. Historical background. In Settipane GA et al. *Nasal polyps: Epidemiology, Pathogenesis and treatment,* Rhode Island: Oceanside Publications; 1997.
16. Bremer B, Behrbohm H, Kaschke O. Differentialdiagnostik des rhinogenen Kopfschmerzes. *HNO akt.* 1996; 4:93–100.
17. Bull TR, Mackay IS. Alar collapse. *Facial Plastic Surgery* 1986; 3:267–276.
18. Cinelli AA. Collapse of the nares. *Arch Orolaryngol.* 1941; 33:683–693.
19. Caldwell GW. Diseases of the accessory sinuses of the nose and an improved method of treatment for suppuration of the Maxillary antrum. *N.Y. med. J.* 1893; 58:526–528.
20. Cottle MH, Loring R, Fischer, Gaynon I. The maxilla-premaxilla approach to extensive nasal septum surgery . *Arch Otolaryng.* 1958; 68:301–313.
21. Da Vinci L. Cited by Skillern (1920).
22. Deron P, Clement PAR, Derde M-P. Septal surgery and tubal function: Early and late results. *Rhinology* 1995; 33:7–9.
23. Dieffenbach JF. *Über das Schielen und die Heilung desselben durch die Operation.* Berlin: A.Förster: 1842.
24. Dieffenbach JF. *Die operative Chirurgie.* 2 Volumes. Leipzig: FA Brockhaus: 1845.
25. van Dishoeck HAE. Inspiratory nasal resistance. *Acta Otolaryngol.* 1942; 30:431–439.
26. Döderlein W. Experimentelle Untersuchungen zur Physiologie der Nasen- und Mundatmung. *Z. Hals-Nas.- u. Ohrenheilk.* 1932; 30:459.
27. Draf W. Die chirurgische Behandlung entzündlicher Erkrankungen der Nasennebenhöhlen. *Arch. Otorhinolaryngol.* 1992; 235: 133–305, 367–377.
28. Eckert-Möbius A. Die Bedeutung der Zunge für die Nasen- und Mundatmung. *Fortsch. Kieferorthopäd.* 1953; 14:229.
29. Farrior RT. Korrigierende und rekonstruktive plastische Chirurgie an der äußeren Nase. In Naumann HH, ed. *Kopf- und Hals-Chirurgie, Vol. 2. Gesicht und Gesichtsschädel,* Stuttgart: Thieme; 1974.
30. Friedman HM, Kern EB. Complications of intranasal ethmoidectomy: A review of 1000 consecutive operations.*Laryngoscope* 1979; 89:421–434.
31. Goldman JB. New technique in surgery of the deviated nasal septum. *Arch Otolaryngol* 1956; 64:183–189.
32. Goode R, Alto P. Surgery of the incompetent nasal valve. *Laryngoscope.* 1985; 95:546–555.
33. von Graefe CF. *Rhinoplastik oder die Kunst, den Verlust der Nase zu ersetzen.* Berlin: In der Realschulbuchhandlung: 1818: 4.
34. Gray L. Deviated nasal septum III—its influence on the physiology and disease of the nose and ear. *J. Laryngol.Otol.* 1967; 81:953–985.
35. Grünwald L. Deskriptive und topographische Anatomie der Nase und ihrer Nebenhöhlen. In Denker A, Kahler O. *Die Krankheiten der Luftwege und der Mundhöhle.* Berlin: Springer: 1–95.
36. Gubisch W. Zwanzig Jahre Erfahrung mit der extrakorporalen Septumkorrektur. *Laryngo-Rhino-Otol.* 2002; 81:22–30.
37. Gudziol H, Förster G. Zur Durchführung präoperativer Riechtests aus medicolegaler Sicht. *Laryngo-Rhino-Otol.* 2001; 81:586–590.
38. Haas E. Allgemeines zur korrektiven Rhinoplastik. *Z. Laryng.Rhinol.* 1973; 52:405.
39. Hajek M. *Pathologie und Therapie der entzündlichen Erkrankungen der Nebenhöhlen der Nase.* Leipzig and Vienna: Franz Deutike: 1926.
40. Hartmann A. Partielle Resektion der Nasenscheidewand bei hochgradiger Verkrümmung derselben. *Dtsch Med Wschr.* 1882;8:691–692.
41. Hauben DJ. Die Geschichte der Rhinoplastik. *Laryng. Rhinol. Otol.* 1983; 62:53–55.
42. Hauben DJ. Jacques Joseph (1865–1934). *Laryng. Rhinol. Otol.* 1983; 62:56–57.
43. Henrici L. Nasenatmung und Mundatmung bei körperlicher Anstrengung. *Z. Ohrenheilk.* 1917; 77:31.
44. Highmore N. Cited by Wendler (1924).
45. Hildebrandt T, Behrbohm H, Jahnke V, Kaschke O. Teil 2: Neue Aspekte der Septumplastik bei Nasenkorrek turen. *HNO akt.* 2000; 6:161–170.
46. Hildebrandt T, Behrbohm H. Functional aesthetic surgery of the nose. The influence of the septum on the aesthetic of the nasal tip. CD-ROM, Mediaservice, Storz, Tuttlingen; 2001.
47. Hill W. External alar collapse. *Proc Royal Soc Med II.*1918; :129–130.
48. Hirschmann A. Über Endoskopie der Nase und deren Nebenhöhlen. Eine neue Untersuchungsmethode. *Arch. Laryngol. Rhinol.* 1903; 14:195–202.
49. Holmquist J. The role of eustachian tube in myringoplasty. *Acta Otolaryngol.* 1968; 66:289–295.
50. Hosemann W. Medicolegale Probleme in der endonasalen Nasennebenhöhlenchirurgie. *Eur. Arch. Oto-Rhino-Laryngol.:* 1992; (Suppl.) 2:284–296.
51. Ingelstedt S, Ivstam B. Study in the humidifying capacity of the nose. *Acta Otolaryngol.* 1951; 39:286–290.
52. JahnkeV. In Pathophysiologie, Differentialdiagnostik und Therapie von Störungen des Geruchsinns. *HNO akt.* 1999; 7:21–29.
53. Junker W, Münker G, Schumann O. Tubenfunktion bei Septumdeviation. *Arch Otorhinolaryngol.* 1977; 216:617.
54. Joseph J. Über die operative Verkleinerung einer Nase (Rhinomiosis). *Berlin. klin. Wochenschr.* 1898; 40:882.
55. Joseph J. *Nasenplastik und sonstige Gesichtsplastik nebst einem Anhang über Mammaplastik und einige wietere Operationen aus dem Gebiete der äusseren Körperplastik,* Leipzig: Curt Kabitzsch: 1931.
56. Kaschke O. Komplikationen bei der endoskopischen Chirurgie der Nasennebenhöhlen. In Behrbohm, Kaschke, Nawka, eds. *Endoskopische Diagnostik und Therapie in der HNO,* Stuttgart: G. Fischer; 1997.
57. Kastenbauer E. Äußere Nase und Nasenscheidewand. *Z. Laryng. Rhinol.*1973; 52:597.
58. Kastenbauer E. Eingriffe an der Nasenscheidewand. *Laryngo-Rhino-Otol.* 1997: A93–A103.
59. Keck T, Leiacker R, Heinrich A, Kühnemann S, Rettinger G. Humidity and temperature profile in the nasal cavity. *Rhinology.* 2000; 38:167–171.
60. Kennedy D. Functional endoscopic sinus surgery. *Arch. Otolaryngol.* 1985; III:643–649.
61. Killian G. *Einleitung zu der Discussion über die operative Therapie der Septumdeviation. Verhandlungen Gesellschaft Deutscher Naturforscher und Ärzte.* Leipzig: FCW Vogel:1899:392–393.
62. Killian G. Die submuköse Fensterresektion der Nasenscheidewand. *Arch Laryng Rhinol (Berl)* 1904; 16:362–387.
63. Killian G. Die Krankheiten der Kieferhöhle. In Heymann. ed. *Handbuch der Laryngologie und Rhinologie, Vol. 3,* Vienna: 1004–1096.
64. Knight LC, Eccles. The relationship between nasal airway resistance and middle ear pressure in subjects with acute respiratory tract infection. *Acta Otolaryngol.* 1993; 113:196–200.
65. Kobal G, Klimek L, Wolfenberger M. Multi-center investigation of 1036 subjects using a standardized method for the assessment of olfactory function combining tests of odor identification, odor discrimination, and olfactory thesholds. *Eur Arch Otorhinolaryngol.* 2000; 257:205–211.

66. Koch U, Herberhold C, Opitz H-J. Mittelohrdruckverhältnisse nach rhinoplastischen Eingriffen. *Laryngol.Rhinol.* 1977; 56:657–681.

67. Koch U, Opitz HJ, Paul W. Tubenfunktion und Mittelohrdruck bei adhäsiven Trommelfellen. *Laryngo-Rhinol-Otol.* 1977; 56:156–159.

68. Koch U. Der Adhäsovprozeß. Teil II: Untersuchungen zur Pathogenese. *Laryngo-Rhinol-Otol.* 1980; 59:655–665.

69. Lavater JC. *Essai sur la Physiognomie.* La Haye: Tome I: 1783.

70. Laszig R. Druckentwicklung im Mittelohr nach Nasenoperation. *HNO.* 1985; 33:187–189.

71. Legler U. Die Lateroposition der unteren Nasenmuschel–ein einfacher Eingriff zur Verbesserung der Luftdurchgängigkeit der Nase. *Z. Laryngol. Rhinol.* 1970; 49:386–391.

72. Lienhardt W. *Compendium der chirurgischen Operationslehre*, Wien: XX; 1867: 554.

73. Luc H. Une nouvelle méthode opérative pour la cuire radicale et Rapide de lèmpyeme chronique du sinus maxillaire. *Arch. int. Laryng.* 1897; 10:273–282.

74. Farrior RT. Korrigierende und rekonstruktive plastische Chirurgie an der äußeren Nase. In Naumann HH., ed. *Kopf- und Hals-Chirurgie: Gesicht und Gesichtsschädel, Teil 1*, 1974.

75. Maelicke A. *Vom Reiz der Sinne*, Weinheim, New York: Verlagsgesellschaft mbH: 1990.

76. Maier W, Krebs A. Ist die Chirurgie der inneren Nase vor Tympanoplastik indiziert? *Laryng. Rhinol. Otol.* 1998; 77:682–688.

77. Mang W-L. Aktuelle Bemerkungen zur funktionell-ästhetischen Rhinoplastik. *HNO.* 1987; 35:274–278.

78. MannW. Nasal surgery in German-speaking countries around the turn of the century. *Rhinology.* 1991; 29:79–84.

79. Masing H. Nasenkorrektur und Atemfunktion. *Z. Laryng. Rhinol.* 1968; 4:277–288.

80. Meyer R. *Secondary Rhinoplasty.* Berlin: Springer; 2002.

81. McKenzie M. *Manual of diseases of the throat and nose.* London: Churchill; 1884:380.

82. McNicoll WD. Submucous resection. The treatment of choice in the Nose-Ear Distress Syndrome. *J Laryngol Otol.* 1979; 93:357–367.

83. Messerklinger W. Über die Drainage der menschlichen Nasennebenhöhlen unter normalen und pathologischen Bedingungen. *Mschr. Ohrenheilk., Wien.* 1967; 101:313–326.

84. Messerklinger W. Die normalen Sekretwege des Menschen. *Arch. klin. Exp. Ohr.-Nas.-u.Kehlk.Heilk.* 1969; 195:138–151.

85. Messerklinger W. Die Endoskopie der Nase. *Mon.schr. Ohrenheik., Wien.* 1970; 104:451–456.

86. Messerklinger W. Das Infundibulum ethmoidale und seine entzündlichen Erkrankungen. *Arch Otorhinolaryngol.* 1979; 222:11–22.

87. Messerklinger W. Die Rolle der lateralen Nasenwand in der Pathogenese, Diagnose und Therapie der rezidivierenden und chronischen Rhinosinusitis. *Laryng. Rhinol. Otol.* 1987; 66:293–299.

88. Mikulicz J. Zur operativen Behandlung des Empyems der Highmorshöhle. *Arch. klein. Chir.* 1887; 34:626–634.

89. Mink PJ. *Physiologie der oberen Luftwege.* Leipzig: Vogel; 1920.

90. Moss ML. The role of the nasal septum cartilage in midfacial growth. In McNamara jr. *Factors Affecting The Growth of the Midface*, Ann Abor: XX; 1976.

91. Mrowinski D. In Pathophysiologie, Differentialdiagnostik und Therapie von Störungen des Geruchsinns. *HNO akt.* 1999; 7:21–29.

92. Müller AH *Lehrbuch der Paläozoologie. Teil 2. Reptilien und Vögel*, Jena: Fischer; 1985.

93. Natvig P. *Jacques Joseph: Surgical sculptor.* Baltimore: Saunders; 1983.

94. Neumann HJ. *Möglichkeiten und Grenzen der ästhetisch-plastischen Gesichtschirurgie.* Reinbeck: Einhorn-Presse; 1992.

95. Nischwitz A, Haake K. *100 Jahre Hals-Nasen- und Ohrenklinik an der Charité zu Berlin.* Berlin: Format Studios; 1993.

96. Nolst Trenité GJ. Trauma reduction in rhinoplastic surgery. *Rhinology.* 1991; 29:111–116.

97. Onody A. *Die Nasenhöhle und ihre Nebenhöhlen. Nach anatomischen Durchschnitten in 12 Holzschnitttafeln dargestellt.* Wien: Hölder; 1893.

98. Peck GC. *Techniques in Aesthetic Rhinoplasty.* New York: Gower Med. Publ. Ltd.; 1984:80–88.

99. Perkins SW, Hamiliton MM, McDonald K. A successful 15-year experience in double-dome tip surgery via endonasal approach. *Arch Facial Plast Surg.* 2001; 3:157–164.

100. Petersen F. Über subperichondrale Resektion der knorpligen Nasenscheidewand. *Berl Klin Wschr.* 1883; 20:329–330.

101. Pirsig W. Die Regeneration des kindlichen Septumknorpels nach Septumplastik. *Acta oto-laryngol.* 1975; 79:451–459.

102. Polzehl D. Das vomeronasale Organ des Menschen. *Laryngo-Rhino-Otol.* 2002; 81:743–749.

103. Ponikau JU, Sherris DA, Kern EB, Homburger HA, Frigas E, Gaffey T, Roberts GD. The diagnosis and incidence of allergic fungal sinusitis. *Mayo Clin Proc.* 1999; 74:877–884.

104. Rasp G. Die eosinophile Entzündung der Nasenschleimhaut. *Laryngo-Rhino-Otol.* 2002; 81:491–498.

105. Rees TD. *(Traumared) Aethetic plastic surgery.* Philadelphia: WB Saunders Co. Vol I; 1989:153–176.

106. Reiter D, Alfor E, Jabourian Z. Traumared. Alternatives to packing in septorhinoplasty. *Archs Otolaryngol Head Neck Surg.* 1989; 115:1203–1205.

107. Rethi L. Die Verbiegungen der Nasenscheidewand und ihre Behandlung. *Wien. Klin Wsch.* 1890; 27:514–516.

108. Rettinger G, Masing H. Rotation of the alar cartilage in collapsed ala. *Rhinology.* 1981; 19:81–86.

109. Rettinger R. Nasenseptumpathologie. In Naumann, Helms, Herberhold, Kastenbauer, eds. *Oto-Rhino-Laryngologie in Klinik und Praxis. Nase, Nasennebenhöhlen, Gesicht, Mundhöhle und Pharynx, Kopfspeicheldrüsen.* XX, 1992:369–374.

110. Riedel F, Verse Th, Hörmann L. Nasenkorrekturen mittels Stirnlappen. *HNO akt.* 2002; 35:274–278.

111. Robin JL. The preplanned rhinoplasty. *Aesthetic Plastic Surgery.* 1979; 3:179–193.

112. Roe JO. The deformity termed "pig nose" and its correction by a simple operation. *The Med. Record.* 1887; 31:621.

113. Rouadi P, Baroody FM, Abbott D, Naureckas E,Solway J, Nacleiro RM. A technique to measure the ability of the human nose to warm and humidify air. *J Appl Physiol.* 1999; 87:400–406.

114. Rüster D. *Alte Chirurgie.* Berlin: Verlag Volk und Gesundheit; 1985

115. Sanden U. Aktuelle Aspekte der chronischen Eosinophilen-assoziierten Erkrankungen der oberen und unteren Luftwege. *HNO akt.* 1998; 6:22–30.

116. Schulz-Coulon H-J. Rhinoplastik–ein überwiegend ästhetischer oder funktioneller Eingriff? *Laryng. Rhinol.* 1977; 56:233–243.

117. Schulz-Coulon H-J. Die Korrektur ausgeprägter Deformitäten des ventro-kaudalen Septumabschnittes bei Kind. *HNO.* 1983; 31:6–9.

118. Siebenmann F. Die Behandlung der chronischen Eiterungen der Highmors-Höhle durch Resektion der oberen Hälfte (Parssuprarurbinalis) ihrer nasalen Wand. *Verhandl. Vereins Süddeutscher Laryng:* 1899.

119. Skillern RH. Accessory sinus of the nose. 2ⁿᵈ edition. Philadelphia: Lippincott; 1920.

120. Stammberger H. Unsere endoskopische Operationstechnik der lateralen Nasenwand—ein endoskopisch-chirurgisches Konzept zur Behandlung entzündlicher Nasennebenhöhlenerkrankungen. *Laryng.Rhinol. Otol.* 1985; 64:559–566.

121. Stammberger H, Wolf G. Headaches and sinus disease: The endoscopic approach. *Ann. Otol. Rhinol. Laryngol.* 1988; 134:3–23.

122. Stammberger H. *Uncapping the egg, Der endoskopische Weg zur Stirnhöhle*, Tuttlingen: Endopress; 2002.

123. Stankiewicz JA. Complications in endoscopic intranasal ethmoidectomie. An update. *Laryngoscope.* 1989; 99:686–690.

124. Tagliacozzi G. *De curtorum Chirurgia per insitionem libro duo*, Venice: G. Bindoni; 1597.

125. Tardy ME. Interdependent dynamics of rhinoplasty: The cadaver revisited. *Trans Am Acad Ophthal Otol.* 1976; 82:432–436.

126. Tardy ME, Denneny JC. *Micro-osteotomies in thinoplasty. Facial plastic surgery.* New York: Thieme-Stratton Inc. Vol. I, No. 2; 1984.

127. Tardy ME, Garner ET. Inspiratory nasal obstruction secondary to alar and nasal valve collapse: Technique for repair using autogenous cartilage. *Oper Tech Otolaryngol Head Neck Surg.* 1990; 1:215.

128. Tardy ME, Patt BS, Walter MA. Transdomal suture refinement of the nasal tip: Long-term outcomes. *Facial Plast Surg.* 1993; 9:275–284.

129. Tardy ME, Brown R. *Surgical anatomy of the nose.* Philadeilphia: Raven Press; 1995.

130. Tardy ME. *Rhinoplasty: The art and the science. Parts 1 and 2*, Philadelphia: Saunders; 1996.

131. Toffel PH. Simultaneous secure endoscopic sinus surgery and rhinoplasty. *Rhinology.* 1992; 31:165–171.

132. Tolsdorf A. Eingriffe an den Nasenmuscheln unter besonderer Berücksichtigung der subperiostalen Conchektomie. *Laryng. Rhinol.* 1981; 60:615–619.

133. Trendelenburg GF. Verletzungen und chirurgische Krankheiten des Gesichtes. In Enke F. *Deutsche Chirurgie*, Stuttgart: XX;1886.

134. Versalius A. *De humani corporis fabrica.* Basel: XX; 1543.

135. Walter C. Plastische und Wiederherstellende Chirurgie: Zum Thema: Nasenflügelkollaps. *Laryng. Rhinol.* 1976; 55:447–449.

136. Wendler D. Nathanael Highmore (1613–1685) und die Oberkieferhöhle. *Anat. Anz. Jena.* 1924; 5:375–380.

137. Wigand ME. Transnasale, endoskopische Chirurgie der Nasennebenhöhlen bei chronischer Sinusitis. I. Ein biomechanisches Konzept der Schleimhautchirurgie. *HNO.* 1981; 29:215–221.

138. Wigand ME. *Endoskopische Chirurgie der Nasennebenhöhlen und der vorderen Schädelbasis.* Stuttgart: Thieme: 1989.

139. Wigand ME. Personal Communication.

140. Ziegelmayer G. Äußere Nase. In Becker PE. *Humangenetik. Ein kurzes Handbuch in fünf Bänden,* Vol.1/2, Stuttgart: Thieme; 1969:56–81.

141. Zuckerkandl E. *Normale und pathologische Anatomie der Nasenhöhle und Ihrer pneumatischen Anhänge. Vol. 1.* Vienna: Wilhelm Braumüller: 1882.

142. Biermann E- Nasale CPAP-Therapie beim obstruktiven Schlafapnoe-Syndrom: Verbessert funktionelle Rhinochirurgie die Compliance? *Somnologie.* 2001; 5:59–64.

143. Dorn M, Pirsig W, Verse T. Postoperatives Management nach rhinochirurgischen Eingriffen bei Patienten mit schwerer obstruktiver Schlafapnoe: eine Pilotstudie. *HNO.* 2001; 49:642–645.

144. Friedman M, Tanyeri H, Lim JW, Landsberg R, Vaidyanathan K, Caldarelli D. Effect of nasal breathing on obstructive sleep apnea. *Otolaryngol Head Neck Surg.* 2000; 122:71–74.

145. Hoffstein V, Mateika S, Metes A. Effect of nasal dilation on snoring and apneas during different stages of sleep. *Sleep.* 1993; 16:360–365.

146. Kawano K, Usui N, Kanazawa H, Hara I. Changes in nasal and oral respiratory resistance before and after uvulopalatopharyngoplasty. *Acta Otolaryngol (Stockh).* 1996; Suppl 523: 236–238.

147. Lavie P, Zomer J, Eliaschar I et al. Excessive daytime sleepiness and insomnia. Association with deviated nasal septum and nocturnal breathing disorders. *Arch Otolaryngol.* 1982; 108:373–377.

148. Lofaso F, Coste A, d'Ortho MP, Zerah-Lancner F, Delclaux C, Goldenberg F, Harf A. Nasal obstruction as a risk factor for sleep apnoea syndrome. *Eur Respir J.* 2000; 16:639–643.

149. Olsen KD, Kern EB, Westbrook PR. Sleep and breathing disturbance secondary to nasal obstruction. *Otolaryngol Head Neck Surg.* 1981; 89:804–810.

150. Pirsig W, Verse T. Long-term results in the treatment of obstructive sleep apnea. *Eur Arch Otorhinolaryngol.* 2000; 257:570–577.

151. Sher AE, Schechtman KB, Piccirillo JF. The efficiency of surgical modifications of the upper airway in adults with obstructive sleep apnea syndrome. *Sleep.* 1996; 19:156–177.

152. Verse T, Maurer JT, Pirsig W. Effect of nasal surgery on sleep-related breathing disorders. *Laryngoscope.* 2002; 112:64–68.

153. Welinder R, Cardell LD, Uddman R, Malm L. Reduced nasal airway resistance following uvulopharyngoplasty. *Rhinology.* 1997; 35:16–18.

154. Bremer B, Seidner, W, Behrbohm, H. *Der Einfluß endoskopischer Nasennebenhöhlenoperationen auf die Klangbildung der Stimme bei Patienten mit Sing- und Sprechberufen,* Manuscript.

155. Dalston RM, Neumann GS, Gonzales-Landa G. Nasometric sensitivity and specifity: A cross-dialect and cross-culture study. *Cleft Palate Craniofac. J.* 1993; 30:285.

156. Fletcher SG. Theory and instrumentation for quantitative measurement of nasality. *Cleft Palate Craniofac. J.* 1970; 7:601.

157. Müller R, Beleites T, Hloucal U, Kühn M. Objektive Messung der normalen Nasalanz im sächsischen Sprachraum. *HNO.* 2000; 48:937.

158. Trenschel W. *Das Phänomen der Nasalität.* Berlin: Akademie-Verlag: 1977.

159. Wendler J, Seidner W, Kittel G, Eysholdt U. *Lehrbuch der Phoniatrie und Pädaudiologie.* Stuttgart: Thieme: 1996.

Contemporary Rhinoplasty: Principles and Philosophy

M. E. Tardy, Jr.

Contents

Introduction and Philosophy

Although the history of modern rhinoplasty surgery extends back only one century, typical, traditional *reduction* rhinoplasty has given way to a nasal reconstructive procedure characterized by tissue *preservation, reconstruction*, and *reorientation*. The most significant advances in rhinoplasty in the past two decades have been characterized by a stronger emphasis upon *exacting anatomical analysis*. Although techniques have certainly been refined and improved, the final result of any rhinoplastic procedure develops as the consequence of the patient's unique anatomy coupled with the surgeon's skill in accurately diagnosing the exact anatomy and variants in anatomical components. Fundamental knowledge of the universal principles and canons of rhinoplasty, coupled with an understanding of the dynamics of the operation itself and the healing changes that inevitably evolve over time, equips the contemporary surgeon best to achieve uniformly excellent results. The surgeon must initially judge, by inspection and palpation, the character and texture of the skin and subcutaneous tissues as they vary from nasal region to region, the influences of facial mimetic musculature, the relative strength and support of the cartilaginous and bony framework and substructure, and the limitations imposed by

the interrelationship of all these structures on the ultimate favorable result. Concomitant creation or preservation of normal airway function is essential. All this must be balanced with the individual surgeon's esthetic judgment, factoring in the surrounding facial features and overall stature of the patient. No *single* surgical technique will suffice to refine every nose to an ideal state, thus a wide repertoire of surgical skills must be employed to manage the plethora of abnormalities encountered. Most importantly, the wishes of the patient create a critical factor in fashioning the ultimate surgical outcome.

The objective of esthetic nasal plastic surgery is to create a nose that draws no attention to itself but enhances the beauty of the eyes, allows for comfortable nasal function, and is in harmony with the other features of the face. This simple statement belies a complex problem. The universal concept of what is "beautiful" or "ideal" remains an age-old question, and the answer involves a multiplicity of emotional reactions and prejudices. In addition, values and assessments of beauty vary within different age groups and social structures. To evaluate what is beautiful entails a study of physical and cultural anthropology, ethnology, psychology, and esthetics.

Beauty of the human face is neither abstract nor absolute; it varies among different ethnic groups and is subject to interpretation by each individual. This attitude is based on a multi-

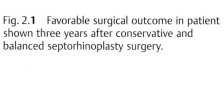

Fig. 2.**1**   Favorable surgical outcome in patient shown three years after conservative and balanced septorhinoplasty surgery.

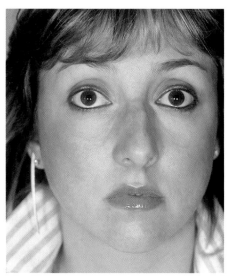
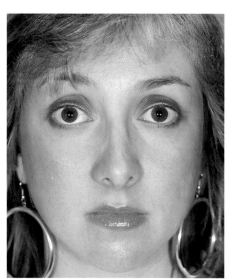
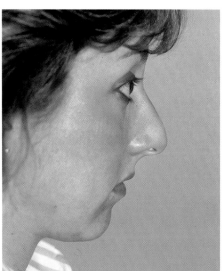
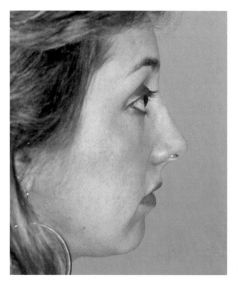

a

b   Fig. 2.**1 c** u. **d**   ▷

plicity of factors varying according to the body image and cultural values of individual conditioning, particularly during the formative years, when it often becomes part of the unconscious mind.

Contemporary rhinoplasty fortunately is characterized by the strong, appropriate concern for conservative and subtle anatomical changes (Fig. 2.**1**). Rather than *excisional* sacrifice of large segments of cartilage or bone, a philosophy of *preservation* and *reorientation* of tissues has developed that largely eliminates the creation of unnecessary tissue voids that too often heal and scar unpredictably. Conservation surgery thereby further extends the surgeon's *control* over the healing surgical result, as an appropriate equilibrium between the corrected nasal skeleton and investing soft-tissue covering is more reliably achieved. Effective methods of autogenous tissue grafting extend the surgeon's control over the final outcome and its long-term stability. Finally, thoughtful nasal surgeons, through accurate anatomical diagnosis, discern which portions of the nasal anatomy are pleasing and satisfactory, striving to avoid disturbing these structures and areas when correcting (or gaining access to) anatomical components in need of correction.

An artistic anatomical concept must be developed by the rhinoplastic surgeon when approaching the study of nasal anatomy (Fig. 2.**2**). The surgeon visualizes the nasal structure not only as static bone and cartilage, but also as muscle tension, skin texture, interconnected relationships with surrounding structures, and the effect of related and interrelated structures on the shape of the nose. He must develop a personal sense of the "ideal normal," altering abnormal nasal anatomical components based on this artistic concept, coupled with the patient's clearly defined expectations.

Indications

Rhinoplasty is traditionally undertaken as the result of a patient's request to surgically correct perceived anatomical nasal abnormalities. A didactic list of surgical indications might include:
1. Nasal esthetic deformity
2. Nasal functional deformity with airway blockade
3. Nasal traumatic deformities, both acute and preexisting
4. Abnormalities from previous nasal operations (revision rhinoplasty)

Fig. 2.**1**

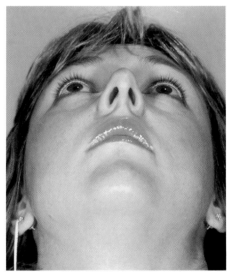
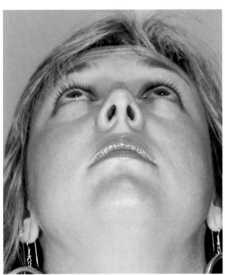
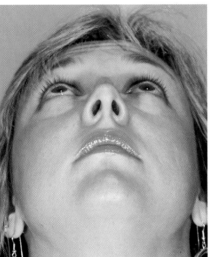

c

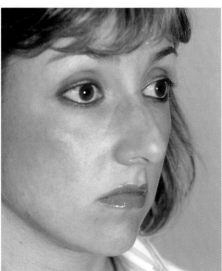
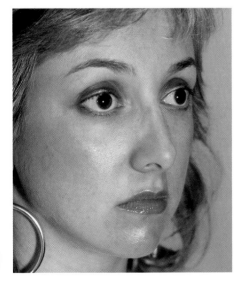

d

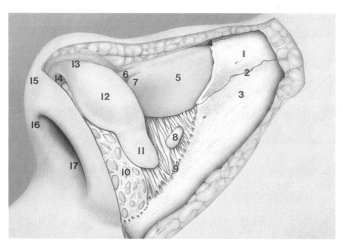

Fig. 2.**2**   Cadaver dissection illustration demonstrating the individual components and subcomponents which characterize the nasal anatomy.
1. Nasal bone
2. Nasomaxillary suture line
3. Ascending process of maxilla
4. Osseocartilaginous junction (rhinion)
5. Upper lateral cartilage
6. Anterior septal angle
7. Caudal free edge of upper lateral cartilage
8. Sesamoid cartilage
9. Pyriform margin
10. Alar lobule
11. Lateral crus of alar cartilage—lateral portion
12. Lateral crus of alar cartilage—central portion
13. Tip-defining point
14. Transitional segment of alar cartilage (intermediate crus)
15. Infratip lobule
16. Columella
17. Medial crural footplate

Contraindications

Absolute as well as relative contraindications to rhinoplasty exist.

Absolute Contraindications
- Bleeding and coagulation disorders which are uncorrectable
- Pregnancy
- Any systemic illness which might be worsened by rhinoplasty surgery
- Significant psychiatric disorder

Relative Contraindications
- Temporary or correctable coagulopathies
- Severe nasal sunburn
- Severe nasal acne
- Psychological and psychiatric disorders which cannot be corrected or stabilized
- Active relapsing polychondritis and similar autoimmune illnesses

Alternative Techniques

Although closed reduction of nasal fractures is not uncommon in acute and subacute nasal fractures, no other true alternatives to elective rhinoplasty exist.

Preoperative Considerations

Whether septorhinoplasty is to be performed as a hospital inpatient or an office (or hospital) outpatient procedure depends on several factors. Although traditionally this operation involved hospitalization for one to two days, increasingly rhinoplasties deemed to be straightforward may be accomplished safely as outpatient or office procedures, provided that no additional compromise to patient safety and well-being is involved. Regardless of the surgical setting, the preoperative evaluation and preparation remain the same, and must be exacting.

Education of the patient by the surgeon and his staff is preeminent. It is essential to guide patients gently through a form of self-analysis and awareness of the interdependent structures of the nose and face, an exercise that catalyzes his/her understanding of the scope of the deformity and operation, and the limitations imposed on the procedures by the imperfect existent anatomy. Utilizing a three-way mirror supplemented by accurate preoperative photographs aids in the patient and surgeon arriving at a joint understanding about the nature and goals of the operation. It is absolutely essential that the patient be able to characterize exactly what outcome is desired. Without this knowledge even a result judged by the surgeon to be superb may fall short of the patient's expectations.

If, in the surgeon's judgement, realistic motivation and understanding is present, plans are made to schedule the desired operation. If any doubt exists, it is propitious to allow a period of reflection and contemplation on the part of the patient, scheduling a second interview and consultation before any firm decision for surgery.

The following is a list of characteristics of potential problem patients:
- Unrealistic expectations
- Obsessive-compulsiveness, perfectionism
- Sudden whims
- Indecisiveness
- Rudeness
- Unkemptness
- Uncooperativeness
- Depression

Patients may also be:
- Overly flattering
- Overly familiar
- Possessed of a minimal or imagined deformity
- A careless or poor historian
- Obsessed of being a "very important person"
- Overly talkative
- A "surgeon shopper"
- A "plastic-surgiholic"

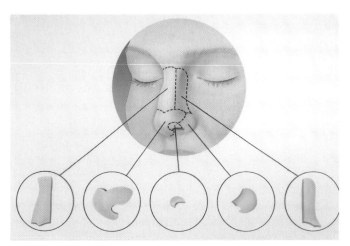

Fig. 2.**3** The fundamental anatomical topographical subunits of the nose, isolated in an exploded illustration for more critical esthetic evaluation. Both nasal reconstructive procedures and rhinoplasty techniques should incorporate an appreciation for and an understanding of the importance of restoring and rendering symmetrical these subunits.

- A price haggler
- Involved in litigation
- Disliked by the surgeon or his staff

Surgeons should be alert to the above characteristics and evaluate such patients more carefully before accepting them for appearance-changing surgery.

Special Surgical Requirements

Standard classical rhinoplasty instrument sets are ubiquitous in operating theaters throughout the world. In addition, a personal preference is strongly held for the following:
1. The Dunning semisharp septal perichondrial elevator
2. Long nasal speculum
3. Rubin guarded osteotomes
4. 2- and 3-mm osteotomes
5. Sharpening stone (hone)
6. Tardy microsurgical rhinobur (Medtronic, Jacksonville, Florida)

Preoperative Analysis

An exacting preoperative analysis and diagnosis of the unique nasal deformity presenting in each patient is arguably more important than surgical skill. Skillful surgeons who fail to accurately understand (and thus correct) the many nasal variants encountered in a rhinoplasty practice stand little opportunity of achieving an excellent long-term outcome. Thus certain aspects of nasal anatomy deserve consideration here. Detailed anatomical descriptions of the nasal anatomy exist in several excellent anatomy textbooks. This description, unlike traditional anatomy discussions, will review the specific features of

nasal anatomy that directly influence the rhinoplasty operation, with emphasis on the philosophy of surgical conservatism and reorientation of the interrelated nasal anatomical components. The commonly accepted anatomical terms in rhinoplasty are illustrated in Figures 2.**2**–2.**5** and will prevail throughout this chapter.

The nose itself represents an esthetic unit located centrally within the other esthetic regional units of the face. On the nasal surface, one can identify several distinct anatomical topographical subunits (Fig. 2.**3**) (1). Individual inherited characteristics render these subunits prominent or unobtrusive. In the reconstruction of external nasal defects, it is often preferable to resect and replace an entire topographical subunit with skin of like color, character, and texture rather than simply fill the existing primary defect with a skin graft or pedicle flap. In similar fashion, during rhinoplasty the surgeon must avoid a sharp, unnatural overemphasis of any one subunit in comparison to a surrounding subunit; each should ideally blend into the other with a gracefulness that draws no attention to the nasal repair. Nasal subunits consist of the nasal dorsum, the nasal sidewalls, the nasal tip (including the infratip lobule and columella), the alar lobules, and the depressions of the supraalar facets (Fig. 2.**3**).

The quality and thickness of the skin and supportive subcutaneous tissues investing the nose exert a major influence on the surgical dissection in rhinoplasty and the ultimate natural appearance of the final healed result. By inspection and palpation, one can judge the character, thickness, elasticity, and overall quality of the skin to accurately estimate how much and what form of surgical correction is possible. Surgeons often prefer patients with thin, delicate skin, as they invariably develop less postoperative edema and heal more quickly. Markedly thin skin with sparse subcutaneous tissue, however, poorly camouflages even minor irregularities in the nasal supporting structures, potentially unveiling bony or cartilaginous highlights, asymmetries, offsets, or irregularities during the early postoperative healing period. Conversely, thick skin, which heals and contracts less quickly, tends toward greater postoperative edema, healing and contracting less quickly. Since subcutaneous scar formation generally is more abundant, the unwary surgeon is exposed to the possibility of one form of postoperative pollybeak deformity; this is particularly true when excessive nasal skeleton is needlessly sacrificed. Smooth draping of skin is less easily accomplished when thick skin exists; therefore, efforts aimed at surgical creation of accentuated definition, particularly at the nasal tip, are largely limited. Excision of excessive subcutaneous tissue in the nasal tip, commonly necessary in thick skin, is usually contraindicated in thin skin, since the maintenance of a pleasing, natural contour demands preservation of interposed soft tissue between skeletal structures and delicate overlying skin. Nasal skin is considerably thinner, more mobile, and more easily repositioned in the cephalic three fifths of the nose, where it is relatively devoid of subcutaneous tissue and sebaceous glands. Progressing caudally toward the nasal tip, the skin assumes a thicker, more glandular quality (Fig. 2.**2**).

An ideal skin type does in fact exist for favorable results in rhinoplasty. Neither too thick nor too thin, this ideal epithelium possesses a minimum of sebaceous glands and wide pores and redrapes well after conservative undermining and elevation. Sufficient subcutaneous tissue is present to

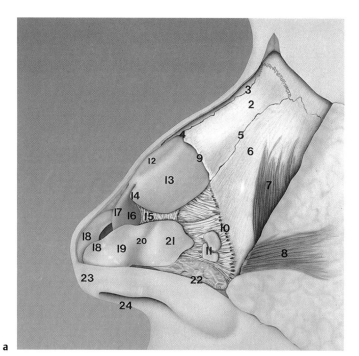

a

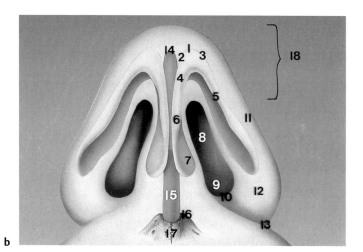

b

Fig. 2.**4**   Additional anatomical landmarks and standard terminology.
1. Nasofrontal suture line
2. Nasal bone
3. Internasal suture line
4. Osseocartilaginous junction (rhinion)
5. Nasomaxillary suture line
6. Ascending process of maxilla
7. Levator labii superioris muscle
8. Transverse nasalis muscle
9. Cephalic portion of upper lateral cartilage (articulates with undersurface of nasal bone)
10. Pyriform margin
11. Sesamoid cartilages
12. Cartilaginous dorsum
13. Upper lateral cartilage
14. Caudal free margin of upper lateral cartilage
15. Intercartilaginous tissue condensation
16. Quadrangular cartilage
17. Anterior septal angle
18. Tip-defining point alar cartilage
19. Lateral crus of alar cartilage
20. Concavity ("hinge") of lateral crus
21. Lateral aspect of lateral crus
22. Alar lobule
23. Infratip lobule
24. Columella

1. Apex of alar cartilage
2. Medial angle of dome
3. Lateral angle of dome
4. Alar cartilage transitional segment (intermediate crus)
5. Lateral crus alar cartilage
6. Medial crus alar cartilage
7. Medial crural footplate
8. Nostril aperture
9. Nostril floor
10. Nostril sill
11. Lateral alar sidewall
12. Alar lobule
13. Alar–facial junction
14. Anterior septal angle
15. Caudal septum
16. Maxillary crest
17. Nasal spine
18. Infratip lobule

cushion the epithelium from underlying osseocartilaginous structures, but a minimum of fat is present. Gentle palpation and rolling of the nasal skin during the physical examination identify this favorable skin condition for the surgeon.

The varying thickness of the skin–subcutaneous tissue sleeve plays a vital role in profile planning in rhinoplasty. The skin covering is usually thin at the rhinion and thick at the nasion and supratip area (Fig. 2.**4**); a slight skeletal hump at the rhinion exists even when the external epithelial profile line is relatively straight and devoid of an external humped appearance. Straight-line removal of the nasal hump (consisting of cartilage and bone) will generally result in an unacceptable profile line. The more abundant and subcutaneous tissue covering the cartilaginous dorsum creates a need for a quantitatively differential profile alignment (as opposed to bony dorsum alignment) to achieve desirable profile contouring. Whereas excessive soft tissue may require reduction in thick-skinned patients, ordinarily every effort must be made to preserve the subcutaneous soft tissues to ensure the most favorable long-term result.

There are definitive tissue dissection planes in the nose and these should be exploited during primary rhinoplasty; in revisional rhinoplasty, favorable dissection planes are commonly obliterated by scar tissue. By sharp knife and scissor dissection in the *immediate supraperichondrial plane* over the upper and lower lateral cartilages and subperiosteal elevation over the bony dorsum, ideal soft-tissue preservation for potential cushioning and camouflage of possible slight irregularities that may develop postoperatively along the nasal profile is maintained (Fig. 2.**5**). Elevation of the soft tissues in this favorable plane not only creates less eventual scarring, it facilitates access to the supportive skeletal substructures of the nose and avoids the vascular and neural structures lying more superficially.

Too much emphasis cannot be placed on this all-important concept of proper nasal dissection planes. Ideally, anesthetic infiltration should be placed precisely in this supraperichondrial (superficial musculoaponeurotic system) plane in the lower half of the nose to aid in avascular dissection.

The ideal base view and the terminology applied to the anatomical components are depicted in Figure 2.**6**.

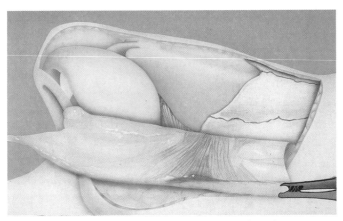

Fig. 2.**5** All-important favorable tissue plane in rhinoplasty surgery, which is found just superficial to the bony–cartilaginous skeleton of the nose, and just beneath the overlying canopy of soft tissue and superficial muculoaponeurotic system (SMAS).

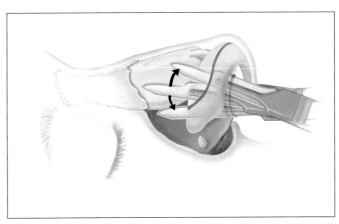

Fig. 2.**6** Favorable tissue plane over nasal skeleton is ideally entered with sharp knife elevation of the overlying skin–subcutaneous canopy during rhinoplasty.

Surgical Techniques

As a bilateral and often difficult operation, rhinoplasty remains the most challenging of all esthetic facial operations because no two procedures are ever identical. Equally importantly, total control of the healing process by the surgeon is not possible. Each patient's nasal configuration and structure require individual and unique operative planning and surgical reconstruction. *Therefore, no single technique, even when mastered, will prepare the surgeon for the varied anatomical patterns encountered.* It is essential to regard rhinoplasty as an operation planned *to reconstitute and shape* the anatomical features of the nose into a new, more pleasing relationship with one another and the surrounding facial features. Rhinoplasty should be approached as an anatomical dissection and exposure of the nasal structures requiring alteration, conservatively shaping and repositioning these anatomical elements. Excision should be kept to a minimum, and cartilage grafting employed when indicated. Many more problems and complications arise from *overcorrection* of nasal abnormalities than from *conservative* correction. An inappropriate technique applied persistently without regard for existing anatomy creates frequent complications. One truism, namely that "it is not what is removed in rhinoplasty that is important but what is left behind," remains valid. Furthermore, one must comprehend clearly the dynamic aspects of operative rhinoplasty because all surgical steps are interrelated and interdependent, *most maneuvers leading to a temporary deformity to be corrected progressively by the steps that follow* (the "dynamics" of rhinoplasty).

Surgery of the Nasal Tip

Sculpture of the nasal tip is regarded, and properly so, as the most exacting aspect of nasal plastic surgery (2, 3). The surgeon is challenged by the bilateral, animate, and mobile nasal anatomical components. Because no single surgical technique may be used successfully in correction of the endless anatomical tip variations encountered, the surgeon must analyze each anatomical situation and make a reasoned judgment about which approaches and tip modifications are indicated and which techniques will result in a predictably natural appearance. Factored into this decision must be consideration of, among other things:

1., 2. The strength, thickness, and attitude of the alar cartilages,
3. The degree of tip projection,
4. The texture and quality of tip skin and subcutaneous thickness,
5. The columellar length,
6. The length of the nose,
7. The width of the tip,
8. The interdomal distance and domal angles, and
9. The tip–lip complex angulation.

One fundamental principle of tip surgery is that normal or ideal anatomical features of the tip should be preserved and, if possible, remain undisturbed by surgical dissection, and abnormal features must be analyzed, exposed, reanalyzed, and corrected by reduction, augmentation, or reorientation and shape modification (3). Surgeons have gradually come to understand that radical excision and extensive sacrifice of alar cartilage and other tip support mechanisms all too frequently result in eventual unnatural or "surgical" tips. What appears pleasant and natural in the early postoperative period may heal poorly because of overaggressive attempts to modify the anatomy more extensively than the tissues allow. Cross-cutting or morselization of the lateral crura may provide an excellent early appearance, but commonly results in asymmetry, bossae, and distortion or loss of tip support as the soft tissues "shrink-wrap" around the weakened cartilages over time. Rhinoplasty is, after all, a *compromise* operation, in which tissue sacrifices are made to achieve a more favorable appearance. It is thus judicious to develop a reasoned, planned approach to the nasal tip *based entirely on the anatomy encountered* coupled with the final result intended. A philosophy of a *systematic incremental anatomical approach* to tip surgery is highly useful in achieving a consistently natural result (Fig. 2.**7**).

Conservative reduction of the volume of the cephalic margin of the lateral crus, preserving a substantially complete, undisturbed strip of residual alar cartilage, is a preferred operation in individuals in whom nasal tip changes are intended to

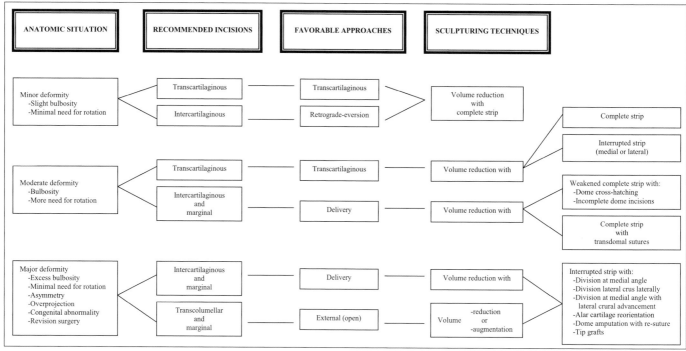

Fig. 2.**7** Algorithm depicting the graduated anatomical systematic approach to nasal tip surgery: As the tip deformity which presents to the surgeon becomes more severe, more invasive and aggressive tip operations are considered than if the tip deformity were modest.

be modest. As the tip deformity or asymmetry encountered becomes more profound, more aggressive techniques are required, from weakened and complete strip techniques to significant *vertical interruption* of the residual complete strip with profound alteration in the alar cartilage size, attitude, and anatomy. Cartilage structural grafts (tip shield grafts, columellor struts, onlay grafts, alar batten grafts, and alar sidewall grafts) to influence the size, shape, projection, and support of the tip are often invaluable.

Tip sculpture cannot be successfully undertaken, let alone mastered, until the *major and minor tip support mechanisms* are appreciated, respected, and preserved or, when indicated, reconstructed (Table 2.**1**). Loss of tip support and projection in the postoperative healing period is one of the most common surgical errors in rhinoplasty. This tip "ptosis" is usually the inevitable result of sacrificing nasal tip support mechanisms.

Table 2.**1**

Major supports of the nasal tip
1. Size, shape, thickness, and resilience of the alar cartilages
2. Upper lateral cartilage attachment to the cephalic margin of the alar cartilages
3. Wrap-around attachment of the medial crural footplates to the caudal septum

Minor supports of the nasal tip*
1. Anterior septal angle
2. Skin of nasal tip
3. Membranous septum
4. Caudal septum
5. Nasal spine
6. Ligamentous sling spanning the paired domes of the alar cartilages
7. Sesamoid cartilage complex extending the support of the lateral crura to the pyriform margin

* Under certain anatomical variant conditions, minor tip supports can contribute major support to the tip

In the majority of patients the major tip support mechanisms consist of :
1. The size, shape, and resiliency of the medial and lateral crura,
2. The wrap-around attachment of the medial crural footplates to the caudal end of the quadrangular cartilage, and
3. The soft-tissue attachment of the caudal margin of the upper lateral cartilage to the cephalic margin of the alar cartilage.

Compensatory reestablishment of major tip support by suture repair, columellar struts, application of tip grafts, etc. should be considered if, during the operation, any or all of these major tip support mechanisms are compromised in any fashion.

The minor tip mechanisms that, in certain anatomical configurations, may assume major support importance include:
1. The dorsal cartilaginous septum,
2. The interdomal ligament,
3. The membranous septum,
4. The nasal spine,
5. The surrounding skin and soft tissues, and
6. The alar sidewalls (4).

Tip projection in every rhinoplasty operation is inevitably *enhanced, reduced,* or *preserved* in its original state (Fig. 2.**8**). Anatomical situations in which each of these outcomes is desirable and intended are regularly encountered in a diverse rhinoplasty practice (5). The desirable surgical goal in every operation is *preservation of the projection already existent,* if, as is true in the majority of rhinoplasty patients, preoperative projection of the tip is satisfactory. Other patients require an *increase in the projection of the tip* relative to the intended new profile line. A predictable variety of reliable operative methods exist for creating or augmenting tip projection; they are discussed later in this chapter. Finally, in a limited but clearly

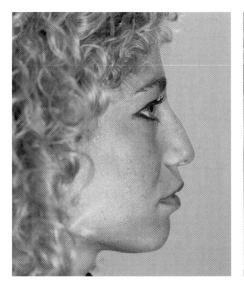 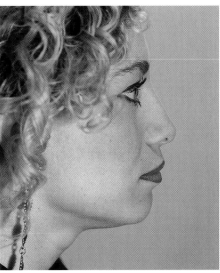

Fig. 2.**8** Ideal tip projection improvement in patient who requires columellar strut associated with an infratip sutured-in-place cartilage tip graft.

definable group of patients with overprojecting tips, a calculated, intentional reduction of excessive tip projection is desirable to *effect intentional retroprojection*. Successfully achieving these diverse surgical results requires an understanding of and a healthy respect for the major and minor tip support mechanisms, seasoned by the recognition of the intraoperative surgical tip dynamic principles that interact in every tip operation (6). It clearly follows that the *appropriate tip incisions and approaches should be planned to preserve as many tip supports as possible.* Alar cartilage sculpturing should similarly respect this principle by conserving the volume and integrity of the lateral crus and avoiding, in all but the most extreme anatomical situations, radical excision and sacrifice of tip cartilage.

The surgeon should differentiate clearly between *incisions, approaches,* and *techniques.* Incisions are simply methods of gaining access to the underlying supportive structures of the nose and in themselves have little importance. Approaches to the nasal tip provide important exposure to the skeletal structures and consist of procedures either to deliver the tip cartilages or to avoid complete delivery or operating on the alar cartilages without removing them from their anatomical beds. Sculpturing techniques are defined as surgical modifications: Excision, reconstruction, or orientation of the alar cartilages calculated to cause significant changes in the definition, size, orientation, and projection of the nasal tip. Because of the amazing complexity of anatomical configurations encountered in nasal tip surgery, further modifications are frequently used to ensure stable refinements. In planning tip remodeling, the surgeon must determine whether or not the tip requires:

1. A reduction in the *volume* of the alar cartilages,
2. A change in the *attitude and orientation of* the alar cartilages,
3. A change in the *projection* of the tip,
4. A cephalic *rotation* with a subsequent increase in the columellar inclination (nasolabial angle),
5. A bilateral narrowing of the angle of the domes, and
6. Reduction of the interdomal distance.

Ideally, conservative reduction of the volume of the cephalic margin of the lateral crus, preserving the majority of the crus

while maintaining a complete (uninterrupted) strip of alar cartilage, is preferred (7). This procedure is satisfactory and appropriately safe when minimal conservational tip refinement and rotation are required. As the tip deformity increases in size and complexity, more aggressive techniques are required. A philosophy of a graduated incremental anatomical approach to nasal tip surgery has proved useful. This implies that no routine tip procedure is ever used; instead, the *appropriate incisions, approaches, and tip sculpturing techniques are selected based entirely on an analysis of the varying anatomy encountered.* Whenever possible, a complete strip operation is used, reserving more complicated and risky interrupted strip techniques for anatomical situations in which more profound refinement changes and significant rotation are desirable.

Surgical Approaches to the Tip

Nondelivery Approaches

In anatomical situations in which the nasal tip anatomy is favorable, only conservative refinements are necessary, and nondelivery approaches are of great value. Less dissection and less disturbance of the tip anatomy are necessary, and this reduces the chance for asymmetry, error, and unfavorable healing. Properly executed (when indicated), nondelivery approaches therefore allow the surgeon to control the healing process more accurately than when more radical approaches and techniques are chosen. The transcartilaginous approach is preferred—*when the presenting anatomy will allow*—because of its simplicity, ease of use, and predictable healing (Fig. 2.**9**). The same tip refinements, however, may be accomplished through the retrograde approach. This approach is chosen in patients whose tip anatomy is fundamentally satisfactory and the domal angles and interdomal distance is normal, requiring only cephalic volume reduction of the lateral crus to accomplish a thinning sculpture reduction (Fig. 2.**10**). Nondelivery approaches with transcartilaginous incisions require that the following anatomical situations exist: Normal domal angles, normal interdomal distance, and reasonable symmetry. When tip projection is to be enhanced by the use of cartilage tip grafts, nondelivery approaches are useful because precise recipient

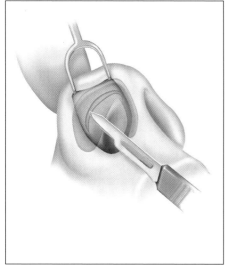

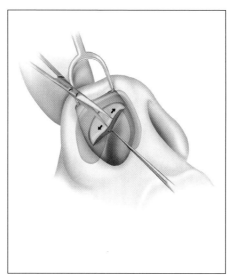

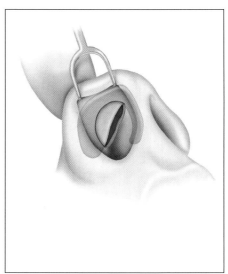

a, b

c

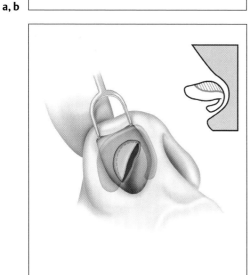

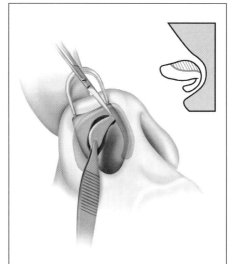

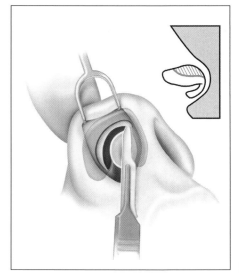

d, e

f

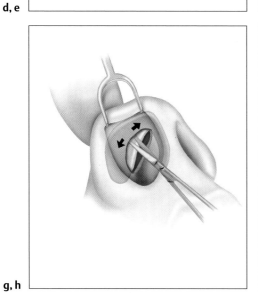

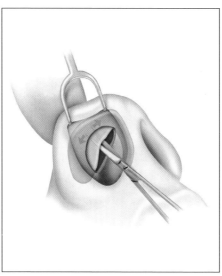

Fig. 2.9 Nondelivery transcartilaginous approach to the nasal tip. (**a**) Knife incision of vestibular skin only. (**b**) Elevation of vestibular skin flap from the cephalic portion of the lateral crus, exposing another favorable avascular tissue plane. (**c**) Direct visualization of anatomy of cephalic margin of lateral crus and dome. (**d**) Conservation excision of cephalic margin of lateral crus. (**e**) Excision of planned amount of lateral crus. (**f**) Removal of planned amount of lateral crus. (**g**) Retrograde approach to cephalic margin of lateral crus: intercartilaginous incision followed by elevation of caudal vestibular skin flap, exposing cephalic margin of cartilage. (**h**) Elevation of soft tissue over the lateral surface of lateral crus to expose cephalic margin of cartilage. Calculated amount of resection can now be effected.

g, h

pockets may be more accurately created in the infratip lobule undisturbed by the minimal dissection inherent in nondelivery approaches. Properly positioned, tip grafts may be sutured in place without the open approach. If complex sutured-in-place tip grafts are planned, a delivery or open approach is preferred.

Delivery Approaches

Delivering the alar cartilages as individual bipedicle chondrocutaneous flaps through intercartilaginous and marginal incisions is the preferred approach when the nasal tip anatomy

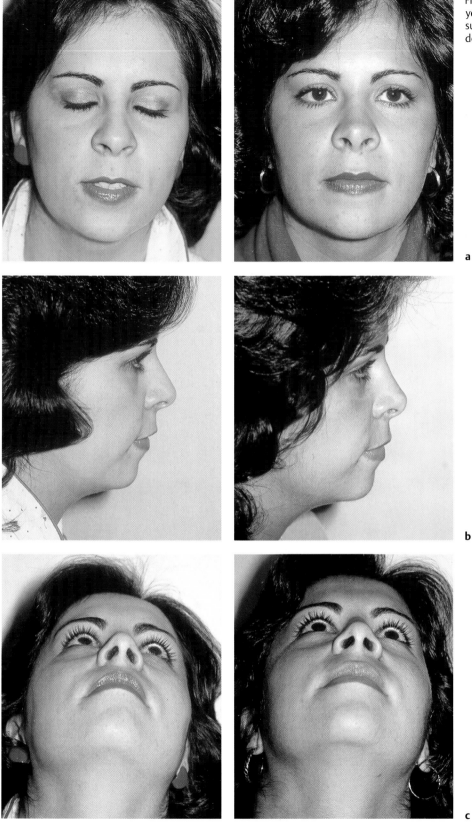

Fig. 2.**10 d** ▷

Fig. 2.**10** Favorable long-term outcome (10 years) in patient requiring conservative surgery, in whom a transcartilaginous nondelivery approach to the nasal tip was ideal.

is more abnormal (broad, asymmetrical, etc.) or when more dramatic tip refinements are necessary. Significant modifications in the alar cartilage shape, attitude, and orientation are more predictably attained when the cartilages are delivered (Fig. 2.**11**). The base photograph is usually helpful in determin-

ing which patients may best be approached in this manner (8). If the triangularity of the tip from below is satisfactory and only modest volume reduction of the lateral crus appears necessary, the nondelivery approach serves well. If, however, on base and frontal view the alar cartilages flare unpleasantly, tip

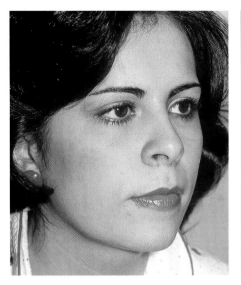

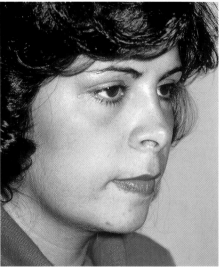

Fig. 2.**10 d**

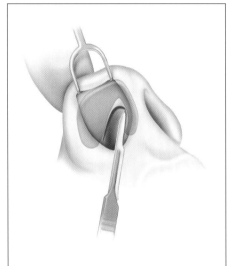

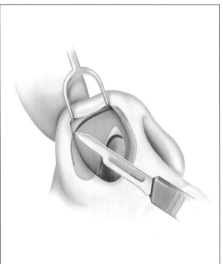

a

b

Fig. 2.**11**   Delivery approach to the nasal tip, effected through bilateral intercartilaginous and marginal incisions, delivering the alar cartilages as bipedicle chondrocutaneous flaps. (**a**) Intercartilaginous incision. (**b**) Marginal incision. (**c**) Freeing and delivery of alar cartilage as a bipedicle chondrocutaneous flap. (**d**) Resection of calculated portion of cephalic margin of lateral crus

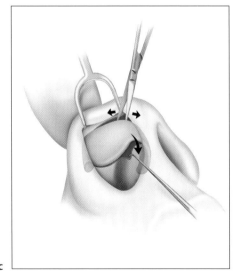

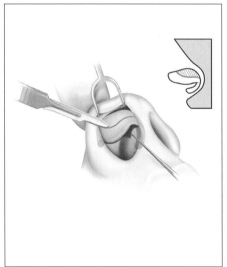

c

d

triangularity is unsatisfactory, or the tip appears too amorphous and bulbous, the domal angles are too wide, and the interdomal distance must be narrowed, a delivery approach is chosen to correct these esthetic deficiencies more thoroughly. Transdomal suture narrowing of broad domes (Fig. 2.**12**), an ef-

fective and preferred technique, is easily effected by means of the delivery approach. In similar fashion, interrupted strip techniques (rarely necessary) for more radical tip refinement and cephalic rotation are more efficiently accomplished when the cartilages are delivered (9). The increased surgical expo-

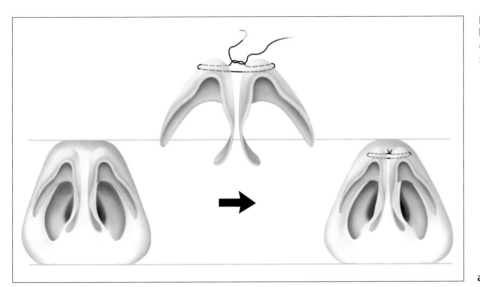

a

Fig. 2.**12**   Transdomal suture narrowing of the broad nasal tip, characterized by a wide inter-domal distance and domal angles. Outcome shown at 11 years following surgery.

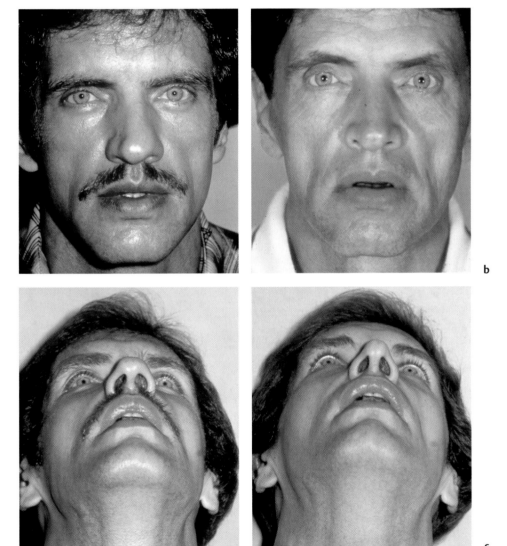

b

c

Fig. 2.**12 d**   ▷

sure provides the surgeon with an improved binocular view of the tip anatomy and affords the added ease of bimanual surgical modifications.

Open (External) Approach

The external or open approach to the nasal tip is in reality a more aggressive form of the delivery approach and is chosen with discretion in specific nasal tip deformities (Fig. 2.**13**).

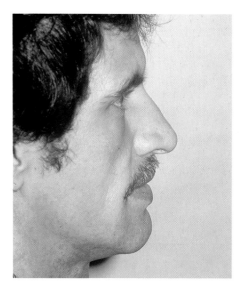
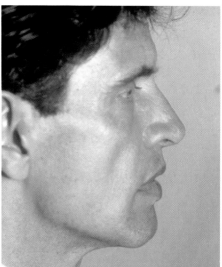

Fig. 2.**12 d**

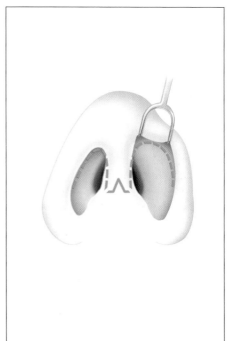

a

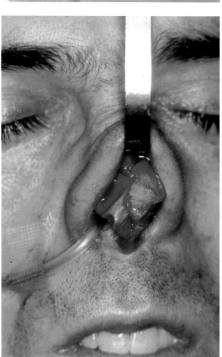

b

Fig. 2.**13** Open approach to nasal tip cartilages. (**a**) Transcolumellar incision connected to paracolumellar and marginal incisions. (**b**) View of exposed nasal tip cartilages utilizing open approach. (**c**) Illustration of one method of repairing the concave lateral crus seen in (**b**): Removal, reversal, and replanting of crus with its convex surface outward.

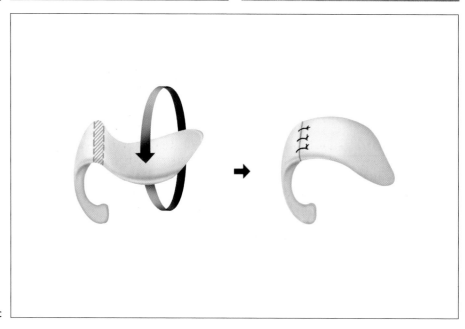

c

When the nasal tip is highly asymmetrical, markedly overprojected, severely underprojected, or anatomically confusing in its form (as in certain secondary revision cases), the open approach is considered. The transcolumellar scar is of negligible importance in this decision because it routinely heals inconspicuously when meticulously repaired. The anatomical view is unparalleled through this approach, affording the surgeon diagnostic information unavailable through traditional closed approaches. These technical virtues must be balanced with the potential disadvantages of an enlarged scar bed, slightly delayed healing with some prolongation of tip edema, and increased operating time. Indications for choosing the open approach might include:

- Asymmetrical tip cartilages
- Severe tip underprojection or overprojection
- Severely deviated nose
- Middle vault deformities requiring grafting
- Nasal tumors
- Cleft lip/nose deformities
- Difficult revision rhinoplasty
- Infantile (tiny) nostrils
- Teaching

Clearly, when subtle and conservative tip surgery is indicated by the patient's existent anatomy, the open approach is unnecessary and even counterproductive.

Alar Cartilage Sculpturing Techniques

The choice of the technique used to modify the alar cartilages and the relationship of the nasal tip with the remaining nasal structures should be *based entirely on the anatomy encountered* and the *predicted result desired*, as defined from the known dynamics of long-term healing. The astounding diversity of anatomical tip variations encountered demands the mastery of a broad diversification of surgical planning and execution.

Three broad categories of nasal tip sculpturing procedures may be identified. Although additional subtle technical variations exist, the three primary categories are:
1. *Volume reduction of the cephalic lateral crus margin with residual complete strip,*
2. *Volume reduction with suture reorientation of the residual complete strip* (dome-narrowing sutures, interdomal sutures, transdomal sutures), and
3. *Volume reduction with interrupted strip.*

Preserving intact the major portion of the *residual complete strip* of the alar cartilage is always preferred when the anatomy of the alar cartilages and their surrounding soft-tissue investments allows. This preservative approach retains the supportive advantage of the intact cartilage strip (thus "mimicking" nature), discourages cephalic rotation when it is undesirable, eliminates many of the potential hazards of more radical techniques, and tends to produce a more natural final result.

Techniques involving a weakened (or suture-reoriented) residual complete strip have all the foregoing positive virtues and in addition allow the surgeon to effect reorientation of the breadth of the domal angle and interdomal projection modification, and narrowing refinement so desirable in the ideal postoperative appearance. The control of favorable healing is enhanced with these techniques, with the risk of complication diminished considerably.

Despite a laudable desire to preserve the integrity of the residual complete strip whenever possible, anatomical situations are occasionally encountered in which the shape, breadth, and orientation of the alar cartilages must be changed more radically by interrupting the complete strip in a vertical fashion somewhere along its extent to refine severe anatomical deficits (Fig. 2.**14**) (9). When significant cephalic rotation is indicated, interrupted strip techniques are considered. The risks of asymmetrical healing are higher when the alar cartilages are divided, however, and initial loss of tip support occurs immediately. The latter problem must be recognized and countermeasures taken during surgery to ensure that sufficient tip support is reconstituted (10). Shoring struts in the columella, infratip lobule cartilage grafts, and transdomal suturing are the most commonly used tip support adjuncts. Almost without exception, interrupted strips should be avoided in patients displaying thin skin with sparse subcutaneous tissue.

Cephalic Trim Preserving Complete Strip Intact

When only modest reduction of the alar cartilages is indicated by the presenting anatomy, symmetrical resection of a conservative amount of the cephalic margin of the lateral crura while preserving a complete intact residual cartilage provides a predictable healing outcome.

Transdomal Suture Repair

In patients who demonstrate a broad, boxy tip characterized by bifidity, broad domal angles, and excessively large alar cartilages, predictable narrowing refinement may be achieved by transdomal suturing of the reduced, residual complete strips with one or more horizontal mattress sutures of 5–0 polydioxanone suture (PDS) (Fig. 2.**15**). Narrowing refinement results, vital tip supports are preserved, and symmetrical healing is facilitated (Fig. 2.**16**). Because a complete strip is preserved intact and only its shape is modified, *the surgical outcome is highly predictable.* Transdomal sutures strengthen tip support and can be used to enhance tip projection slightly. We rely strongly on this narrowing technique when the proper anatomy is encountered. When indicated to further narrow an excessively broad domal angle, individual dome narrowing sutures are positioned in each dome.

Tip Projection and Cartilage Tip Grafts

In addition to the creation of narrowing refinement and symmetry of the nasal tip, most evident in the frontal view, *appropriate projection* must be preserved or newly created to result in the most natural appearance possible. Clearly, the most attractive and elegant noses are those in which anterior projection is sufficient to set the tip subtly but distinctly apart from the nasal supratip areas. Ptotic or poorly projected tips produce a snubbed and indistinct appearance (10).

Ideally on profile view, the nasal tip should be slightly elevated above the cartilaginous dorsum by 1–2 mm, blending gently rather than abruptly into the supratip. If the preoperative projection of the tip is normal and adequate, lowering the cartilaginous dorsum into proper alignment will achieve a satisfactory esthetic appearance, provided no loss of tip support occurs during the operative or postoperative periods. Preserving the major and minor tip support structures increases likelihood of this, whereas their sacrifice without compen-

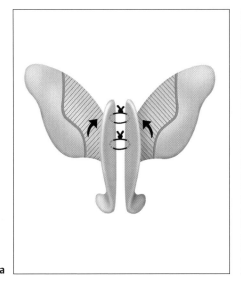

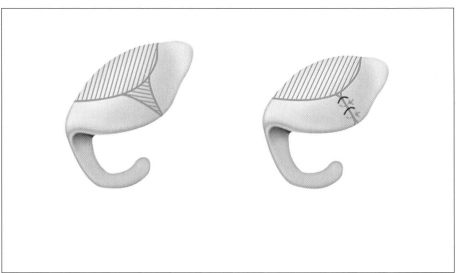

a

b

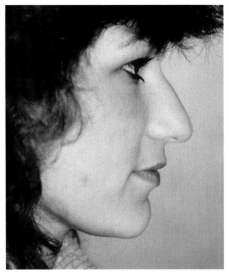

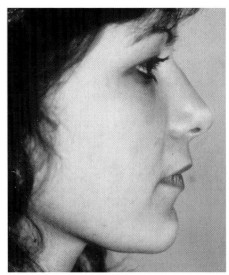

Fig. 2.**14** (**a**) Interrrupted strip procedure, utilized only when more conservative procedures are not indicated or sufficient to gain significant tip projection and tip narrowing. (**b**) Lateral interrupted strip technique, resecting a triangle base upward to effect significant upward tip rotation, created when the cut edges of the lateral crus are reconstituted by fine suture. (**c**)

c

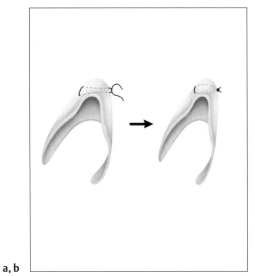

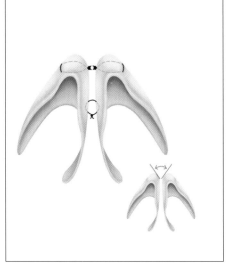

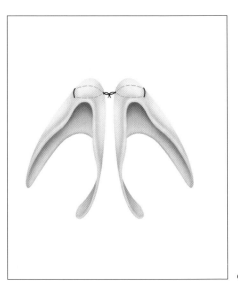

a, b

c

Fig. 2.**15** (**a**) Narrowing refinement of broad boxy tip characterized by wide domal angles and excessive interdomal distance, created by a horizontal mattress suture passed through both domes and tied without undue tension between the domes. (**b**) Single-dome sutures utilized to narrow the overwide domal angle found in some patients with overwide tips. (**c**) Interdomal suture placed in conjunction with transdomal or single-dome sutures to bring tip-defining points closer together. Care should be taken not to overnarrow tip, resulting in an abnormal "unitip" appearance.

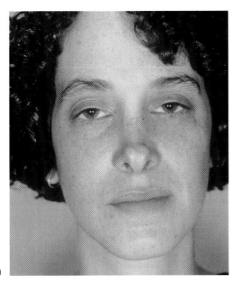
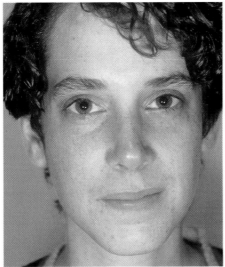

a

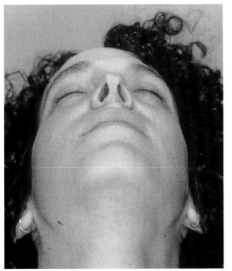
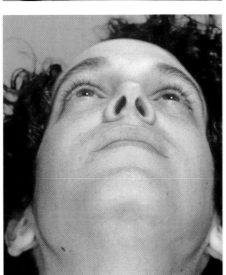

b

Fig. 2.**16**   Narrowing refinement of boxy nasal tip created, following removal of the abnormal bossae, by transdomal suturing. (**a**) Frontal view. (**b**) Basal view, demonstrating improved triangularity and symmetry.

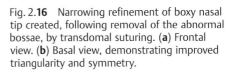

satory reestablishment of support inevitably leads to eventual tip ptosis. If preoperative tip projection is inadequate, attempts to overreduce the supratip cartilaginous dorsum to produce pseudoprojection of the tip are inadvisable and lead to apparent flattening or widening of the middle third of the nose.

If tip projection is inadequate, several reliable methods may be used singly or in tandem to establish permanent improvement. All involve reorientation of the alar cartilages or addition of autogenous cartilage grafts to strengthen or sculpture the projection and/or attitude of the tip and infratip lobule. Because the long-term viability and stability of sutured-in-place cartilage tip grafts are well established, they are regularly and successfully used if the surgical modification of existing alar cartilage configuration is not adequate to produce the desired degree of projection (Fig. 2.**17a, b**) (2, 3). In revision rhinoplasty in particular, tip cartilage grafts are irreplaceable in skeletal reconstruction beneath scarred skin and asymmetrical topography. Such grafts are routinely used to camouflage and provide more symmetry to nasal tips whose alar cartilages have been badly damaged. Two distinct varieties of tip grafts are preferred: Those that directly overlie the dome profile of the alar cartilage, and those that redefine and contour the skeletal anatomy of the infratip lobule. Because these grafts (single or laminated) lie in intimate subcutaneous pockets, exacting sculpture of their size and shape is mandatory. Harvested from septal or auricular cartilage, they are ideally inserted with or without suture fixation into small pockets dissected to accommodate exactly the dimensions of the graft(s). Bilateral marginal incisions beneath the anatomical dome area facilitate precise graft positioning.

Onlay and Stiffening Supportive Tip Grafts

Onlay Grafts

Patients are commonly encountered who present with asymmetrical tip anatomy, unilateral or bilateral lateral crural concavity, or even unequal development of the alar cartilages. If the asymmetry or deformity is not overly profound, onlay cartilage grafts may be fashioned from resected segments of the lateral crus, septal cartilage fragments or curved contoured cartilage grafts from the auricle (preferred). One or two layers of grafts may be sculpted and sutured together and in place to camouflage irregularities, provide needed projection, and reconstruct tip defects (Fig. 2.**18**).

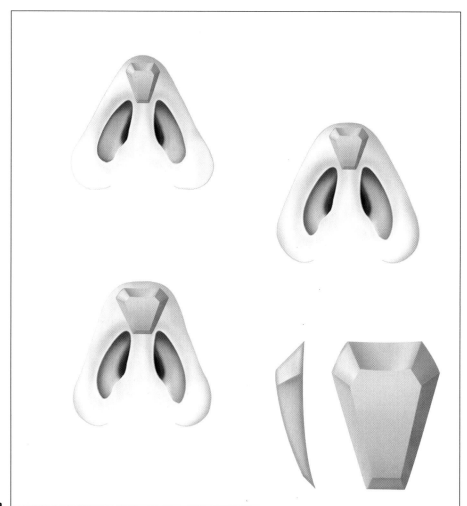

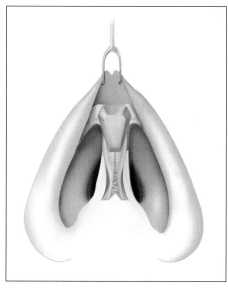

Fig. 2.**17** (**a**) Various sized and shapes of cartilage tip grafts used for improving nasal tip projection in patients with inadequate projection (grafts are generally best avoided in patients with extremely thin skin). (**b**) Sutured-in-place tip graft placed through an open approach to the nose.

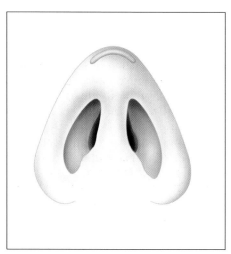

Fig. 2.**18** Contoured auricular projection (CAP) graft placed directly over the nasal domes to camouflage irregularities and effect increased tip projection.

Lateral Crural Strut Grafts

Patients are encountered with nasal tip variants that are characterized by thin, frail, and delicate alar cartilages that support the nasal tip poorly, leading to asymmetry, tip irregularities, and even inspiratory alar sidewall collapse. Such frail lateral crura may be strengthened by lateral crural strut grafts, fashioned to stiffen, straighten, and support weak lateral crura. By dissecting a pocket between the undersurface of the lateral crus and the underlying vestibular skin, thin supportive grafts may be sutured to the crus, offering stiffening and straightening characteristics (Fig. 2.**19**).

Tip Rotation

In many patients undergoing rhinoplasty, *cephalic rotation* of the nasal tip complex (alar cartilages, columella, and nasal base) assumes major importance in the surgical event, whereas in other individuals, the *prevention* of upward rotation is vital. Certain well-defined and reliable principles may be invoked by the nasal surgeon essentially to calibrate the degree of tip rotation (or prevention thereof). The dynamics of healing play a critical role in tip rotation principles; the control of these postoperative healing changes distinguishes rhinoplasty from less elegant procedures. In the past, overrotation of the nasal tip created an unhealthy stigma regarding the rhinoplasty procedure. Most individuals recognize and prefer the es-

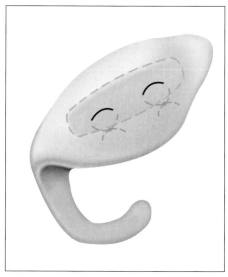

Fig. 2.**19**   Lateral crural cartilage strut grafts may be effectively utilized to stiffen and favorably reshape irregular, concave, or excessively convex lateral crura. Grafts are sutured between the undersurface of the lateral crus and the vestibular skin.

thetic advantages of a stronger nose possessed of sufficient length to impart character and suitable proportions to the face.

The planned degree of tip rotation depends on a variety of factors, which often include:

1. The length of the nose
2. The length of the face
3. The length of the upper lip
4. Facial balance and proportions
5. The patient's esthetic desires
6. The surgeon's esthetic judgment.

An important distinction must be drawn between *tip rotation* and *tip projection* (11). Although certain tip rotation techniques may result in desirable increases in tip projection, the converse is not true. Tip rotation and projection, in fact, complement each other, and their proper achievement in individual patients is constantly interrelated. A classic example of this interdependent relationship is illustrated by the almost inevitable loss of tip projection when interrupted strip techniques are chosen to enhance cephalic rotation; steps must be planned to restore adequate long-term tip projection by one of the several methods recommended.

Finally, a distinction must be drawn between *true* tip rotation and the *illusion* of tip rotation achieved by contouring cartilage grafts placed in the infratip lobule, columella, and nasolabial angle. Favorable modifications in the tip–lip complex profile areas with autogenous implants may obviate the need for any actual tip rotation, thus preserving a long, and at times more desirable, nasal appearance. Reduction of the nasal profile, particularly the supratip cartilaginous pyramid, may also impart the illusion of rotation and a shortened nose, although occasionally at the expense of a strong and narrow dorsum.

Nasal tip rotation results fundamentally from planned surgical modifications of the alar cartilages, but increments of rotation may also be realized from additional adjunctive procedures on nasal structures adjacent to the alar cartilages, which exert a favorable influence on calibrated tip rotation methods used to enhance the effects of a planned degree of tip rotation. Shortening *of the caudal septum, excision of overlong caudal upper lateral cartilages, and septal shortening with a high transfixion incision* (11) are regularly used to enhance the effects of a planned degree of tip rotation.

Because tip rotation is only one of the many objectives of rhinoplasty, decisions regarding rotation and planning for tip volume reduction, alar cartilage thinning reduction, and modifications in the attitude and angulation of the alar cartilages must be interrelated (12).

The techniques and healing dynamics described are not absolute, but are reasonably predictable. Most tip rotation techniques may be incorporated into an organizational scheme that involves three procedures to preserve a complete, intact strip of alar cartilage (Fig. 2.**20**) and three additional procedures involving interrupted strip techniques (Fig. 2.**21**). Unique anatomical situations are regularly encountered that require modifications of this scheme to achieve a more refined result, but the fundamental principles elaborated remain constant. In addition, the thickness and strength of the alar cartilages, along with the character of their enveloping soft tissue and skin, dictate, to a degree, which techniques may safely and predictably be used in each anatomical situation.

Complete strip techniques are always preferable tip procedures when the nasal anatomy permits, and the goals of the surgical procedure may be met without resorting to the less predictable interrupted strip procedures. Preserving a complete, uninterrupted segment of alar cartilage remnant contributes to a more stable and better supported nasal tip that tends to *resist* cephalic rotation during healing (13).

Interrupted strip techniques combined with volume reduction of excessive alar cartilage tend to result in a more substantial degree of cephalic rotation of the tip complex. Once the complete strip of residual alar cartilage is divided (interrupted), the result is relative instability of the nasal tip, on which the forces of upward scar contraction create a variable degree of cephalic rotation, underscoring the principle that during scar contracture tissues are generally moved from areas of instability (in this case, the unstable nasal tip cartilages) toward areas of stability (the bony–cartilaginous nasal pyramid). Generally suture-reconstitution of the divided lateral crus after removal of a base-up triangle achieves predictable and reliable rotation from repositioning of the attitude of the alar cartilages (Fig. 2.**22**). Caution must be exercised constantly in the use of interrupted strips in patients with thin skin and/ or more delicate cartilages because the absence of good tip supporting structures sets the stage for loss of projection, alar collapse, notching, pinching, and asymmetry.

Correcting the Overprojecting Tip

Profound facial and nasal disharmony may result from the anatomical facial feature variant termed "the overprojecting nose." Because the entire nose, and especially the normal nasal tip, are composed of distinct, interrelated anatomical components, any one or a combination of several of these components may be responsible for a tip that projects too far forward of the anterior plane of the face. The guidelines for determining appropriate and inappropriate tip projection are now well accepted. When numerous patients with overprojecting

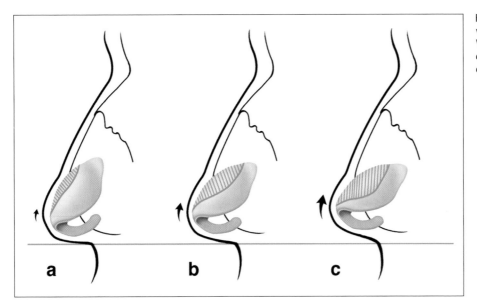

Fig. 2.**20**   Principles applicable to tip rotation when a complete strip procedure is utilized. Within limits, as slightly more cephalic margin of the lateral is removed, slightly more cephalic rotation occurs.

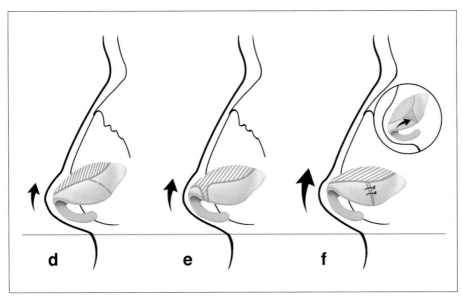

Fig. 2.**21**   General principles applicable to tip rotation when an interrupted strip procedure is utilized. The degree and amount of cephalic rotation are affected by other maneuvers as well, such as caudal septal resection, resection of the caudal aspect of the upper lateral cartilages, and even moderate resection of excessive vestibular skin.

tips are analyzed, it becomes apparent that no single anatomical component of the nose is consistantly responsible for overprojection; therefore, no single surgical technique is uniformly useful in correcting all the problems responsible for the various overprojection deformities (3, 4). Accurate anatomical diagnosis allows preoperative development of a logical individualized strategy for correction and tip repositioning. In almost every instance, *weakening or reduction of normal tip support mechanisms is required* to achieve normality, supplemented by reduction of the overdeveloped components. The following anatomical variants are commonly responsible individually or collectively for overprojection of the nasal tip.

Overdevelopment of the alar cartilages, commonly associated with thin skin and large nostrils, is frequently encountered in the overprojecting nose. The junction between the medial and lateral crura may form an overlarge dome of significant convexity, or the anatomical dome area may be sharply angulated, twisted, or even buckled, frequently demonstrating significant asymmetry of the entire tip and its tip-defining points. The hypertrophied cartilages must be delivered, their abnormalities visually diagnosed, and overall volume reduction of both the lateral and medial crura accom-

plished. Portions of the medial crus may require resection to reposition the nasal tip satisfactorily.

Overprojection and obliteration of a definitive nasolabial angle may be the result of *overdevelopment of the caudal quadrangular cartilage*. The nasal spine may in fact be of normal size, but if it is even slightly overlarge, it compounds the problem of overprojection. In effecting repair, the caudal septal margin abutting the nasal spine should always be inspected and shave reduced to normal proportion before sacrificing any of the nasal spine.

A *high anterior septal angle* caused by an overdeveloped quadrangular cartilage component may spuriously elevate the tip to an abnormally forward-projecting position, even when associated with otherwise perfectly normal tip anatomy (12). This condition tends to "tent" the tip away from the face and "tether" the upper lip, producing an indefinite nasolabial angle and, on occasion, creating abnormal exposure of the maxillary gingiva, particularly on smiling. Correction demands a departure from the normal operative sequence of correcting the tip first. The initial surgical steps are planned to lower the cartilaginous profile first, releasing the tip from an abnormal overprojected influence. Further tip refinement measures can

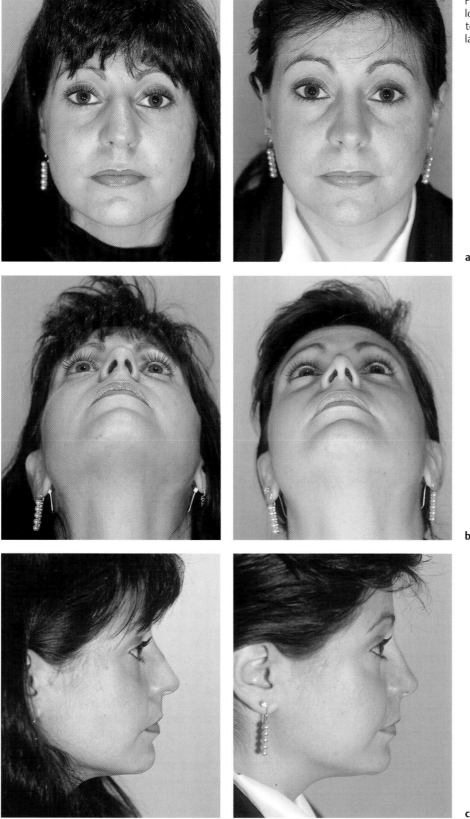

Fig. 2.**22**   Favorable outcome three years following tip-narrowing rhinoplasty with dome interruption procedure, borrowing from the lateral crural to increase tip projection.

a

b

c   Fig. 2.**22 d**   ▷

then be carried out as desired and indicated by the alar cartilage anatomy.

A less common cause of excess nasal tip projection is an *overlarge nasal bony spine*, which seemingly imparts an upward thrust of the tip components (which may otherwise be of normal dimensions). Compounding this abnormal appearance

is often a coexistent blunting of the nasolabial angle, which may appear full, webbed, and excessively obtuse, with no obvious demarcation between the tip and columella. The upper lip may appear short, tethered, and tense, often exposing excessive gingiva in facial repose as well as in animation. Rongeur or osteotome reduction of the overlarge spine and associated

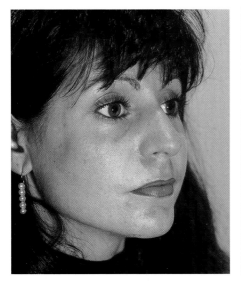
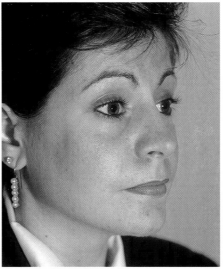

Fig. 2.**22 d**

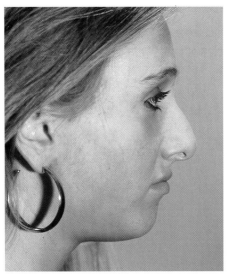
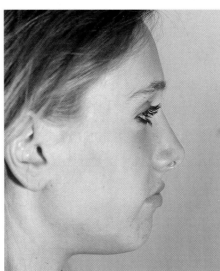

Fig. 2.**23** Favorable reduction of overprojection of the nasal tip by utilization of a complete transfixion incision to reduce the tip support created by the attachment of the medial crural footplates to the nasal septum. Because of hypertrophy, the medial crural footplates were excised in this patient.

caudal quadrangular cartilage and soft tissue is a surgical prerequisite to tip retrodisplacement.

Tip overprojection may occur as a result of an *overly long columella* associated with excessively long medial crura. In this deformity, the infratip lobule is commonly insufficient, creating the effect of extremely large and disproportionate nostrils. This deformity suggests the use of an external approach to the nasal tip to shorten the columellar length as well as that of the medial crura.

Various *combinations* of the foregoing hypertrophic anatomical problems may contribute to the overprojecting tip problem. In preoperative analysis, each nasal component must be identified and analyzed; only then can a definitive plan for natural correction be conceived. Generally, a combination of

weakening of the major tip support mechanisms associated with reduction of the components responsible for the tip overprojection is carried out incrementally and as conservatively as possible to achieve the desired normal final result in a progressive fashion. The various components capable of creating or contributing to overprojection of the nose are shown in Table 2.**2**.

Iatrogenic overprojection may occur when surgeons intent on profoundly increasing tip projection produce an unnaturally sharp and projected tip configuration (often with associated overrotation of the tip) (4). These misadventures commonly result from overaggressive tip surgery in which portions of the lateral crus are borrowed and rotated medially to increase medial crus projection.

Table 2.**2** Anatomical causes of tip overprojection

1. Hypertrophy of alar cartilages
   a. Enlarged alar cartilages
   b. Elongated medial crural
2. Hypertrophy of dorsal septum (anterior septal angle)
3. Hypertrophy of caudal septum (midseptal and caudal septal angle)
4. Hypertrophy of nasal spine
5. Combined components (combinations of above)

Profile Alignment

Three anatomical nasal components are responsible for the preoperative profile appearance: The *nasal bones, the cartilaginous septum,* and *the alar cartilages* (14). Generally, all three must undergo modification to create a pleasing and natural profile alignment. If the nose is overlarge with a convex

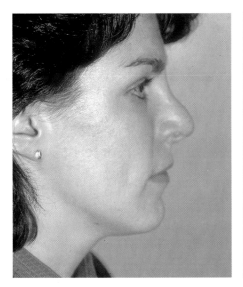 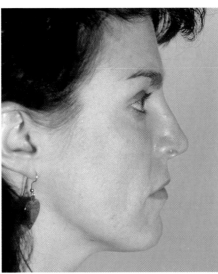

Fig. 2.**24** Maintenance of a strong, high profile generally leads to a more normal, nonoperated appearance of the nose.

profile, reduction of the three segments is required. Less commonly (except in revision rhinoplasty), profile *augmentation* with autograft materials must be accomplished.

The surgeon visualizes the ultimately intended profile, extending from the nasofrontal angle to the tip-defining point, and then on around the infratip lobule and columella to the nasolabial angle. The extent of reduction of bone, cartilage, and soft tissue always depends on and should be guided by stable tip projection; *therefore, positioning the projection of the tip at the outset of the operative procedure is beneficial.* Because the thickness of the investing soft tissues and skin varies at different areas of the profile and from patient to patient, dissimilar portions of cartilage and bone must be removed to ultimately create a straight or slightly concave profile (14). Strong, high profiles generally suit the patient best in the long term, contributing to a more elegant nose on profile and oblique views and also a more narrow nasal appearance on frontal view (Fig. 2.**24**). Overreduced profiles result in a washed-out, indefinite, and widened appearance from the front, inadequately separating the eyes and poorly reflecting light.

In planning profile alignment, the two stable reference points are the existing (or planned) *nasofrontal angle* and the *tip-defining point* (15). Esthetics are generally best served when profile reduction results in a high, straight-line profile in men and with the leading edge of the tip just slightly higher in women. A gentle slope of no more than 2–3 mm should exist between the caudal part of the cartilaginous dorsum and the most anteriorly projecting aspect of the nasal tip. Reversal of the usual preoperative tip–supratip relationship is required to achieve this esthetic ideal. The degree and angulation of the "hump removal" depends on various factors, the most important of which are the size of the various anatomical components involved and the surgeon's confidence in the stability of postoperative tip projection (14). These must be balanced with the personal preference for profile appearance combined with the surgeon's value judgment of facial esthetics.

Surgical access to the nasal dorsum is gained through the transcartilaginous, intercartilaginous, or transcolumellar incision, depending on which approach was used during tip refinement. In endonasal approaches, a complete transfixion incision for exposure is unnecessary and may compromise tip support by sacrificing the attachment of the medial crural footplates to the caudal septum.

The plane of tissue elevation over the nasal dorsum is important for several reasons. A relatively avascular potential plane exists intimate (superficial) to the perichondrium of the cartilaginous vault and just below the periosteum of the bony vault (3, 6). Elevating the soft-tissue flap in this important plane (Fig. 2.**6**) preserves the thickest possible ultimate epithelial–soft-tissue covering to cushion the newly formed bony and cartilaginous profile. Generally, only sufficient skin is elevated to gain access to the bony and cartilaginous profile, and therefore wide undermining is unnecessary in the typical rhinoplasty. In older patients with redundant and less elastic skin, or when access is needed for major autograft augmentation, wider undermining is carried out (15). Even in the latter instance, the periosteal–soft-tissue layer over the intended site of the low lateral osteotomies is preserved intact to help stabilize the mobile bony pyramid after in-fracture osteotomy maneuvers.

The soft tissues over the cartilaginous dorsum are elevated by means of scalpel dissection with a No. 15c blade, and the periosteum over the bony pyramid is lifted from its stable bony attachment with the knife and sharp Joseph elevator. Because the periosteum inserts into the internasal suture line in the midline, the periosteum is lifted on either side of this suture and the space brought into continuity with the sharp scissors. Little or no bleeding should ensue.

Either of two methods of profile alignment is preferred: *incremental* or *en bloc* (14). In the first method, the cartilaginous dorsum is reduced by incrementally shaving away the cartilaginous dorsum until an ideal tip–supratip relationship is established " followed by sharp osteotome removal of the residual bony hump. If only minimal hump removal is contemplated, the knife is positioned at the osseocartilaginous junction and plunged through this area, then advanced caudally to and around the anterior septal angle of the caudal septum (Fig. 2.**25**). In large cartilaginous reductions, a portion of the upper lateral cartilage attachment to the quadrangular cartilage must be removed with the dorsal septum, but leaving these two cartilaginous components attached by the intact underlying mucous perichondrial bridge.

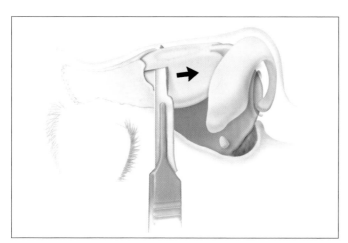

Fig. 2.**25**   Knife reduction of the cartilaginous dorsum, creating a "fish-mouth" mortis joint for the acceptance of the osteotome which will continue hump resection by final removal of the bony hump, thus removing the hump as an en-bloc segment.

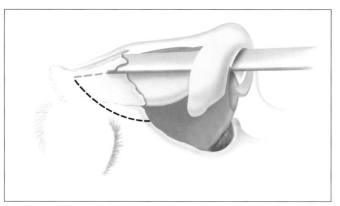

Fig. 2.**26**   Guarded Rubin osteotome completing removal of the bony hump.

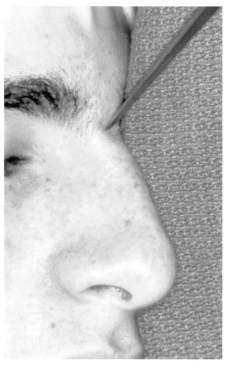

Fig. 2.**27**   Transcutaneous osteotomy at the nasion to deepen the naso-frontal angle.

A Rubin osteotome, honed to razor sharpness for each procedure and seated in the opening made by the knife at the osseocartilaginous junction, is advanced cephalically to remove the desired degree of bony hump in continuity with the cartilaginous hump (Fig. 2.**26**).

Any remaining irregularities are corrected under direct vision with a knife and sharp tungsten-carbide rasp. Palpating the skin of the dorsum with the examining finger moistened with hydrogen peroxide often provides clues to unseen irregularities, as does intranasal palpation of the profile with the noncutting edge of the No. 15 blade. Except in large or severely twisted noses, it is unnecessary and potentially harmful to separate the upper lateral cartilages from the septum by cutting through the mucoperichondrial bridge of tissue connecting them at the nasal valve (16). Redundant soft tissue around the anterior septal angles may be trimmed away to achieve improved tip–supratip definition. The caudal septum, assessed by stretching the partial transfixion incision posteriorly, lies exposed for geometric shortening or repositioning.

In patients in whom the nasofrontal angle is poorly defined or in need of retropositioning, weakening of the bone in the desired area is accomplished before bony hump removal. At the exact site in the midline where nasofrontal angle is desired, a 2-mm osteotome is plunged transcutaneously into the midline of the nasal bone (Fig. 2.**27**) (3). By angulating this small osteotome laterally on either side, the exact cephalic extent of bony hump removal may be controlled by *scoring the bone* in a horizontal line at the nasofrontal angle. During the bony hump removal phase of profile alignment, the nasal bones fracture cephalically where this weakening maneuver has established a bony dehiscence, allowing the surgeon some additional control over the ultimate site of the nasofrontal angle. Creating a more caudally placed angle provides the illusion of a shorter nose without actually shortening, whereas establishing a more cephalically placed angle creates the appearance of a longer nose.

In patients in whom the nasofrontal angle is overly deep, augmentation with a radix graft composed of residual septal cartilage or remnants of the excised alar cartilages provides a beneficial esthetic refinement (Fig. 2.**28**).

Further profile enhancements may be favorably developed with contouring cartilage grafts positioned along the dorsum, supratip area, infratip lobule, columella, and nasolabial angle (16). In the last site, so-called plumping grafts are commonly used to open an otherwise acute or unsatisfactory nasolabial angle and thereby contribute to improved profile appearance (17). The illusion of tip rotation and nasal shortening results from this maneuver, reducing the degree of actual shortening required and preserving a longer and often more elegant nose.

Bony Pyramid Narrowing and Alignment

Significant advances have been made over the past two decades in the reduction of osteotomy trauma in rhinoplasty surgery. Osteotomies, the most traumatic of all nasal surgical maneuvers, are best delayed until the final step in the planned surgical sequence, when vasoconstriction exerts its maximal influence and the nasal splint may be promptly positioned (3, 18, 19). Profile alignment in typical reduction rhinoplasty in-

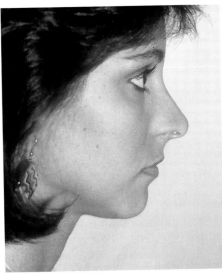

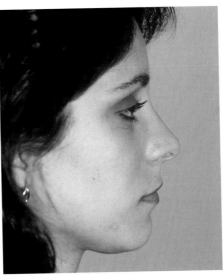

Fig. 2.**28** Improved profile 6 years following retropositioning of an overprojected tip, enhanced by an onlay radix graft to the overdeep nasofrontal region.

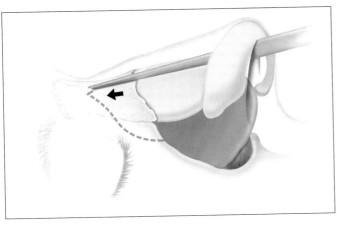

Fig. 2.**29** Medial–oblique osteotomy is sited and created 15–20° from the midline to create a weakened segment of bony for the lateral osteotomy to encounter.

evitably results in an excessive plateaulike width of the nasal dorsum, requiring narrowing of the bony and cartilaginous pyramid to restore a natural and more narrow frontal appearance to the nose. The lateral bony sidewalls (consisting of the nasal bones and maxillary ascending processes) must be completely mobilized by nongreenstick fractures and moved medially (exceptions may exist in older patients with more fragile bones in whom greenstick fractures may be acceptable or even preferable). The upper lateral cartilages are also moved medially because of their stable attachment cephalically to the undersurface of the nasal bones.

To facilitate atraumatic low lateral osteotomy execution, medial–oblique osteotomies angled 15–20° laterally from the vertical midline are preferred (Fig. 2.**29**) (19). By creating an osteotomy dehiscence at the intended cephalic apex of the lateral osteotome, the surgeon exerts added control of the exact site of backfracture in the lateral bony sidewall. A 2- to 3-mm sharp micro-osteotome is positioned intranasally at the cephalic extent of the removal of the bony hump (if no hump removal has been necessary, the site of positioning is at the caudal extent of the nasal bones in the midline). The osteotome is advanced cephaloobliquely to its intended apex at an angle of 10–15°, depending on the shape of the nasal bony sidewall. Little trauma results from medial–oblique osteotomies, which prevent the ever-present possibility of eccentric or asymmetrical surgical fractures from developing when lateral osteotomies alone are performed. In addition, bony narrowing to accomplish desired in-fracture as a consequence of lateral

osteotomies combined with medial–oblique osteotomies occurs without strong manual pressure exerted on the nasal bones, a traditional but unnecessary traumatic maneuver.

Trauma may be significantly reduced in lateral osteotomies if 2- or 3-mm micro-osteotomies are used to accomplish a controlled fracture of the bony sidewalls (3). There is no need for elevation of the periosteum along the pathway of the lateral fractures because the small osteotomies require little space for their cephalic progression. Appropriately, the intact periosteum stabilizes and internally splints the complete fractures, facilitating stable and precise healing. The low curved lateral osteotomy is initiated by pressing the sharp osteotome through the vestibular skin to encounter the margin of the pyriform aperture at or just above the inferior turbinate. This preserves the bony sidewall along the floor of the nose, where narrowing would achieve no favorable esthetic improvement but might compromise the inferior nasal airway without purpose. The pathway of the osteotome then progresses toward the base of the maxilla, curving next up along the nasal maxillary junction to encounter the previously created small medial–oblique osteotomy (Fig. 2.**30**). A complete, controlled, and atraumatic fracture of the bony sidewall is thus created, allowing in-fracture without excessive traumatic pressure. Immediate finger pressure is applied bilaterally over the lateral osteotome sites to forest all further extravasation of blood into the soft tissues. *In reality, little or no bleeding occurs during micro-osteotomies because the soft tissues embracing the bony sidewalls remain essentially undamaged.*

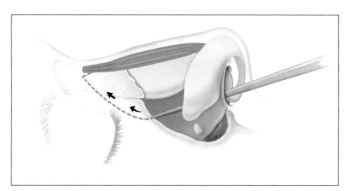

Fig. 2.**30**   Curved low lateral osteotomy, beginning higher on the ascending process at the level of the inferior concha, coursing lower onto the ascending and finally curving upward toward the medial–oblique osteotomy site.

In most rhinoplasty procedures, controlled nasal fractures as the result of osteotomy should cause slight but definite mobility of the bony sidewalls stabilized by the internal and external periosteum (19), which bridges the nasal fragments on either side of the osteotome pathway. Large guarded osteotomies destroy this vital periosteal sling, potentially rendering the bony fragrnents unstable and susceptible to eccentric or asymmetrical healing. In addition, trauma from large osteotomes may produce increased bleeding, edema, and unnecessary ecchymosis. In the elderly, however, greenstick fractures are preferred because of the tendency for the brittle nasal bones to become unstable.

Alar Base Reduction

Appropriate retroprojection of the projecting nose typically requires diminishing the various major and minor tip support mechanisms to reposition the tip closer to the face. A concomitant reduction of the alar component length and lateral flare (occasioned by tip repositioning) is usually required to improve nasal balance and harmony. Alar wedge excisions of various geometric designs and dimensions are necessary to balance alar length and position (see Chapter 9, Alar Reduction and Sculpture). The exact geometry of these excisions is determined by the present and intended shape of the nostril aperture, the degree and attitude of the lateral alar flare, the width and shape of the nostril sill, and the thickness of the alae. It is axiomatic that the surgeon creating alar reduction by excision of alar or nostril floor tissue should always err on the side of conservatism and strive for symmetrical repair, since overaggressive and asymmetrical tissue resection leads to an almost irreversible situation of disharmony and even nostril stenosis.

Dressings and Bandages

Nasal dressings are now applied. No intranasal dressing or packing is necessary in routine rhinoplasty. If septoplasty has been an integral part of the operation, a folded strip of Telfa is placed into each nostril along the floor of the nose to absorb drainage. If septoplasty has been incorporated into the operation, the previously placed *transseptal quilting mattress suture* (Fig. 2.**31**) acts as a sole internal nasal splint for the septum (3),

completely obliterating the submucoperichondrial dead spaces and fixing the septal elements in place during healing. The external splint consists of a layer of compressed Gelfoam placed along the dorsum and stabilized in place with flesh-colored Micropore tape, extending over and laterally beyond the lateral osteotome sites. A small aluminum and Velcro splint applied firmly over the nasal dorsum completes the operation.

Key Technical Points

1. Exacting preoperative analysis
2. Profound hemostasis (anesthesia injected into favorable tissue planes)
3. Dissection in favorable tissue planes
4. Atraumatic surgery with sharp instruments
5. Streamlined, efficient surgical technique
6. Preservation of normal tissues
7. Avoidance of overreduction of nasal skeletal structures
8. Disciplined, accurate suture repair of all incisions
9. Application of quilting transseptal mattress sutures rather than nasal packing

Postoperative Care

Care of the postrhinoplasty patient is directed toward patient comfort, reduction of swelling and edema, patency of the nasal airway, and compression with stabilization of the nose.

Whether the patient is discharged on the afternoon of or the morning after surgery, all intranasal dressings are removed from the nose before the patient leaves. A detailed list of instructions is supplied for the patient or accompanying family member; the important aspects of these do's and don'ts are emphasized. Prevention of trauma to the nose is clearly the most important consideration. Oral decongestant therapy is helpful, but the value of corticosteroids and antibiotics in routine rhinoplasty is conjectural.

The external splint is removed five to seven days after surgery. An important consideration should be gentle removal of the tape and splint by bluntly dissecting the nasal skin from the overlying splint with a dull instrument without disturbing or tenting up the healing skin. Failure to follow this policy may lead to disturbance of the newly forming subcutaneous fibroblastic layer over the nasal dorsum, with additional unwanted scarring and even abrupt hematoma.

Complications

Early complications following well-performed rhinoplasty by experienced surgeons are uncommon; any of the well-recognized complications of surgery (and anesthesia) are certainly possible. Since most patients undergoing this surgery are ordinarily youthful and healthy, serious complications are rare. The most important (and still all too common) complication is

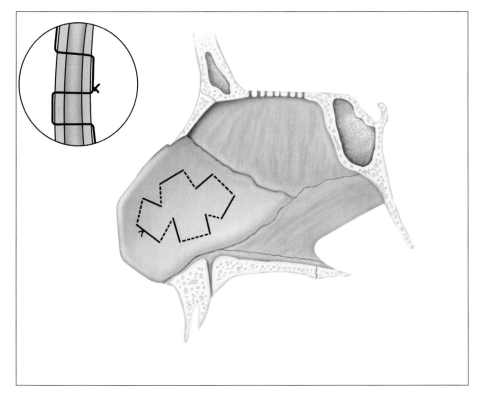

Fig. 2.**31**   Quilting mattress suture of 4–0 chromic catgut suture courses back and forth through the entirety of the septum, closing the dead space created when the mucoperichondrial flaps are elevated and further helping to splint the septum for the healing period.

patient dissatisfaction. Complications may be categorized as follows:

Early Postoperative Complications
- Epistaxis
- Hematoma
- Airway obstruction
- Patient trauma and injury to nose
- Infection (nasal, sinus, skin)
- Excess swelling

Late Postoperative Complications
- Patient dissatisfaction
- Recurrence of deformity
- Development of new deformity or asymmetry
- Tip support loss with ptosis
- Airway blockade
- Contour abnormalities

Summary

Contemporary rhinoplasty is characterized by increased preservation of the presenting anatomy, and reorienting and reshaping the abnormal anatomical components. An intimate knowledge of the variant anatomy encountered in patients, supplemented by accurate detailed analytical and diagnostic skills, sets the stage for superior surgical outcomes generated through tried and tested surgical techniques designed to produce superior long-term outcomes.

References

1. Burget GC, Menick FJ. *Aesthetic reconstruction of the nose.* St. Louis: CV Mosby: 1994.
2. Johnson, CM, Toriumi, DM. *Open structure rhinoplasty.* Philadelphia: WB Saunders: 1990.
3. Tardy, ME. *Rhinoplasty: The art and the science.* Philadelphia: WB Saunders: 1997.
4. Sheen JH, Sheen A. *Aesthetic Rhinoplasty* (2nd edition). St. Louis: CV Mosby: 1987.
5. Goin JM, Goin MK. *Changing the body.* Baltimore: Williams and Wilkins: 1981.
6. Tardy, ME. *Surgical anatomy of the nose.* New York: Raven Press: 1991.
7. Tardy ME, Thomas JR, Brown RJ. *Facial aesthetic surgery.* St. Louis: CV Mosby: 1995.
8. Tardy ME, Brown RJ, Childs C. *Principles of photography in facial plastic surgery.* New York: Thieme: 1992.
9. Goldman IB. Nasal tip correction with special reference to the medial crura. *Trans Am Acad Ophthalmol Otolaryngol.* 1964; 68:854.
10. Tardy ME. Rhinoplasty tip ptosis: etiology and prevention. *Laryngoscope.* 1973; 83:923.
11. Parkes ML, Brennan HG. High septal transfixion to shorten the nose. *Plast Reconstr Surg.* 1970; 45:487.
12. Aiach G, Levignac J. *Aesthetic rhinoplasty.* London: Churchill-Livingstone: 1991.
13. Nolst-Trenité G. *Rhinoplasty.* The Hague: XX: 1993.
14. Wright WK. Study on hump removal in rhinoplasty. *Laryngoscope.* 1967; 77:508.
15. Smith TW. The selection of patients for rhinoplasty. *Arch Otolaryngol.* 1971; 94:56.
16. Frye H. Interlocked stresses of cartilage. *Br J Plast Surg.* 1966; 19:276.
17. Walter C. Composite grafts in nasal surgery, *Arch Otolaryngol.* 1969; 90:622.
18. Wright WK. Lateral osteotomy in rhinoplasty. *Arch Otolaryngol.* 1963; 78:680.
19. Farrior RT. Corrective surgery of the nasal framework. *J Fla Med Assoc.* 1968; 45:276.

3 Facial Proportions and Esthetic Ideals

I. D. Papel, R. B. Capone

**"Beauty is Nature's brag, and must be shown
In courts, at feasts, and high solemnities,
Where most may wonder at the workman-
ship…"**
John Milton (1608–1674)

Contents

Introduction

Beauty is the aggregate of human features that produces a sense of pleasure in the beholder. Among the earliest records of history are Paleolithic stone carvings displaying the human form as art (Figs. 3.**1**, 3.**2**). Such works are thought to represent the standard of beauty at the time they were created.

Artwork from successive civilizations illustrates not only the persistent desire to create beauty, but also the dynamic nature of beauty's perception (Figs. 3.**3**, 3.**4**). Over a period of 27 000 years, the human form as depicted in art serves as a historical record for the standard of beauty.

This reveals a fundamental anthropological principle: Human features deemed attractive change with time, but the social, reproductive, and evolutionary advantages they convey do not. This principle, in part, provides the motivational basis for facial plastic surgery. Facial plastic surgery has established the human face as an additional medium with which to create and display beauty, enabling the procurement of those advantages beauty commands. Of the surgical repertory, rhinoplasty has assumed a preeminent role. This chapter will examine facial proportions, esthetic ideals, and analysis of nasal deformity in the modern era of rhinoplasty.

> **"[T]he qualities of measure and proportion invariably…constitute beauty and excellence."**
> **Plato (427–347 BC)**

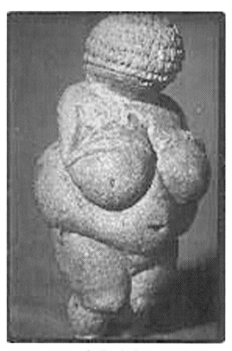

Fig. 3.**1** Venus of Villendorf, ca. 25 000 BC (*Naturhistorisches Museum*, Vienna, Austria.)

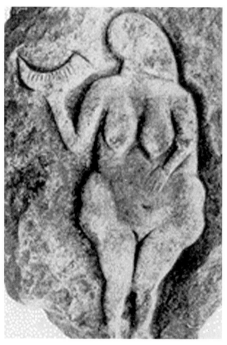

Fig. 3.**2** Venus of Laussel, ca. 20 000 BC (*Musee d'Aquitaine*, Bordeaux, Dordogne, France)

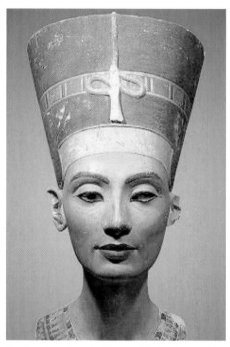

Fig. 3.**3** The head of Queen Nefertiti, ca. 1365 BC (Berlin State Museum, Berlin, Germany.)

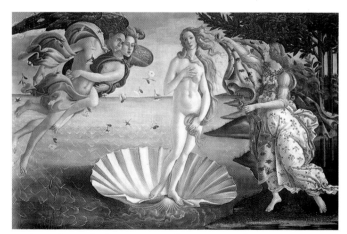

Fig. 3.**4** The Birth of Venus, Boticelli, ca. 1480. (Uffizi Gallery, Florence, Italy.)

Facial Proportions

The exact awareness of beauty cannot be placed in the historical record. Self-ornamentation with jewelry has been dated to the genus *Homo neandertalensis* in the Upper Pleistocene Epoch (ca. 32 000 BC), well before the Gravettian Venuses (1). It is unknown, however, whether this practice was for personal adornment or superstitious protection from evil. This is an important distinction, as the former purpose implies a concern for appearance and perhaps an acknowledgement of beauty. Despite the possibility that these ancient hominids had such concerns, history documents with certainty that the academic study of beauty and the first principles of facial analysis arose many years later in Ancient Greece.

The word esthetic derives from the Greek *aisthesis,* meaning to have a sense of or devotion to beauty. Greek philosophers felt that beauty was an essential part of the ideal universe and attempted to define it with the same mathematical principles and geometric relations that were thought to define the laws of nature (2). Chief among them was the great philosopher Plato, much of whose work concentrated on harmony, beauty, and mathematic proportions. His philosophy likely influenced Greek sculptors including Polykleitos (ca. 450–420 BC) and Praxiteles (400–330 BC), whose works defined the ideal beauty that influenced perceptions of subsequent generations (3).

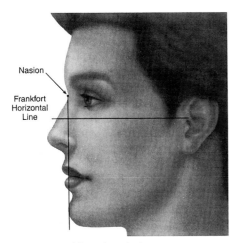

Fig. 3.5 Frankfurt plane (19)

Standard of Reference

Despite centuries of endeavor, there is no universal algorithm for the creation of beauty. Beauty is achieved when an individual's features combine to produce an esthetically pleasing result. This quality is more accurately described by a set of geometric conditions, or *rules of facial proportion,* which when met, tend to yield an attractive visage. As with all descriptive constructs, a universal standard of reference is necessary. A line connecting the superior aspect of the external auditory canal to the inferior aspect of the infraorbital rim placed parallel to the plane of the floor defines the standard plane of reference known as the Frankfurt horizontal plane (Fig. 3.5). This plane defines the patient position in which facial analysis and photography should occur. Since the landmarks defining the Frankfurt plane are bony landmarks that would require radiographic determination, corresponding surface anatomy is used. The tragion (Greek *tragos,* goat) marks the supratragal notch and approximates the superior aspect of the external auditory canal. The point of transition between the skin of the inferior eyelid and the skin of the cheek approximates the infraorbital rim.

Recognized topographical facial landmarks are shown in Figure 3.6.

Golden Proportion

An interesting rule of historical significance is known as the Golden Proportion. This mathematical phenomenon was probably first recognized by the Ancient Egyptians, and subsequently utilized by the Ancient Greeks. It is found in their architecture as well as in their art and results in a proportion especially appealing to the human eye. The Golden Proportion is defined as the ratio of two unequal segments of a line, where

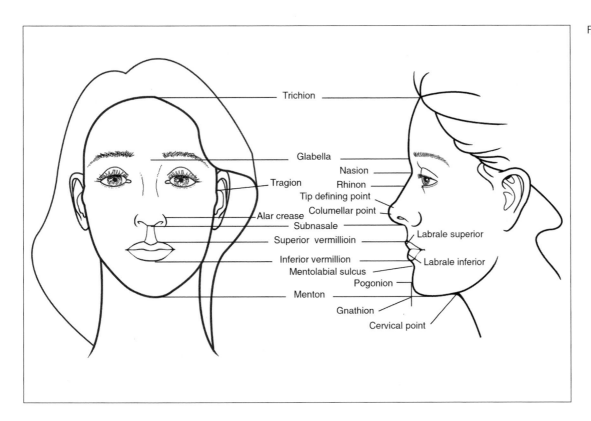

Fig. 3.6 Facial landmarks

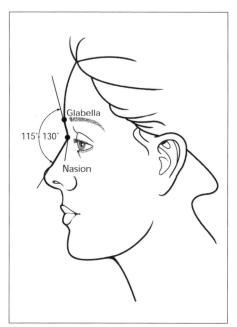

Fig. 3.**7** Nasofrontal angle

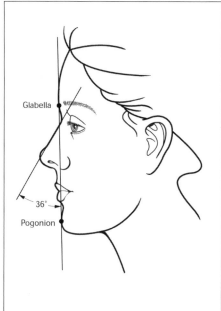

Fig. 3.**8** Nasofacial angle

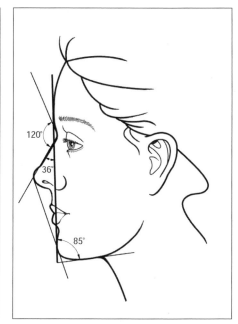

Fig. 3.**9** Nasomental angle

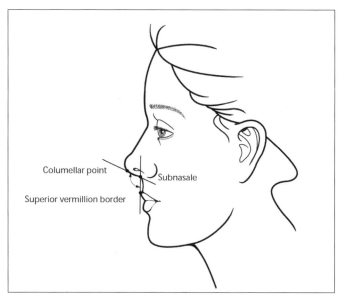

Fig. 3.**10** Nasolabial angle

the ratio of the shorter segment to the longer segment is equal to the ratio of the longer segment to the whole line (4). Represented by the Greek letter φ, after the Greek sculptor Phidias (500–432 BC), the numerical value of the Golden Proportion equals 1.61803.... An example of the Golden Proportion in nasal analysis is the ratio of nasal projection to nasal length (nasion to tip). If this ratio is Golden, then the nasofacial angle falls within the esthetic ideal (36–38°).

The Facial Angles

The face is a complex set of surfaces with tremendous variability. One goal of facial analysis is to provide a straightforward framework to compare preoperative and postoperative results. The facial angles describe such a framework and are especially important in evaluation of the rhinoplasty patient. The lines connecting the nasion (Latin *nasus*, nose) to the glabella (Latin *glaber*, smooth) and the nasion to the tip-defining point form the *nasofrontal angle* (Nfr). Ideally this angle is 115–130° (Fig. 3.**7**). The *facial plane* (fp) is a two-dimensional coronal section including the glabella and the pogonion (Greek *pogon*, beard). The *nasofacial angle* (Nfa) is formed by the angle between the facial plane and the line tangent to the nasal dorsum (Fig. 3.**8**). The ideal nasofacial angle is 36–40°. The *nasomental angle* (Nme) is formed by the line tangent to the nasal dorsum and the line connecting the tip-defining point to the pogonion (Fig. 3.**9**). Its esthetic range is 120–132°. The *nasolabial angle* (Nla) is defined by the line from the subnasale to the superior vermillion border and the columellar tangent from the subnasale (Fig. 3.**10**). It ideally is between 90° and 100° in males and 100° and 110° in females. The facial plane and the line connecting the cervical point to the menton (Latin *menton*, chin) define the *mentocervical angle* (Mce). It ideally lies between 80° and 95° (Fig. 3.**11**).

Use of the five facial angles collectively was outlined by Powell and Humphries and is known as the Esthetic Triangle (5). Incorporation of the individual facial geometric relations into this single construct allows for simultaneous evaluation of facial proportions and emphasizes the interdependence of the facial elements (Fig. 3.**12**).

The Face

The Ancient Greeks taught that the ideal human head is one eighth the height of the body and twice the length of the neck, as measured from the sternal notch to the chin and from the chin to the vertex (6). The face can be divided into horizontal thirds (Fig. 3.**13**) on frontal inspection. The superior third is the forehead from the trichion (Greek *trich-*, hair) to the glabella. The middle third, or midface, extends from the glabella to the subnasale, and the inferior third, or lower face, is the region from the subnasale to the menton. These divisions are less ap-

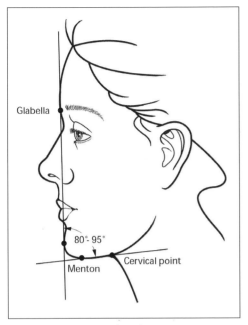

Fig. 3.**11**   Mentocervical angle

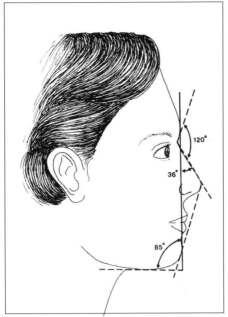

Fig. 3.**12**   Esthetic triangle (Powell and Humphreys)

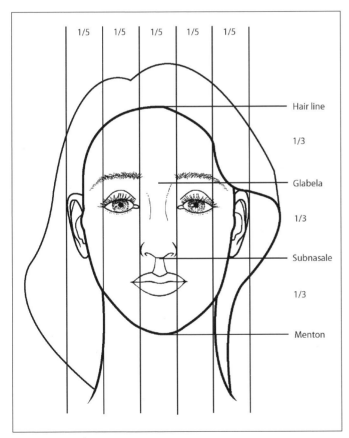

Fig. 3.**13**   Facial proportions

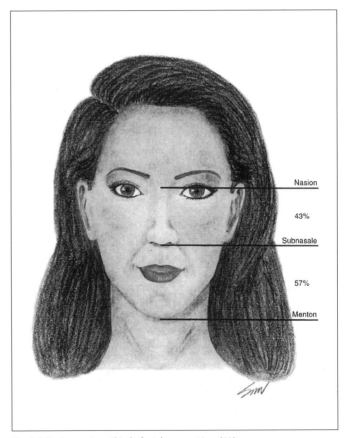

Fig. 3.**14**   Lower two thirds facial proportion (19)

plicable if the trichion is high, as in male pattern baldness, or unusually low. In such instances, division of the lower two thirds of the face liberates facial analysis from the position of the hairline (Fig. 3.**14**). The superior landmark becomes the nasion, the middle point the subnasale, and the lowest the menton. Using this method, the upper division (n–sn) is ideally three fourths the height of the lower division (sn–me).

The face also can be divided vertically into equal fifths. The width of one eye should equal the intercanthal distance, and this width should equal one fifth the facial width. Lines dropped from the outer canthi should approximate the width of the neck. The lateral fifths of the face extend from the lateral canthi to the furthest lateral points of the pinnae (Fig. 3.**13**).

The Forehead

Division of the face into its constituent anatomical features yields the esthetic units.

The forehead is the prominent region of the face located superior to the brows and inferior to the hairline. It ideally comprises the upper third of the face and has a gentle sloping convexity. The glabella is the most anterior point of the forehead and is located at the nose–forehead transition, just superior to where the paired nasal bones about the frontal bone. As with nearly all facial units, the forehead and nose maintain an esthetic interdependence. Differing contours of the forehead influence nasal appearance by either accentuating the nasal profile, as in the case of a retrusive forehead, or diminishing it with a protrusive forehead.

The Brow

Part of the frontal bone, the brow is the supraorbital bony prominence that separates the upper and middle thirds of the face and serves as the face's prime horizontal buttress. Just anterior to the frontal sinuses, the brow serves to protect the orbits and cranial vault from the forces of blunt trauma. It is accentuated by the presence of eyebrows, two paramedian strips of hair-bearing skin. The eyebrows ideally begin 1 cm above the medial canthus, directly superior to the lateral aspect of the ala nasi. In females, the eyebrows should have an arched shape peaking above the supraorbital rim at the level of the lateral limbus. Males should have less of an arched shape with the eyebrows located at the level of the supraorbital rim. The eyebrow terminus should occur laterally at an oblique line that passes from the lateral aspect of the ala nasi through the lateral canthus.

Eyes

Inferior to the brow lay the eyes. With variegated color and size, the eyes are perhaps the most individualized part of the human face. They are frequently described as the seat of human expression; however, the intrinsic muscles of the pupil and iris are under involuntary autonomic control, incapable of commanding outward affect. A simple series of expressions performed in the mirror quickly reveals that emotion is conveyed, in fact, by the muscles surrounding the eyes. Aging is also conveyed by the appearance of the eyes' surrounding skin and soft tissues. Blepharochalasis and blepharoptosis project a worn look, often incongruous with the actual state of the patient's physical and mental health.

The distance from the medial to lateral canthus is the width of the eye. In the well-proportioned face, this distance equals one fifth the facial width as well as the intercanthal distance. This distance should equal one half the interpupillary distance, which ideally is the distance from the nasion to the vermillion border of the upper lip.

The structure of the ideal orbit has the supraorbital rim projecting anterior to the infraorbital rim with the head in the Frankfurt plane. The lateral canthus is located slightly superior to the medial canthus, and it's attachment is posterior to the medial canthal attachment. Eyelids cover the eyes, and their edges of opposition are lined by a row of protective eyelashes. The distance from the lash line to the supratarsal crease in the upper eyelid varies from 7–15 mm, depending mostly on skin thickness and ethnicity. The upper eyelid normally covers a portion of the iris (but not the pupil), whereas the lower eyelid lies within 1–2 mm of the iris.

Cheeks

The cheeks are rounded soft-tissue regions lateral to the nose and inferolateral to the eyes. Bounded by the preauricular region, the infraorbital rim, the nasojugal groove, the nasolabial fold, and the melolabial fold, their projection to the facial plane is caused by the prominent malar eminence underlying facial musculature, fat, and thick skin. Aging causes a loss of fat in the cheeks, frequently with a sunken midfacial appearance. Concomitant inferior migration of the remaining cheek soft tissue toward the mandible and the appearance of the jowl occur. Malnutrition also can cause a hollowed appearance of the cheeks. Maxillary hypoplasia or trauma can cause flattened, retrusive cheeks whose projection is located posterior to the facial plane.

Ears

The ears are a pair of ovoid cartilaginous appendages on the lateral aspect of the face with a complex yet consistent geometry. Part of the hearing organ, the auricles collect and localize sound with resonance in the vicinity of 4500 Hz (7). To do this effectively, the ear prescribes an auriculocephalic angle of roughly 15–20°. Ear length should equal the distance between the orbital rim and the root of the helix. Ear width is roughly 55 % of its length. The dome of the ear should be located at the level of the lateral eyebrow margin. The long axis of the ear should parallel the nasal dorsum, or 20–25° off vertical.

Lips

The lips are the only vertically paired esthetic unit of the face. Fullness of the lips with a pronounced vermillion border and strong philtrum define a provocative and youthful appearance. Ideal lip length occurs when the oral commissures are located at a vertical dropped from the medial limbus. Lip posture can be referred to as procumbent or recumbent and is largely dependent on the underlying dentition. On profile, lip posture can be analyzed by drawing a line from the subnasale to the pogonion. The distance along a perpendicular from this line to the most anterior point of each lip defines its position. The upper lip should rest 3.5 mm anterior to this line and the lower lip 2.2 mm (8).

Chin

The chin is one of the most overlooked facial esthetic units, and failure to properly evaluate the nasal–chin relationship is a common error in assessment of the rhinoplasty patient. Chin deformities occur in multiple varieties, including chin asymmetry or any combination of horizontal micro-/macrogenia and vertical micro-/macrogenia. The ideal chin is proportionate in both the vertical and horizontal dimensions and should fit harmoniously with the remaining units of the face. A properly positioned pogonion with a labiomental sulcus of 3–4 mm in depth is important for maintaining proper balance of the lower facial third with the remainder of the face. Several methods of chin analysis have been devised, but none is universally accepted (8, 9, 10, 11). Most of these address the projection of the chin in the horizontal dimension, but ignore the vertical dimension. Retrognathia and prognathia are terms

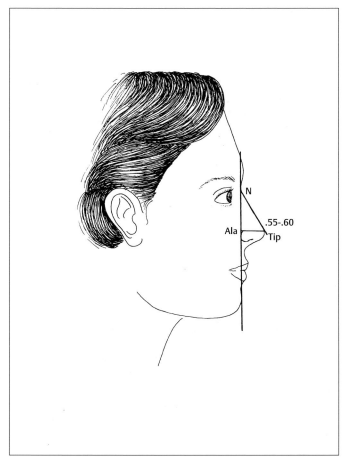

Fig. 3.**15**   Goode's ratio for nasal projection (19)

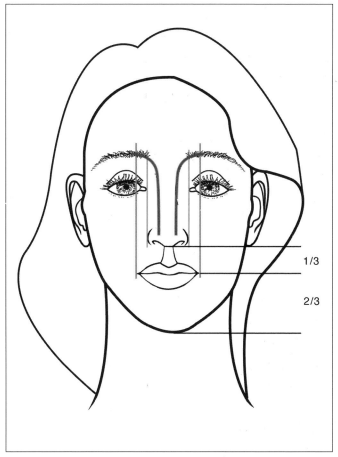

Fig. 3.**16**   Radix contours

that describe the position of the mandible, not the mentum. In these instances, orthognathic surgery, not mentoplasty, may be required depending on the patient's occlusion.

Dentition

Although not traditionally considered an esthetic unit, dentition is of significant esthetic importance. It should be examined as any other facial esthetic subunit. Dental deformities include various eruption asymmetries and imperfections, increased gingival show, and occlusal disturbances originally described by Angle (12). All of these will hinder the appearance of the rhinoplasty patient.

The Nose

Of all the facial esthetic units, the nose plays perhaps the most critical role in proportion and facial harmony. A single, unpaired anatomical unit occupying the central face, it serves to balance the facial thirds and fifths as well as those structures surrounding it. Seemingly small changes to the nose can affect dramatic changes in facial appearance and the other esthetic units. The nose has been divided into subunits, which helps with surgical planning and description of both cosmetic and reconstructive procedures. These units include the dorsum, sidewalls, tip, alae, columella, and soft-tissue triangles. The subunits' borders define natural demarcations and shadows that allow for the placement of incisions or scars, less easily seen on inspection.

The nose projects anteriorly from the face, and this forward thrust is ideally orthogonal to the facial plane and parallel to the midsagittal plane. Quantifying nasal projection is a critical component of rhinoplastic evaluation and several methods have evolved. The simplest method, described by Simons, defines projection as the distance from the subnasale to the tip-defining point and postulates that it should equal the length of the upper lip (13). Baum described a method based upon a line connecting the vertices of the nasolabial and nasofacial angles, and a second perpendicular line to the nasal tip (14). He suggests ideal projection occurs when the former line has a 2:1 ratio to the latter. Powell modified the Baum method and using the same parameters suggested the ideal ratio of nasal height to projection was 2.8:1 (7). Alternatively; Goode's method measures the distance from the alar crease to the tip-defining point as projection, and relates this to dorsal length. Using this method, ideal projection is between 0.55 and 0.6 of the dorsal length (Fig. 3.**15**). He found that when the ratio of projection to height to length was 3:4:5, the nasofacial angle is an ideal 36° (15). Crumley found the most consistent method of determining tip projection related a line from the nasion to the vermilion border to a perpendicular line to the nasal tip. Ideal projection is formed when projection is 0.2833 of the facial height (18).

On frontal view, the nasal dorsum should follow a gentle curve from the medial brow to the ipsilateral tip-defining point. Any irregularities in this contour will quickly be noted as different from the contralateral side, thereby contributing to asymmetry and an unsightly appearance (Fig. 3.**16**). Nasal

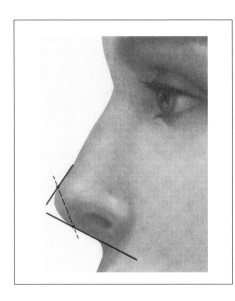

Fig. 3.**17**   Nasal profile (19)

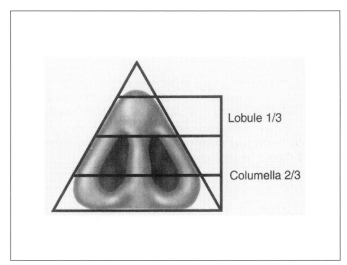

Fig. 3.**18**   Nasal base proportions (19)

width varies along its length, and is widest at the base and narrowest at the nasion. Perpendicular lines dropped from the medial canthi describe the ideal nasal base width and the width at the nasion is approximately the height of the palpebral fissure. In addition, frontal view should reveal the paired tip-defining points and a gull-wing appearance of the alae blending with the columella.

On lateral view, the dorsum should be straight and lie at or slightly posterior to a line connecting the nasion to the tip. The nasal ala to tip lobule ratio should be nearly equal. The ideal tip has a double break where the infratip lobule descends into the columella, and there should be 2–3 mm of columellar show (Fig. 3.17).

The view from the nasal base should resemble an isosceles triangle with the infratip lobule comprising one third and the columella and nostrils two thirds. The nostrils should be symmetrical, pear-shaped and with a long-axis orientation at 45° with respect to the columella. Each nostril should approximate the width of the columella. The columella is narrowest at its midportion, flaring anteriorly to meet the infratip lobule and posteriorly as the medial crural feet of the lower lateral cartilages splay apart (Fig. 3.18).

> **"A great nose indicates a great man—
> genial, courteous, intellectual,
> virile, courageous."**
> **Edmond Rostand (1868–1918)**

Analysis of Patients with a Nasal Deformity

As the keystone feature of the human visage, slight changes in the nose can produce dramatic improvements in facial harmony and the perception of the surrounding esthetic units (5). Critical to the success of any rhinoplasty, therefore, is a thorough preoperative facial analysis and nasal examination, performed by a surgeon with a precise understanding of nasal anatomy and a clear vision of the desired outcome.

General Considerations

Like all medical encounters, the initial assessment begins with the history. The facial plastic surgeon should elicit the chief concern and motives that bring the patient to the office, as well as expectations of the visit. Past medical history should identify high-risk patients with disorders that could confound anesthesia (e.g., family history of malignant hyperthermia) or nasal surgery (e.g., coagulopathy, progeria). Medications, allergies, and social habits (e.g., alcohol or tobacco abuse) should also be elicited. By the conclusion of the interview, the surgeon should also be able to comment on the patient's personality traits (e.g., narcissistic).

While the patient–doctor relationship is being established, initial assessment of the facial skin, subcutaneous tissue, and underlying facial skeleton should occur. Rhinoplasty has been described as the redraping of skin and soft tissue over an underlying bony–cartilaginous framework, and making note of these features is critical. Skin thickness, Fitzpatrick's sun-reactive skin type, the presence of nevi, rhytids, scars, or other lesions should be noted. Facial fat distribution, particularly regions of excess or atrophy, should also be noted. The surgeon should assess facial musculature for atrophy (e.g., temporal wasting in anorexia nervosa) or other abnormalities (e.g., depressor septi nasi, type I) (16). Additionally, the surgeon should document bone structure and the presence of any craniofacial deformities or asymmetries (e.g., hemifacial microsomia). All of these features can be determined during the interview simply by observation of the patient's static and dynamic visage.

The next step in examination of the patient with nasal deformity should be anterior rhinoscopy and nasal endoscopy to fully determine the status of the nasal valves, septum, and turbinates. Palpation is also critical to determine the degree of tip support, underlying dorsal irregularities, and skin thickness. A comprehensive head and neck exam should always accompany a directed evaluation of facial proportions and esthetic units, as should standard six-view nasal photodocumentation (17).

Nasal Deformity

The nose is a multipurpose organ whose functions include respiration, olfaction, immune defense, and cosmesis. Although nasal pathology can result in defects involving any of these functions, septorhinoplasty usually only corrects anatomical deformities causing any combination of nasal airway obstruction, hyposmia, and patients unhappy with their appearance. The chart below lists many of the deformities the rhinoplastic surgeon should be familiar with.

Nasal Deformities
- Congenital
  - Dermoids, encephaloceles, gliomas
  - Hemangiomata
  - Craniofacial nasal anomalies, e.g., cleft deformity, hemifacial microsomia, arhinia, proboscis lateralis
- Acquired
  - Nasal trauma, e.g., lacerations, septal hematoma, fractured nose, traumatic rhinectomy
  - Dorsal hump
  - Twisted nose
  - Asymmetrical nares
  - Nare stenosis
  - Overprojection
  - Underprojection
  - Overrotation
  - Underrotation
  - Wide nasal base
  - Excessive columellar show ("hanging columella")
  - Columellar insufficiency ("hiding columella")
  - Septal deviation
  - Saddle nose
  - Septal perforation
  - Paradoxical lower lateral cartilages, e.g., convex domes, double dome break
  - Tension Nose
  - Iatrogenic imperfections, e.g., bossae, alar retraction, polly beak, retrousse supratip, open roof, bony pyramid irregularity, inverted V deformity, visible grafts, alar scars
  - Moh's defects
  - Rhinophyma
  - Rhinoscleroma

**"Cleopatra's nose, had it been shorter,
The whole face of the world would have been changed."
Blaise Pascal (1623–1662)**

Ethnic Variations

In the modern age of rhinoplasty, it is important that the rhinoplastic surgeon understand the characteristic features of the ethnic nose as well as the motivations and desires of those patients belonging to various ethnic groups. Surgeons should strive to respect ethnic nasal variation and realize that patients typically wish to refine their nasal appearance, yet preserve their ethnic features. This respect serves to maintain facial harmony among the esthetic units and tends to achieve a natural, unoperated look.

The Caucasian Nose

The Caucasian, or *leptorrhine* (‚tall and thin'), nose is associated with patients of Euro-American descent. For purposes of this discussion, it provides the basis for nasal analysis and comparison. The typical features of the ideal leptorrhine nose have been outlined above (Fig. 3.**19**).

The African Nose

The *platyrrhine* nose (‚broad and flat') is associated with patients of African descent. It is typically characterized by a low radix, a short concave dorsum, an illusory widened intercanthal distance, a bulbous and underprojected tip, flared alae with round nostrils, and extremely thick skin. The nasofrontal angle is frequently as large as 130–140°. Hyperpigmentation or hypopigmentation and hypertrophic scarring or keloids can occur as a result of rhinoplasty in these patients. As a result of racial intermingling, subclassifications of the platyrrhine nose have been described (18). In contrast to the African type, the Afro-Caucasian nose typically has a longer and more prominent dorsum, an occasional dorsal hump, modest alar flaring, and a more refined tip. A prominent dorsum, a bulbous tip, wide alae, and an occasional dorsal hump describe the Afro-Indian nose (Fig. 3.**20**).

The Asian Nose

The *mesorrhine* nose (‚intermediate') is characterized as sharing features common to both the Caucasian nose and the African nose. Examination of an Asian patient will typically reveal a nose with moderately thick skin, a low broad dorsum, short nasal bones, a rounded underprojected and underrotated tip, columellar recession, and somewhat rounded nostrils. A short columella is typical, causing the major axis of the nostrils to be oriented at a more acute angle with respect to the facial plane when viewed from the base (Fig. 3.**21**).

Ethnic variation is challenging to rhinoplastic surgeons. Improving form and function while preserving ethnicity requires thorough preoperative analysis, an understanding of the patient's desires, and facility with the various techniques of rhinoplasty. As races continue to intermingle, strict classifications will be less meaningful, and as with any rhinoplastic procedure, the surgery must be individualized.

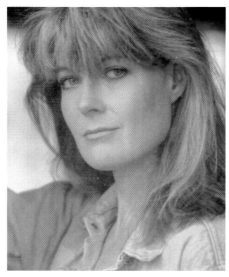

Fig. 3.**19**   Caucasian characteristics *

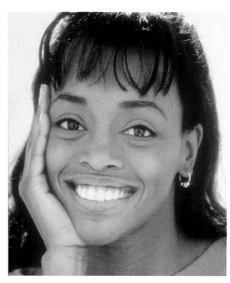

Fig. 3.**20**   African-American characteristics *

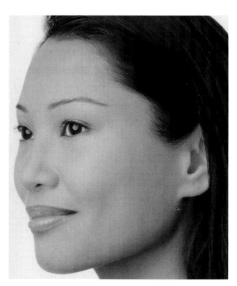

Fig. 3.**21**   Asian characteristics *

Summary

Modern facial analysis is vital to the success of any facial plastic surgery procedure, especially rhinoplasty. It serves to define qualitative standards for facial beauty while providing a framework within which to quantify operative results, thereby providing a basis for comparison between surgeons, and improving the consistency of nasal surgery results. Modern facial analysis also aids communication between the patient and surgeon, which leads to more realistic expectations. With meticulous examination, the surgeon who encounters the patient with nasal deformity or a displeasing anatomical variation will be able to offer the correct rhinoplasty procedure, and hopefully restore or create that complex interplay of outward appearance and perception that is called beauty.

Thanks to Dr. Edward Riggio for his assistance with etymology.

* Photos courtesy of The Face Book published by the American Academy of Facial Plastic and Reconstructive Surgery.

References

1. Spoor F. *Nature.* 1996;16 May.
2. Romm S. *The changing face of beauty.* St. Louis: Mosby-Year Book: 1992.
3. Ridley MB, VanHook SM. Aesthetic facial proportions. In Papel ID, ed. *Facial plastic and reconstructive surgery.* New York-Stuttgart: Thieme: 2002:96–109.
4. Livio M. *The golden ratio.* New York: Broadway Books: 2002.
5. Powell N, Humphries B. *Proportions of the aesthetic face.* New York: Thieme-Stratton: 1984.
6. Seghers MJ, Longacre JJ, de Stefano GA. The golden proportion and beauty. *Plast Reconstr Surg.* 1964; 34:382.
7. Stach BA. *Clinical audiology.* San Diego: Singular: 1998.
8. Burstone CJ. Lip posture and its significance in treatment planning. *Am J Orthod.* 1967; 53:262.
9. Steiner CC. Cephalometrics as a clinical tool. In Kraus BS, Reidel RA, eds. *Vistas in orthodontics.* Philadelphia: Lea & Febiger: 1962.
10. Rickets RM. Divine proportion in facial esthetics. *Clin Plast Surg.* 1982; 9:401.
11. Gonazles-Ulloa M, Stevens E. The role of chin correction in profile plasty. *Plast Reconstr Surg.* 1968; 41:477.
12. Angle EH. Classification of malocclusion. *Dent Cosmos.* 1899; 41:248.
13. Simons R. Nasal tip projection, ptosis, and supratip thickening. *Ear Nose Throat J.* 1982; 61:452.
14. Baum S. Introduction. *Ear Nose Throat J* 1982; 61:426.
15. Crumley R. Quantitative analysis of nasal tip projection. *Laryngoscope.* 1988; 98:202.
16. Rohrich RJ, Huynh B, et al. Importance of the depressor septi nasi muscle in rhinoplasty: anatomic study and clinical application. *Plast Reconstr Surg.* 2000; 105(1):376–383.
17. Kontis TC Photography in Facial Plastic Surgery. In Papel ID, ed. *Facial Plastic and Reconstructive Surgery.* New York-Stuttgart: Thieme: 2002:116–124.
18. Ofodile FA, Bokhari FJ, Ellis C. The Black American nose. *Ann Plast Surg.* 1993; 31:209–218.
19. Papel ID, ed. Facial Plastic and Reconstructive Surgery. 2nd ed. New York-Stuttgart: Thieme: 2002

4 Physiology and Pathophysiology of Nasal Breathing

G. Mlynski

Contents

Introduction

The nose is not only the gateway between the airways and the environment. One of the main roles of the nose is its respiratory function. During inspiration, the air has to be tempered, humidified, and cleaned. These are important prerequisites for an undisturbed exchange of gas in the lungs. Alveolar air temperature should be of body temperature and 100 % humidity. Additionally, the air must be cleaned for protection of the lower airways.

The respiratory performance of the nose is an enormous commitment since, during breathing at rest, six liters of air per minute flow at a local speed of up to 20 m/s through it (1) and have to be conditioned and cleaned in the meantime.

In order to fulfil this task, the nose has a specific shape. Sufficient knowledge of the interaction between shape and function of the nose helps the rhinosurgeon to not only improve air passage of the nose, but also to maintain and reconstruct structures that are important for the respiratory function of the nose. On the basis of experiments on fluid dynamics (2, 3) we shall now review the structure of the nose from a functional point of view.

Preconditions for the Respiratory Function of the Nose

The most important precondition for nasal function is an undisturbed passage. High airway resistance consequently leads to mouth breathing and thus bypasses the nose. The reason for high airway resistance is a loss of energy due to friction of the streaming molecules with the wall and between each other. In a narrow section, molecules stream closer together and to the wall, thereby increasing the friction.

Another reason for high resistance is friction caused by turbulence. Turbulent streaming particles not only flow forward but sideways as well. Therefore, the molecules frequently hit each other and the wall, releasing kinetic energy. For that reason, strong turbulence provokes high airway resistance.

The resulting high nasal airway resistance can be caused by narrowness as well as a pathologically increased degree of turbulence. Both factors induce airway resistance to varying degrees.

The second precondition for the respiratory function is contact between the streaming particles and the mucosa. In laminar flow (i.e., all particles streaming parallel to the wall), only the particles flowing nearest to the wall have contact with the mucosa. More central streaming particles are neither warmed, nor humidified, nor cleaned. Not until sideways movement arises, as in turbulent flow, do particles close to the wall leave their place and give way to particles moving from the center toward the mucosa. On the other hand, high degrees of turbulence extract too much thermal energy and moisture of the mucosa, causing sicca symptoms. The nasal airflow, therefore, should neither be overly laminar nor intensely turbulent. A well-balanced turbulent behavior as a warrant for sufficient air–mucosa contact is a prerequisite for the respiratory function of the nose.

The mucous surface of the nose is especially enlarged by the turbinates, which provide effective exchange of thermal energy and humidity.

Surgical consequence: As little mucosa reduction as possible!

Contact between air and this large mucous surface is maintained by distribution of the inspired air over the entire cross section of the nasal cavum. Moreover, functional efficiency is increased by deceleration of local flow velocity at the nasal turbinates.

The third precondition is that the mucosa be supplied with thermal energy and fluid for humidification. These prerequisites are fulfilled by the blood circulation and are in coherence with the nasal cycle. The erectile tissue enables the turbinates to cyclicly swell. One side of the nose is in its working phase, with an unimpeded air passage and increased turbulence, conditioning the air. At the same time, the contralateral side, in its resting phase with high airway resistance and low turbulence, stores energy and moisture.

Surgical consequence: One main target of functional rhinosurgery is to create adequate space for the physiological congestion and decongestion of the turbinates during the nasal cycle.

The Correlation between Shape and Function of the Nose

In order to understand the correlation between shape and function of the nose, Bachmann assigned common structural elements with familiar effects on flow, known from the physics of fluid dynamics, to discrete sections of the nose. Bachmann's synopsis (4) can be enhanced by additional experiments on fluid dynamics (2, 3) (Fig. 4.**1**).

The actual functional area of the nose is its center, which contains the largest mucosal surface. There the nose serves its respiratory function.

Inspiration

The nasal vestibule, the internal ostium (isthmus nasi) and the anterior cavum are upstream of the functional area (Fig. 4.**1 a**). This part is termed the inflow area. The posterior cavum, including the choana and the nasopharynx, is located downstream of the functional area. This part is named the outflow area.

The *nasal vestibule* has the shape of a bend with a decrease in cross-sectional area like a nozzle (Fig. 4.**1 a**). The first effect is to direct the lateral and bottom-up approach of air toward the functional area of the nose (Fig. 4.**2 a**). Therefore, the correct bearing of the vestibule to the cavum is of great importance. This is the case if the angle between nose and lip is 90–100°. A downward rotated vestibule (nasolabial angle < 90°) directs inspired air toward the upper cavum (Fig. 4.**2 b**). The lower turbinate has no contact with the air and thus is not available for respiratory function. An oversized nasolabial angle (> 100°) guides the air through the lower nose while not ventilating the upper parts (Fig. 4.**2 c**).

Surgical consequence: Preservation and reconstruction of a nasolabial angle between 90° and 100° should be aspired to in functional rhinosurgery.

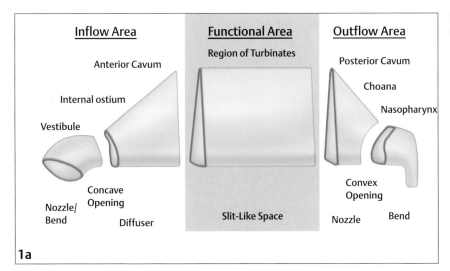

Fig. 4.**1** Structural elements of the nose. Inspiratory (**a**), and expiratory (**b**) flow direction.

Inflow Area   **Functional Area**   **Outflow Area**

Region of Turbinates

Anterior Cavum

Posterior Cavum

Internal ostium

Choana

Nasopharynx

Vestibule

Concave Opening

Convex Opening

Nozzle/ Bend

Diffuser

Slit-Like Space

Nozzle   Bend

1a

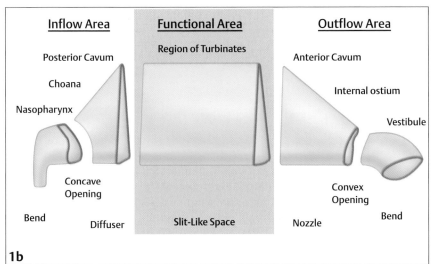

Inflow Area   **Functional Area**   **Outflow Area**

Region of Turbinates

Posterior Cavum

Anterior Cavum

Choana

Internal ostium

Nasopharynx

Vestibule

Concave Opening

Convex Opening

Bend

Diffuser   Slit-Like Space   Nozzle   Bend

1b

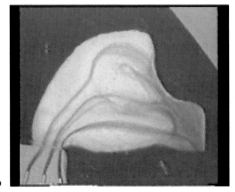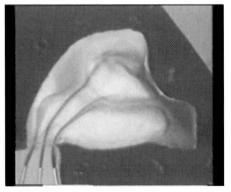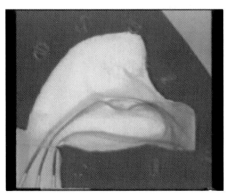

a, b   c

Fig. 4.**2** Airstream in nose model with normal (**a**), too small (**b**), and too large (**c**) nasolabial angle.

The constriction of the cross-sectional area from the outer to the inner ostium of the nose produces a nozzle effect in the vestibule (Fig. 4.**1 a**). The degree of turbulence is reduced in a nozzle. This effect is important because the inspired air has to pass through the narrowest part of the nose, the ostium internum, next. In this narrow sector, turbulent flow leads to very high flow resistance. Figure 4.**3** shows the flow in inspiratory direction in a nose model. Due to the forward movement of air molecules parallel to the wall during laminar flow, a sharp border between the flowing color particles and the flowing medium can be seen. During turbulence, additional sideward movements lead to a mixing of color and medium and thereby yield a diffuse coloring. In Figure 4.**3**, laminar flow in the narrowest part of the nose, the isthmus, is shown. In the region of turbinates flow is turbulent.

Expansion of the ostium internum reduces or suspends the nozzle effect of the vestibulum. Consequently, the flow entering the cavum nasi is turbulent ("ballooning phenomenon").

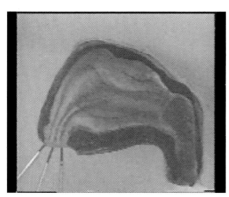

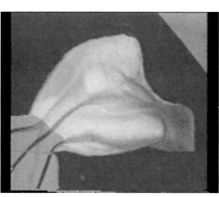

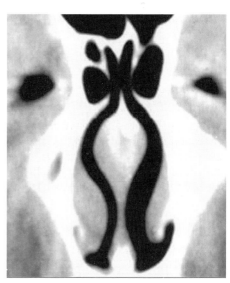

Fig. 4.3   Flow in the model of a nonpathological nose. Laminar flow in the vestibulum and inner ostium (sharp border between color and flowing medium) and turbulent flow in the region of turbinates (diffuse coloring due to mixture).

Fig. 4.4   Nose model without vestibule. Diverging flow lines in the cavum after perfusion of the concave internal ostium.

Fig. 4.5   CT scan through the end of the diffuser with the head of the inferior turbinate and the septum's erectile body as a regulating mechanism for the cross-sectional area expansion and, therefore, adjusting the turbulence behavior.

Surgical consequence: In surgery of the inner ostium the expansion must not be made too great.

In the inspiratory direction, the *internal ostium* is of a concave shape (5) (Fig. 4.1). As is known from fluid dynamics, the effect of a concave opening on flow course is the same as a concave lens acting on beams of light (2). Thus, a diverging of the flow lines within the functional area is achieved, which has a positive impact on flow distribution all over the cross-sectional area of the functional area. Figure 4.4 shows the flow in a nose model without a vestibule. The diverging flow lines after perfusion of the inner ostium can be seen.

Surgical consequence: Due to the fact that at its upper area the inner nostril is made of the caudal margin of the triangular cartilage, it is important to perform surgical procedures in the area of the inner nostril in such a way that when making resections at the caudal margin of the triangular cartilage the concave shape of the ostium internum is maintained.

As a result of the expansion of the cross-sectional area from the ostium internum to the beginning of the concha region, the *anterior cavum* is shaped and acts like a diffuser (Fig. 4.1 a). In a diffuser, the local flow velocity is reduced and turbulence arises. Both effects are important preconditions for sufficient mucous membrane contact with the flowing particles in the functional area. The slowing of the flow as well as the arising turbulence is dependent on the dimensions of cross-sectional area expansion in the diffuser. With growing expansion of the cross-sectional area, the degree of turbulence increases, while the local flow velocity decreases.

There is a mechanism in the nose to regulate such effects. The expansion of the cross-sectional area alters with the swelling of the septum's erectile body and the erectile head of the inferior turbinate (Fig. 4.5). When swelling is at a minimum (right side in Fig. 4.5), the expansion of the cross section is great. This corresponds to the working phases in the nasal cycle. The flowing air becomes increasingly turbulent while the local flow velocity decreases. These are the preconditions for the warming up, moistening, and cleaning of the air. During the resting phase the increase of the cross-sectional area diminishes due to the swelling of the septum's erectile body and the head of the inferior turbinate (left side in Fig. 4.5). The predominantly laminar flow allows the mucous membrane to accumulate thermal energy and moisture.

As a result of external nose deformations and septal deviations, the diffuser is often deformed. In such cases the diffuser cannot fulfill its turbulence-regulating function.

Surgical consequence: One task of functional rhinosurgery is the reconstruction and/or maintenance of the diffuser. The important structures regulating turbulences (head of the inferior turbinate, septum's erectile body) must be preserved.

In terms of flow physics, the *region of turbinates* is a slitlike space that increases mucous membrane surface area. A slitlike space is important in order to keep the flow path of particles close to the mucous membrane. An important precondition for the flow distribution over the entire cross-sectional area is a constant slitlike space. If partial or total resection of the turbinates in a small section is done, then a wider space is created. The flow yields to the narrow portion of the cavum and instead flows exclusively through this wide portion following the principle of least resistance (compare Figs. 4.3 and 4.6). This induces a decrease in the respiratory function of the nose because in the area of the healthy respiratory mucous membrane there is hardly any flow left.

Surgical consequence: In functional rhinosurgery large volumes should not be formed but instead a continuous slitlike space ought to be created.

Due to a decrease in cross-sectional area, the *posterior cavum* works like a nozzle (Fig. 4.1 a). A similar function exists in the vestibule and turbulence is thus decreased here also. This is important since now the air must perfuse the bronchial and alveolar pathway with the least flow resistance possible.

In the inspiratory direction the *choana* is a convex opening (Fig. 4.1 a). A convex opening leads to converging streamlines. This constricts the air streamline and prepares it for the following more narrow breathing pathway.

The *nasopharynx* is an almost rectangular bend (Fig. 4.**1 a**) which redirects the air flowing out of the nose to the lower breathing pathways.

Expiration

In order to keep enough thermal energy and moisture available for the respiratory function of the nose it is important that the nasal mucous membrane regains energy and moisture from the airflow, which is 37 °C and has 100% humidity on expiration. Lacking this process of regaining energy, the nose could keep up its respiratory function only over a short time period. Accordingly, sufficient contact between airstream and mucous membrane is necessary during expiration as well.

In the expiratory direction (Fig. 4.**1 b**), the posterior portion of the nose with the choana and the nasopharynx becomes the inflow area. It is equipped with similarly shaped functional elements as the inflow area in the inspiratory direction.

Due to its bending effect, the *nasopharynx* redirects the air emerging from the lower airways to the functional area. A nozzle effect is not required, since there is no constriction in the expiratory inflow area.

In this direction, the *choana* is a concave opening, which promotes diverging of streamlines.

With its increase in cross-sectional area, the *posterior cavum* has a diffuser effect and therefore leads to a slowdown in flow velocity and increases turbulence. With this, mucous membrane contact of the flowing particles is ensured.

The actual exchange of energy and moisture takes place in the *area of turbinates*, but now in the direction from the air to the mucous membrane.

For the expiration flow, the *anterior cavum* becomes a nozzle, which leads to a decrease in turbulence. With it, laminar flow can perfuse the narrowest opening, the ostium internum.

In expiration direction, the *internal ostium* is of concave shape, which promotes the converging of streamlines. This reduces the broad airstream to the smaller size of the cross-sectional area of the vestibule.

The bending effect of the *vestibule* causes the air to be blown out of the nose in a narrow beam in a lateral downward direction during expiration.

General Remarks

The shape of the nose is almost completely symmetrical (Fig. 4.**1**). Upstream of the functional area is an inflow area consisting of a bend, a concave opening, and a diffuser in each flow direction. Downstream is an outflow area with a nozzle, a convex opening, and a bend. As a result, during expiration the inspiratory inflow area can function as an outflow area, just as the inspiratory outflow area can take over the function of the expiratory inflow area.

The inspiratory inflow area is situated within the external nose. Thus, deformities of the external nose may lead to an altered shape of the inspiratory inflow area. Thereby an increased resistance, an impaired distribution of the airstream over the cross-sectional area of the cavum, and pathological turbulence behavior result. In many cases, this explains the frequent impairment of respiratory function due to deformi-

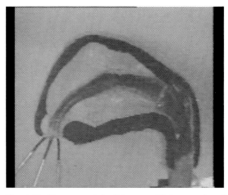

Fig. 4.**6**   Nose model without middle concha. Flow only in area of the considerably expanded middle nasal duct.

ties of the external nose, although the functional region is configured normally.

Surgical consequence: In external nose surgery, the inspiratory inflow area is to be preserved and/or reconstructed.

The Problem of Septal Deviation with Compensatory Turbinate Hyperplasia in Terms of Flow Dynamics

Nature is able to fit turbinates into almost any form of septal deviation that exists. This causes hyperplastic turbinates on the concave side of the deviation and hypoplastic turbinates on the convex side of the deviation. Given these properties, nature attempts to establish a continuous slitlike space with a constant width (Fig. 4.**7**). In functional terms, the hindrance of the hypoplastic turbinate within the nasal cycle is apparent. This side of the nose cannot take over a working phase. Thus, there is no resting phase for the opposite side.

The flow dynamics become evident in flow experiments done using functional models in the shape of small boxes (Fig. 4.**8**). One notes that on the side constricted by deviation, the streamlines are being considerably pushed together (Fig. 4.**8 a**). This explains the increased resistance due to increased friction on the deviated side.

Many patients complain about obstruction on the opposite side as well. The flow experiment shows that on the opposite wide side there is no diverging of streamlines. The part of the area being perfused is relatively narrow. Laterally from here, a so-called dead-water area arises, in which a slow creep-flow turns retrograde. In this area, particles carried with the flow are deposited at the lateral wall. This causes crust formation in significantly expanded areas in the nose.

The simulation of a compensatory turbinate hyperplasia demonstrates that the turbinate fills out the dead-water area and thereby eliminates the problem (Fig. 4.**8 b**).

Computed tomography (CT) scans prove that, due to asymmetries, a straight septum would lead to two very unequal nasal sides (Fig. 4.**9**). The turbinates on the deviated side would have to be considerably augmented in size to meet its compensatory purpose. In the opposite side the turbinate would have

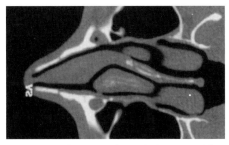

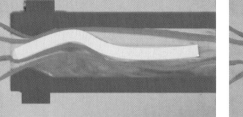

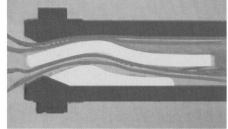

b

Fig. 4.**7**   Axial CT scan through the nose with septum deviation and compensatory hyperplasia/hypoplasia of the turbinates.

Fig. 4.**8**   Box model with septum deviation (**a**) and additional compensatory concha (**b**).

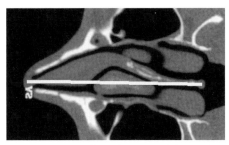

Fig. 4.**9**   CT scan through a nose with septal deviation. The line illustrates the position of a straight septum.

to be significantly reduced in size. Here, a decrease and increase in swelling within the nasal cycle would not be sufficiently possible.

Surgical consequence: The objective of septum surgery should not be a straight septum. The septum should rather be located in the middle of the space between the two lateral nasal walls. (Only in the area of the external nose should the septum be straight as the basis for a straight external nose.)

Inspiratory Nasal Wing Collapse

So far, we have considered the nasal breathing tube as being rigid. In fact, the soft parts in a healthy nasal cavum are not deformed by the airflow during breathing. The alterations in pressure during the breathing process are too small. The polyposis mucous membrane can change its position as a result of the airflow and thereby produce a change in resistance.

The vestibulum must not be seen as a rigid structure. The lateral wall of the anterior part of the inflow area is elastically deformable.

Elastic plasticity means a change in form by an external force, which returns to the original state when the external force decreases. With inspiratory nasal wing collapse, such forces may be explained by means of Bernoulli's law: The sum of static and dynamic pressure is constant. That means that with increasing dynamic pressure due to increasing flow velocity the static pressure decreases. Thus, the pressure in the vestibulum during deep inspiration is so low that the atmospheric pressure outside the nose predominates. If the negative static pressure within the vestibulum exceeds the elastic forces of the mobile lateral wall of the vestibule, the nasal wing collapses.

The nasal wing collapse during high inspiratory breathing velocity is physiologically important because it prevents very high perfusion of the nose and with this it protects the mucous membrane. At a decreased level of elastic forces on the lateral wall of the vestibule as well as increased local flow velocity in the vestibule, due to constriction of the stream course, an inspiratory nasal wing collapse at physiological breathing velocities can be observed.

Surgical consequence: In such cases, either the elasticity of the lateral wall of the vestibulum must be increased or the local flow velocity must be decreased by expanding the flow course.

Rhinological Functional Diagnostics

Unfortunately, insufficient scientific attention has been devoted to rhinological functional diagnostics so far. No method is yet clinically and routinely available for measuring the warming up, moistening, and cleaning of the inspired air in the nose.

The rhinomanometric assessment of the nasal airflow is an important condition for objectifying nasal obstructions. This method does not allow any essential assessment beyond these measurements. Therefore this technique has not been used much to indicate and plan procedures in functional rhinosurgery. Additionally, since the introduction of the method only little has been done to develop it further.

There follows an overview of currently available methods of diagnostics for the respiratory functions of the nose.

Rhinomanometry

In rhinomanometry, the nasal airflow as well as the transnasal loss of pressure during respiration are measured. The transnasal loss of pressure results from the difference between prenasal and postnasal pressure. Two methods for measuring the postnasal pressure are known. During "anterior rhinomanometry" (Fig. 4.**10 a**) the pressure tube is fixed hermetically at the ostium externum on the side opposite to the side of the nose which has to be measured. Thus, this side of the nose acts as a lengthening of the pressure tube up to the choana. It is not possible to do anterior rhinomanometry while the used side of the nose is being totally obstructed or while the patient has a septal perforation. In such cases we recommend the use

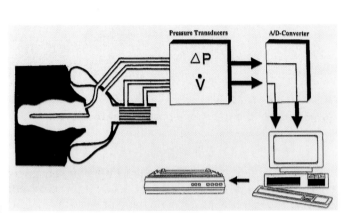
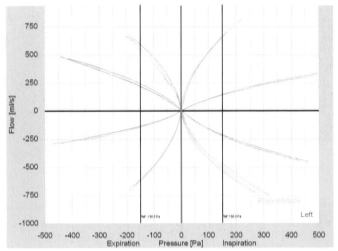

a

b

Fig. 4.**10** Block diagram "anterior rhinomanometry" (**a**) and mirror image x–y description of the measurement curves for both sides of the nose (**b**).

of "posterior rhinomanometry." In this instance, the pressure tube is located in the mouth, tightly enclosed by the lips. The cavum oris serves as the backward elongation of the pressure tube so that the oropharyngeal pressure can be measured. This shows that posterior rhinomanometry does not only measure the transnasal loss of pressure, but the epipharyngeal pressure loss as well. Since the position of the soft palate has a significant influence on flow resistance in this area, the method for evaluating the nasal obstruction is often likely to produce false results.

The Standardization Committee on Objective Assessment of the Nasal Airway (6) recommends registering the measured data in a coordinate system (Fig. 4.**10 b**). Pressure data is assigned to the x-axis and flow data to the y-axis. Pressure–flow curves for the right and left side of the nose are shown as mirror images, with the inspiration of the right side of the nose running in the upper right quadrant, and the inspiration of the left side of the nose running in the lower right quadrant. Accordingly, the expiration phases for the right side of the nose are in the lower left quadrant, while phases for the left side of the nose are in the upper left quadrant.

An inspiratory flow of 150 Pa is used for the evaluation. Most of the available rhinomanometers nowadays offer the option of computer-aided data processing. They calculate the corresponding flow and resistance data at pressure levels of 75, 150, and 300 Pa for each side of the nose as well as for both sides together.

In rhinomanometry an objective method for measuring the nasal airflow has been used to assess the dimensions of nasal obstruction. It is not possible to evaluate the causes of nasal obstruction using this method. Due to the fact that the respiratory function of the nose is not only dependent on the dimensions of nasal airflow, the rhinomanometric measurements may result in a false assessment.

Rhinoresistometry

Rhinoresistometry is a further development of the rhinomanometry (7). In rhinoresistometry, the transnasal pressure difference and the breathing airflow are measured simul-

taneously to the breathing, just as in rhinomanometry. Based on the measured data, functionally important parameters for the nose are calculated on the basis of physical flow laws.

On the arithmetic chart (Fig. 4.**11**), the right side of the nose is marked in red and the left side of the nose blue. The lightly colored curves were previously measured and the brightly colored curves were measured after decongestion of the mucous membrane. The flow resistance, dependent on flow velocity (Fig. 4.**11**, upper curves), is graphically depicted in the inspiratory as well as the expiratory directions for the dimensions of a nasal obstruction can be seen at once. The continuously lined curves correspond to the extent of the patient's breathing during measurement. The dotted lines are extrapolated by the computer and represent the breathing curve during very deep breathing and a rigid lateral wall of the vestibule.

As a result of inspiratory suction of the lateral vestibulum wall, the measured resistance curve may take a steeper course during inspiration than that shown by the extrapolated curve (Fig. 4.**16**). The higher the loss of elasticity of the lateral vestibulum wall, the smaller the flow velocity at which the collapse begins to occur. The dimensions of the collapse can be seen by the dimensions of the diverging of the measured and the extrapolated curve.

The turbulence behavior of the nasal breathing airstream that is dependent on the flow is graphically depicted in Figure 4.**11** (lower curves). Only at very low breathing velocity is the flow completely laminar. The area of turbulent flow (blue–green bar) can be reached only at very high breathing velocities. This means that the normal nose works within the so-called transitional area between laminar and turbulent flow.

The hydraulic diameter is calculated as a measurement for the width of the nose. The friction coefficient λ must be determined as a characteristic value for the configuration of the wall relating to its effect on the triggering of turbulences.

In this way, causes for an increased resistance, a constriction, and/or an increased development of turbulences can be differentiated and assessed.

In a nonpathological nose (Fig. 4.**11**), after the mucous membrane swells down (corresponding to the working phase of the nasal cycle), the nasal breathing resistance at a flow of

Before Decongestion:

Resist. (at 250 cm³/s):	0.24	0.51	[sPa/cm³]
Hydr. diameter:	5.2	4.2	[mm]
Frict. coeffic. λ:	20	15	· 10⁻³

After Decongestion:

Resist. (at 250 cm³/s):	0.20	0.13	[sPa/cm³]
Hydr. diameter:	5.8	6.0	[mm]
Frict. coeffic. λ:	24	28	· 10⁻³

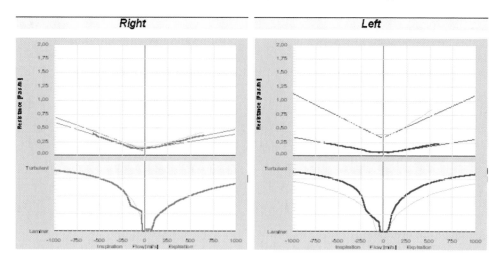

Fig. 4.**11** Rhinoresistometric findings of a nonpathological nose.

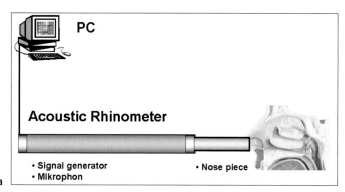
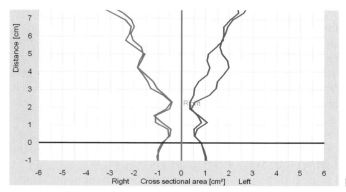

Fig. 4.**12** Acoustic rhinometry. Block diagram (**a**) and measurement curves (**b**) of a nonpathological nose.

250 cm³/s is < 0.3 sPa/cm³, the hydraulic diameter > 5 mm, and λ > 0.025. Purely turbulent flow may already occur at a flow < 750 cm³/s.

In the state of physiological swelling during the resting phase of the nasal cycle, the resistance becomes higher than 0.3 sPa/cm³, the hydraulic diameter < 5 mm, and λ > 0.025. Turbulent flow can be seen only at a flow velocity > 750 cm³/s.

Acoustic Rhinometry

The method for calculating the cross sections of the breathing path taken from pulmonology has now also become established in rhinological diagnostics (Fig. 4.**12**). It is based on the physical phenomenon of sound reflection. A sound wave is conducted into the nose and is reflected there. Amplitude and frequency change depending on the cross-sectional area of the nose. This method allows measurement of the cross-sectional

area in the nose (x-axis) in relation to its distance to the ostium externum (y-axis) in 0.3-cm increments.

The curves for the right (red) and the left (blue) side of the nose are shown as mirror images.

With wide access from the paranasal sinus into the cavum nasi, the measurement data of the cross-sectional area is falsely calculated as being too large (8, 9). Therefore, it is recommended that only the first 4–5 cm of the curve for assessment of the nasal cavum is used. Characteristic cross-sectional areas are to be found in the area of physiological constriction (minimal cross-sectional areas = MCA). They are described as MCA 1 (ostium internum) and MCA 2 (constriction by the head of the inferior turbinate and the erectile body of the septum). The volume of the nasal cavum can be calculated between any two borders.

The expanded cross-sectional area after MCA 1 explains the shape of the diffuser and consequently the arising turbulences (Fig. 4.**12 b**). Additionally, the length of the diffuser is

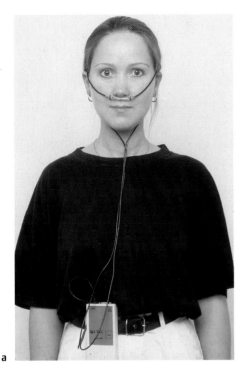

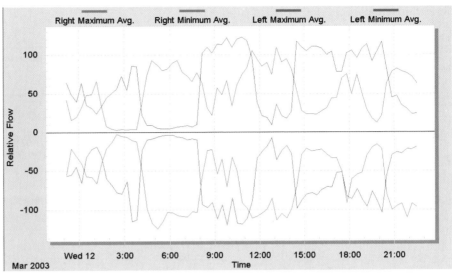

Fig. 4.**13**   Female patient with measuring device for long-term rhinoflowmetry (**a**) and long-term rhinoflowmetry measurement curve (**b**). A nasal increase and decrease in swelling in cyclic phases of three to five hours is considered normal.

a classification number for the dimensions of arising turbulences.

Therefore, this method can be applied to making a diagnosis concerning 'the dimension and location of a narrowness. The curve course after the MCA 1 up to the highest point after MCA 2 explains the shape of the diffuser and thereby the arising of turbulences (Fig . 4.**12 b**).

Long-Term Rhinoflowmetry

The rhinological measurement methods named thus far explain the state of the nose only at the moment of measuring. However, many patients complain at specific instances during the day or in certain situations. The aforementioned methods do not allow a complete assessment of the nasal cycle. This is the motivation for developing long-term rhinoflowmetry. This technique has made it possible to measure the airflow in each side of the nose separately over a period of time of up to three days using a portable, battery-powered device (Fig. 4.**13**). The method allows new insights into the functioning of the nose and disturbances of the nasal cycle and therefore leads to innovative indications for rhinosurgery.

Figure 4.**13** shows a female patient with a measuring device for long-term rhinoflowmetry (**a**) and long-term rhinoflowmetry measurement curve (**b**). A nasal increase and decrease in swelling in cyclic phases of three to five hours is considered normal.

Combination of Rhinoresistometry, Acoustic Rhinometry, and Long-Term Rhinoflowmetry

The combination of these three measuring methods allows a differentiated assessment of functional disturbances of the nose. This will be shown by means of diagnostics of nasal obstructions. In every case a rhinoresistometrical and acoustic rhinometrical measurement has to be performed. Long-term rhinoflowmetry is only used if there are appropriate complaints.

Nasal obstructions may be caused by constriction or by disturbed turbulence behavior. Rigid (septum deviation) and changeable (nasal wing collapse, changes in swelling) are distinguished. Figure 4.**14** schematically shows how these three measuring methods contribute to the assessment of the dimensions and to the cause of a nasal obstruction.

Firstly, the dimensions of the obstruction are rated by the rhinoresistometrically determined resistance. Secondly, the causes for the obstruction are proportionately depicted. The differentiation of the causes is an essential basis for planning surgical procedures.

A *permanent nasal obstruction* results in increased airway resistance even after decongestion. Acoustic rhinometry locates the position and extent of the narrowness. However, the extent of the narrowness does not necessarily correlate with the extent of flow resistance. The shape of the constriction additionally influences the extent in loss of energy. Different shapes of the same cross-sectional area can cause different flow resistance. Circular areas imply lower resistance than slit-like spaces. Therefore, the rhinoresistometrically measured hydraulic diameter should be considered for flow dynamic assessment of narrowness.

Pathological turbulence is assessed by a high reading of the friction coefficient and by interpreting the curve describing the

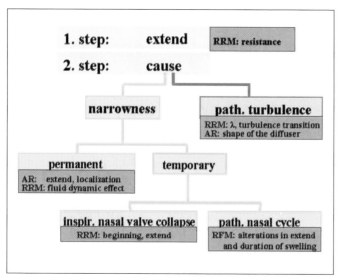

Fig. 4.**14** Schematic diagram of the diagnostics of a nasal obstruction through combination of rhinoresistometry (RRM), acoustic rhinometry (AR), and long-term rhinoflowmetry (RFM).

flow-dependent transition of laminar to turbulent flow. The acoustic rhinometry curve between MCA 1 and the highest point after MCA 2 serves to identify the cause of pathological turbulence onset.

Temporary obstruction due to impaired cyclic congestion and decongestion of the erectile tissue in both sides of the nose can be detected by long-term rhinoflowmetry.

Inspiratory nasal wing collapse is diagnosed using the rhinoresistometric resistance curve. The flow at which the measured curve separates from the extrapolated curve matches the onset of the nasal wing collapse. The degree of separation corresponds to the extent of collapse.

In the following, typical functional diagnostic findings for the different causes of nasal obstructions will be described. Often, there is not only one cause, but two or three causes that act as obstructions.

Case 1: Permanent Narrowness and Arising Turbulences

Figure 4.**15** shows the findings of a patient complaining of permanent nasal obstruction in the right side of the nose.

The resistance curves of the right side show a high-grade obstruction before decongestion and a middle-grade obstruction after decongestion. In acoustic rhinometry, a constriction of the anterior cavum is seen as the cause for this. Even after decongestion, the hydraulic diameter is still seen as the cause for considerable energy dissipation due to constriction. The λ value is high before decongestion and flow within the nose is pathologically turbulent. That in a swollen state the diffuser does not begin at MCA 1 is seen as the cause for this in acoustic rhinometry. The diffuser is deformed; its entry is shifted to the inside.

Apparently, the left side of the nose was in the working phase at the time the measurement was made. Therefore, only little change in resistance, change of the hydraulic diameter, change in the friction coefficient, and change in the turbulence behavior after decreased swelling was observed.

Long-term rhinoflowmetry shows that the left side of the nose has to take over the working phase almost continuously since, due to its constriction, the right side is not in the position to do so. Only during rest and at night, due to the reduced need for air, can the left side swell a little and have a resting phase.

These findings result in the indication for septum plastic with elimination of the narrowness and reconstruction of the right diffuser.

Before Decongestion:

Resist. (at 250 cm³/s):	2.26	0.37	[sPa/cm³]
Hydr. diameter:	3.7	4.2	[mm]
Frict. coeffic. λ:	48	29	· 10⁻³

After Decongestion:

Resist. (at 250 cm³/s):	0.42	0.19	[sPa/cm³]
Hydr. diameter:	4.5	5.0	[mm]
Frict. coeffic. λ:	18	30	· 10⁻³

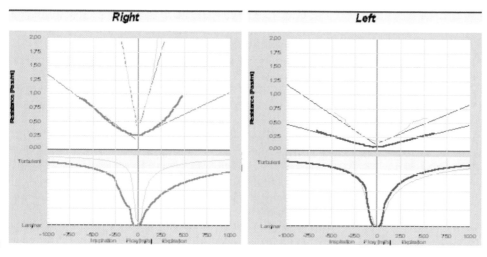

Fig. 4.**15** Rhinoresistometric (**a**), acoustic rhinometric (**b**), and long-term rhinoflowmetry results (**c**) of a patient with septal deviation to the right side.

a

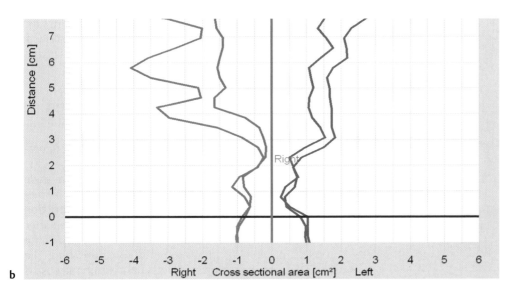

Fig. 4.**15 b** and **c**

b

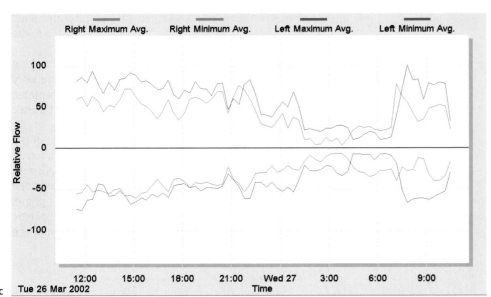

c   Tue 26 Mar 2002

Case 2: Temporary Stenosis Due to Inspiratory Nose Wing Collapse and Permanent Stenosis of the Isthmus with the Arising of Pathological Turbulences in a Tension Nose with Septum Deviation to the Right

Figure 4.**16** shows the findings of a patient with nasal obstruction on both sides.

The rhinoresistometric resistance curves indicate an obstruction in the two nasal sides. A characteristic separation of the measured resistance curve from the extrapolated resistance curve is evident. The inspiratory curves run visibly steeper. Before decongestion, the nose wing starts collapsing; at 120 cm³/sec, a flow equivalent to breathing at rest. The distinct separation between the extrapolated curve and the measured curve indicates a considerable collapse, especially before decongestion. The nose wings are being pushed slightly outward during expiration.

Even after decongestion, the resistance on both sides does not normalize. Causes for this are additional permanent stenoses on both sides, which can be located in the isthmus area with acoustic rhinometry on the right side rather than on the

left side. The low hydraulic diameter proves that the stenoses are flow-dynamically relevant.

Additionally, fully developed turbulences at low flow and high values for the friction coefficient λ can be found on the right side rather than on the left side. The curves for the acoustic rhinometry show that the cause is that the diffuser has a very small opening.

During long-term rhinoflowmetry, an impaired nasal cycle can be found. Due to the obstruction on both sides, both sides are in working phase throughout the day. Only during rest at night is the left side in a resting phase, taking over a working phase in the morning time.

The findings show that a septoplasty itself would not be sufficient to eliminate the deviation because it could lead to neither a sufficient decrease in resistance nor to a normalization of the strong turbulences nor to a solution to the problem of the inspiratory collapse. An additional widening of the nasal valve region is necessary. In this manner, the stenosis of the isthmus and thus the resistance must be sufficiently reduced. Simultaneously, the problem of pathological turbulences would be solved because, with a slightly widened entrance, the diffuser would be able to take on normal shape. Also, the problem of the inspiratory nose wing collapse could be consider-

Before Decongestion:

Resist. (at 250 cm³/s):	5.21	2.48	[sPa/cm³]
Hydr. diameter:	3.6	3.9	[mm]
Frict. coeffic. λ:	37	35	· 10⁻³

After Decongestion:

Resist. (at 250 cm³/s):	1.08	0.47	[sPa/cm³]
Hydr. diameter:	4.0	4.7	[mm]
Frict. coeffic. λ:	32	29	· 10⁻³

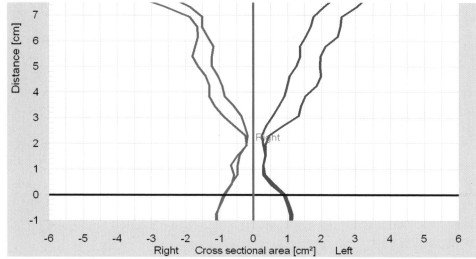

a

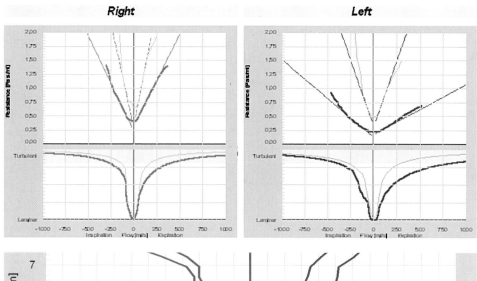

b

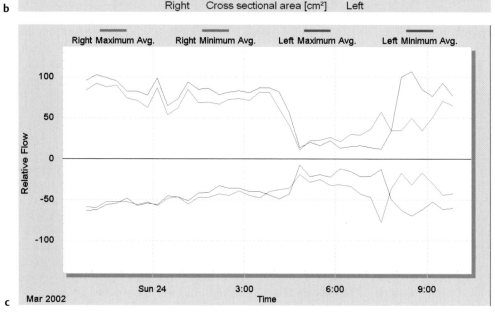

c   Mar 2002

Fig. 4.**16**   Rhinoresistometric (**a**), acoustic rhinometric (**b**), and long-term rhinoflowmetric findings (**c**) of a patient with tension nose as well as septum deviation to the right.

ably improved by this, since due to a greater cross-sectional area within the isthmus the local flow velocity is reduced and thereby the suction effect decreased according to Bernoulli's law.

Concluding Remarks

Precise preoperative diagnostics are part of a surgeon's responsibilities. This not only includes the detailed exploration of the patient's medical history and a subtle clinical examination but also the use of all possible functional diagnostic means. For ear surgeons, this has been a self-evident duty for a long time. Poor rhinomanometric data leads to the fact that for rhinosurgery preoperative functional diagnostics has been optional up to now. We, as rhinosurgeons, should change such regrettable circumstances as soon as possible, because new techniques in rhinological functional diagnostics lead to new indications as well as to a new functional view. Consequently, in some cases, new surgical procedures are the result.

References

1. Fischer R. Das Strömungsprofil der Respirationsluft in der Nase (Modellversuch). *Arch klin exp Ohr-Nas-Kehlk-Heilk.* 1967; 188:404.
2. Mlynski G, Grützenmacher S, Plontke S, Grützmacher W, Mlynski B, Lang C. A method for studying nasal airflow by means of fluid dynamic experiments. *Z Med Phys.* 2000; 10:1–10.
3. Mlynski G, Grützenmacher S, Plontke S, Mlynski B, Lang C. Correlation of nasal morphology and respiratory function. *Rinol.* 2001; 39:197–201.
4. Bachmann W. *Die Funktionsdiagnostik der behinderten Nasenatmung.* Berlin–Heidelberg–New York: Springer:1982.
5. Bachmann W. Die Topographie des anatomischen ostium internum der Nase im Hinblick auf seine funktionelle Bedeutung. *Z Laryng Rhinol.* 1969; 48:263.
6. Clement P. Committee report on standardization of rhinomanometry. *Rhinology.* 1984; 22:151–155.
7. Mlynski G, Loew J. Die Rhinoresistometrie—eine Weiterentwicklung der Rhinomanometrie. *Lar-Rhin-Otol.* 1993; 72(12):608–610.
8. Hilberg O, Jensen FT, Pedersen OF. Nasal airway geometry: comparison between acoustic reflexes and magnetic resonance scanning. *J appl Physiol.* 1993; 75:2811–2819.
9. Mlynski RA, Gruetzenmacher S, Lang C, Mlynski G. Acoustic rhinometry and paranasal sinuses: a systematic study in box models. *Laryngoscope.* (Accepted for publication 2002); 8:27.

5 Preoperative Management

H. Behrbohm

Contents

Evaluation of the Face and External Nose

The First Impression

Analyzing the features of the patient's face and nose starts with something that is difficult to put into words: the *first impression*. Although the first impression takes but a moment, it conveys a variety of information on the rhinoplasty candidate, which the physician perceives mostly intuitively but interprets very quickly. This includes personality, warmth or antipathy, and the patient's "manner," which may be amiable or reserved.

The physician notices how the patient presents his/her desire for corrective surgery. It may be expressed clearly and emphatically, or the patient may be less communicative and withdrawn, and the physician has to "probe" to learn whether the patient is introverted or extroverted.

The first impression will inevitably include the patient's body posture (erect or slumped) and body language, handshake (firm or limp), the patient's voice (loud or soft, hoarse, clear, or dysphonic), and language (expression, grammar, vocabulary, humor).

Socrates once said to one of his pupils, "Speak so that I can see you." Besides the general inspection and clinical examination, the physician should glean as much information about the candidate as possible. He should listen and observe attentively, because the key question—*"Should I operate on this patient?"*—can be answered in some cases before the facial anatomy is even analyzed.

By talking with the patient, the physician can tell whether he/she has an optimistic or pessimistic nature. It is important for the physician to learn what is motivating the patient to seek nasal surgery and find out what expectations the rhinoplasty candidate has for the proposed operation.

Openness and the willingness to cooperate with the treatment are expressed by firm eye contact, while fleeting looks and lack of concentration in the interview signify communication problems.

Besides all of this general information, the physician also looks for evidence of underlying diseases that may or may not relate to the reason for the consultation. Signs of illness are often reflected in the patient's face. These may include cyanosis of the lips due to ischemic heart disease, jaundice due to liver disease, xanthelasmas due to hypercholesterolemia, the flushed complexion of the hypertensive, and palsies, spasms, or tics of the facial musculature.

The Preoperative Consultation

The consultation, or initial interview, should take place in a quiet, stress-free environment with no time pressure. A full waiting room creates a pressured atmosphere that hampers open communication between the physician and patient. The best way to do this in a busy practice is to schedule patients for a special appointment before and after rhinoplasties. A surgical office visit in a general hospital otorhinolaryngology department may lead the patient to conclude that "The doctor has other problems; he obviously doesn't have time for my nose."

In our experience, it is best not to have a telephone in the consultation room, because being interrupted by phone calls during the consultation would serve to reinforce that fear. A computer in the office can also be problematical. By remaining riveted to a data screen, the physician may miss the chance to glean as much information on the patient as possible.

The basis for doctor–patient communication in esthetic surgery must be openness and honesty on both sides. Surgeons must know what the patient really wants. They must honestly convey to the patient what can be done and what is unrealistic or impossible. This is the best way to correct false expectations and preconceptions and avoid failures. The basis for trust is that the physician has time for the patient. He should explain the proposed operation in nontechnical language and address any problems that may arise. If a trusting relationship can be established between the physician and patient before the surgery, it may be easier for the patient to tolerate any touch-ups that may be needed after the primary operation. The patient must go into the operation with the knowledge that the surgeon has addressed his/her problem with time and dedication and will do everything necessary to carry out the jointly discussed plan of operation.

Conducting the Consultation

The interview should be conducted with open-ended questions, which invite patients to express themselves more fully. Examples of open-ended questions are: "What brings you to me?" and "What bothers you about your nose?" Yes-or-no questions make it more difficult to sustain a dialogue. By conducting the interview in this way and listening attentively, the surgeon will learn why the patient desires a rhinoplasty. At the same time, he will gain an impression of the motivation and psychological makeup of the patient.

The goal of every rhinoplasty is a satisfied patient. A successful operation will do much toward achieving this goal. A good result, however, does not necessarily mean a happy patient because the surgeon and patient may evaluate the result differently. Ultimately, the preoperative consultation is designed to answer two questions:

- Can I solve the problem of the nose?
- Will the operation solve the patient's problem?

While the first question can usually be answered after a detailed interview and examination, the second question is more difficult. It requires psychological insights and sensitivity on the part of the surgeon. Unlike a psychologist, he has only a short time in which to make his judgment. He need not make a precise psychological evaluation of the candidate, but he must be able to answer the two key questions as a basis for deciding, *"Should I operate on this patient, or are his/her complaints 'inoperable'?"*

The physician should explain the effects of the desired changes on the face. A simple hump removal can result in a long nasal dorsum and may even worsen the overall appearance and "personality" of the face. Some patients require extra help in understanding the complex effects of rhinoplasty. Many patients also lack appreciation for small morphological variants such as a bifid tip, minor tip asymmetries, or an indistinct nasolabial angle. A smaller percentage have a very finely developed sense for all of the details in their own face.

Starting from these very diverse wishes and demands for the outcome of an esthetic rhinoplasty, the physician can counsel and work with the patient to plan an individualized or even perfect result. Ultimately, however, the plan of operation is determined by the patient's own desires.

Analysis, Clinical Geometry

During the preoperative consultation, the surgeon has already had a good opportunity to inspect the patient's facial features. The nose should be assessed in relation to the overall appearance. A long nose is appropriate for a tall stature. A high nasal dorsum emphasizes individual characteristics more than miniaturized forms. The nose is evaluated within the context of the facial features from the front, from the sides, and from below.

Proportions and Symmetry

Polycleitus (ca. 450–410 BC) was the most important Greek sculptor next to Phidias. Many of his bronze statues, preserved as marble copies, are major works from the Classical era of Greek art (14). *Doryphoros* is perhaps his best-known statue and embodies the principles set forth in his treatise *The Canon* (preserved only in fragments) on the proportions of the human body. *The Canon* begins with a detailed system defining the ideal relative proportions of the various parts of the body, known in classical antiquity as *symmetry*. This symmetry of the human body became a guiding principle for painting, sculpture, and architecture and a hallmark of *esthetics*. The classical teachings on body proportions received renewed attention during the Renaissance. The monk Fra Pacioli di Borgo worked extensively with proportions and esthetics in medieval Venice. In 1509 he published a book in which he announced the discovery of the *golden section:* If we are asked to divide a line asymmetrically, we can do so at any number of points, but there is one section that is most esthetically pleasing to the eye. This section divides the line into two segments called a and b. The ratio of the shorter segment to the longer segment (a/b) is the same as the ratio of the longer segment to the whole line:

$$a/b = b/a + b$$

This principle is reflected in the branches of trees, for example, and in the ratio of the longitudinal and transverse axes of an egg. It demonstrates that proportionality and esthetics follow geometric laws (2).

The practice of dividing the face into equal thirds was introduced by Leonardo da Vinci (1452–1519) and was later modified by Powell and Humphreys (16). Defining ideal proportions for the human face is an important aid for the facial surgeon (see Chapter 3, Facial Proportions and Esthetic Ideals). A much more common goal in any given case, however, is to restore or preserve the harmony of the face with due regard for personal as well as ethnic characteristics (3, 8, 13).

As Naumann (15) put it, "The face must be viewed as a unit, and the nose should have a good structural relationship to the overall balance of the face."

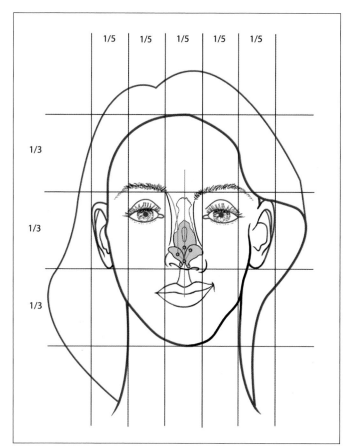

Fig. 5.1 Facial proportions and symmetry. (**a**) The face is divided horizontally into fifths (Leonardo da Vinci). (**b**) The face is divided vertically into thirds (Powell and Humphreys). *Right half of the face.* Symmetry is defined by the eyebrow–tip line, the facial midline, and the rhomboid shape of the nasal tip. *Left half of the face.* Asymmetry is often due to an asymmetrical eyebrow–tip line (pseudodeviated nose), maxillary, midfacial, or mandibular hypoplasia (usually with a crooked mouth), an oblique nasal base (cleft lip and palate), or asymmetry of individual structural elements (upper lateral or alar cartilages).

The Face from the Front

There is a certain hierarchy of facial features. The personality radiates chiefly from the eyes. The nose should be "subordinate" to the eyes, i.e., it should form a smoothly curved line from the medial point of the eyebrow to the tip-defining point. This line should highlight the eyes and not distract from them.

The nasal tip is defined by a roughly equilateral rhomboid. It is formed by the tip-defining points and by the supratip and infratip areas. The basal contour of the alae should form a gently curved line ("gull in flight") (Fig. 5.**1**).

Every face has two slightly different halves and shows some degree of physiological *asymmetry*. This becomes clear when photos of the right and left halves of the same face are assembled in a montage. Marked facial asymmetry, facial scoliosis, or unilateral hypoplasia may affect individual or multiple portions of the midface, for example, or may affect the maxilla or mandible.

Midfacial asymmetries often result in dysgnathia and are associated with axial deformity of the nose. The correction of

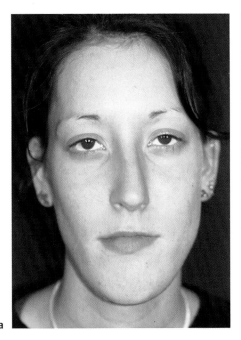
a

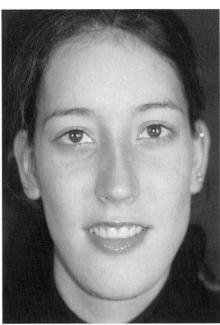
b

Fig. 5.**2**   Woman with marked facial scoliosis and a deviated nose (**a**). Following axial correction, the asymmetry is less conspicuous (**b**).

combined facial deformities and asymmetries requires particularly careful planning (Fig. 5.**2a, b**).

Axial deformities of the nose may affect the bony or cartilaginous part of the nose or may affect both parts simultaneously, producing an S-shaped *twisted nose*. Two different *eyebrow–tip lines* create the impression of a pseudo-deviated nose. Saddle nose is marked by typical deformities that adversely affect facial symmetry. The dorsum and supratip area are broad and depressed. The nasal base is broadened. The columella is low, and the nostrils have a transverse oval shape.

Skin and Connective-Tissue Type

The skin and connective-tissue type has an important bearing on the anticipated tissue reaction and wound healing, making it an important factor in preoperative planning.

Thick, seborrheic skin is advantageous in that it can cover small irregularities in the osseocartilaginous supporting structures of the nose. Onlay grafts, tip grafts, and shield grafts can be used. Suture techniques are also available.

Thick skin is more susceptible to wound healing problems than thin skin. An example is the postoperative *pollybeak* deformity, which is most common in patients with a thick skin type.

Thick skin and thin cartilage are an unfavorable combination for rhinoplasty.

Thin skin is advantageous for wound healing. Graft techniques should not be used on the nasal tip. In cases where a *bifid tip* is present due to prominent alar cartilages, perichondrium or small fascial flaps can be placed beneath the skin of the nasal tip.

The ideal skin type for septorhinoplasty is moderately thick skin.

Besides interindividual differences, the thickness of the skin varies from the glabella to the tip. It measures 2–5 mm at the level of the paranasion, approximately 3.2 mm over the bony dorsum, and 2–2.2 mm over the rhinion. Lang reports a thickness of 7 mm over the alae and 5 mm over the tip (13).

The skin is thinnest, then, over the rhinion. It is thickest and most glandular over the nasal tip, especially in persons with seborrheic skin.

The connective-tissue type is indicated by skin wrinkling, tissue tension, and the elasticity and mobility of the skin. A less firm connective-tissue type is often associated with an increased tendency for hematoma formation. The skin is loose and mobile.

Any cutaneous scars from previous operations (e.g., goiter surgery) should be inspected to gain information on individual scar formation and possible keloid formation. Preexisting scars would be a reason to avoid an open approach.

Profile Analysis

Numerous geometric points and lines can be used to assess the facial profile. They are used to evaluate the relative positions or displacements of specific structures, depending on the points that are emphasized in a given specialty. For example, an orthognathic surgeon will use completely different reference planes than an otorhinolaryngologist or facial surgeon. We are always dealing with *one* profile, however, and therefore we shall focus on several interdisciplinary landmarks.

The *nasion* corresponds to the *nasofrontal suture* and should be located at the approximate level of the supratarsal fold. The *paranasion* is located at the deepest point of the *sella nasi*. The *nasofrontal angle* between the glabella, nasal root, and nasal tip should be between 125° and 135°.

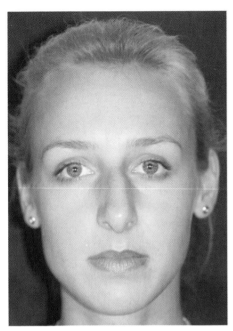
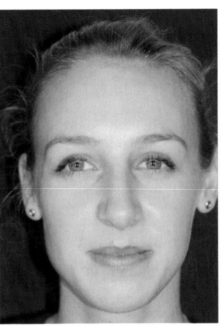

Fig. 5.**3 a**   Woman with a predominantly bony nasal deviation, a bony dorsal hump, and an overprojected nasal tip. The infratip triangle is too long.

Fig. 5.**3 b**   Appearance three years after axial correction of the nose and shortening of the infratip triangle.

The *nasal dorsum* consists of the *bony dorsum* and *cartilaginous dorsum*. The *rhinion* is located at the junction of the nasal bones and upper lateral cartilages. This region is called the *keystone area* because of its key importance in stabilizing the nasal dorsum. It marks the cranial point of attachment of the cartilaginous nose at the center of the face.

The nasal dorsum should be high and straight, or perhaps slightly convex, with the rhinion as its point of maximum prominence. From there the nasal profile descends straight to the *pronasale* in males, while in females it should form a slight depression at the level of the anterior septal angle, called the *supratip break*. From the pronasale, or *tip-defining point*, the profile curves smoothly to the *subnasale*, interrupted by a small break at the level of the columella–lobule junction. Thus, a *double break* exists in the nasal profile between the pronasale and subnasale. The size of the nasolabial angle determines the cranial or caudal position of the nasal tip and thus the length of the nose from the paranasion to the pronasale. The nasofrontal angle should be > 95° (19).

The length of the upper lip should equal the length of the columella. Ideally, the columella describes a slightly convex line several millimeters below the slightly concave alar margin.

We use our own modification of the "facial circle" described by Baud to define the three most important points for general profile analysis and evaluate their relationship in the facial profile. Instead of the external auditory canal, we use the upper border of the tragus (corresponding to the *porion*) for measuring the radius to the pronasale. This point corresponds to the reference point for the Frankfurt horizontal (canthomeatal plane) in the Krönlein system (Fig. 5.4).

The line from the porion to the pronasale forms the radius of a circular arc about the face. Ideally, the *trichion* and *pogonion* are located on the periphery of that circle.

Overprojection of the nose is characterized by a posterior displacement of the chin (soft-tissue pogonion) and the frontal hairline. A relative retrusion of the chin or forehead can also be recognized. This type of analysis provides guidelines for the best way to achieve an harmonious profile.

The goal of a septorhinoplasty is not just to alter the nose but to match the nose to the chin and forehead in a way that produces an esthetically pleasing profile. The esthetic impact of a sloping forehead or receding chin, for example, can be improved by nasal surgery alone (Fig. 5.**3 a–f**).

The nasal dorsum consists of a bony and cartilaginous portion. The relationship of these two components influences preoperative planning. Long nasal bones will adequately stabilize the nose. Short nasal bones are an indication for *spreader grafts*. These grafts will prevent stenosis of the nasal valve and pinching of the alae (Fig. 5.**5 a–d**).

Dentition and Profile

Besides nasal shape, the profile is critically influenced by the position of the maxilla and mandible and by the typical deviations that occur with gnathic anomalies.

Schwarz has identified nine different profile types in orthognathic surgery. The following reference lines are used (17):
- Canthomeatal plane (Frankfurt horizontal)
- Nasal perpendicular of Dreyfuss
- Orbital perpendicular of Simon

Three typical variants are distinguished based on the relationship of the subnasale to the nasal perpendicular:
- Average face: Subnasale is anterior to a vertical line through the nasion.
- Protruded face: Subnasale is posterior to a vertical line through the nasion.

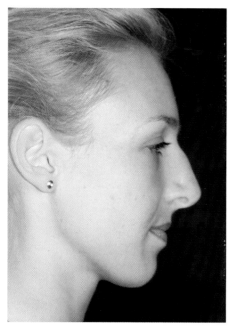

Fig. 5.**3 c** Preoperative profile. Overprojection, bony hump, effaced nasolabial angle, relative retrusion of the chin, vestibular skin show.

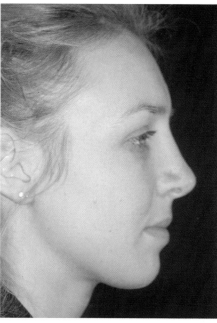

Fig. 5.**3 d** Postoperative profile. The nasal dorsum has been lowered, and a supratip break has been created. The tip has been rotated upward and the upper lip lengthened. There is also a *relative advancement* of the chin.

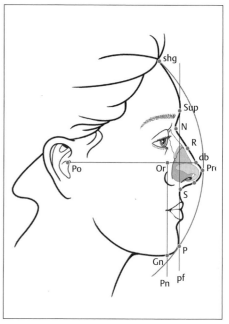

Fig. 5.**4** Geometric points and lines used in analyzing the facial profile. Po = porion, Gn = gnathion, S = subnasale, N = nasion, Sup = supraorbitale, R = rhinion, Pro = pronasale, db = double break, pf = frontal plane, shg = frontal hairline, line between Po and Or = Frankfurt horizontal, **Pn** = orbital perpendicular, P = pogonion

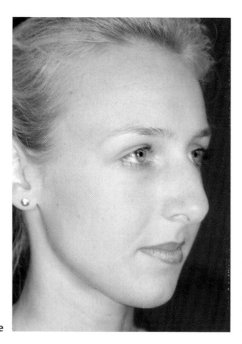

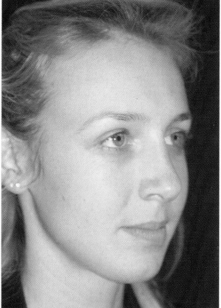

Fig. 5.**3 e, f** Preoperative and postoperative three-quarter profile views.

- With a straight or retruded face, the pogonion shows the same degree of displacement as the subnasale. Anterior or posterior sloping facial types are distinguished according to the displacement of the soft-tissue pogonion.

Two facial reference lines are used in distinguishing between straight, convex, or concave profile types:

- A straight line from the forehead to the margin of the upper lip
- A straight line from the margin of the upper lip to the soft-tissue pogonion

Straight profile: Both reference lines form a straight line.
Convex profile: Relative retroposition of the pogonion.

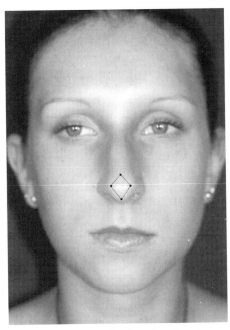

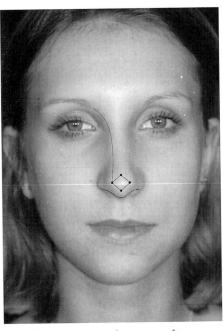

Fig. 5.**5a**   Woman with a functional tension nose. The infratip triangle is too long, and the eyebrow–tip line is imprecise.

Fig. 5.**5b**   Appearance three years after septorhinoplasty. Note the symmetrical rhomboid tip shape, the harmonious eyebrow line, and the "gull-in-flight" line of the alar base.

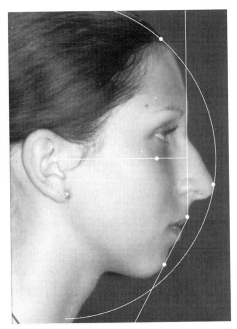

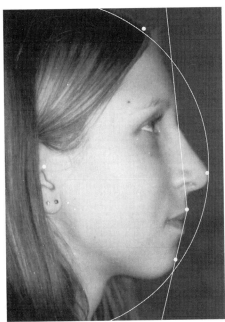

Fig. 5.**5c**   Recessed chin with an overprojected tip.

Fig. 5.**5d**   Profile corrected by septorhinoplasty and mentoplasty.

Concave profile: Relative anteroposition of the pogonion (Fig. 5.**6**).

The classic Angle classification of sagittal malocclusions was introduced in 1907 (1). A concave soft-tissue profile signifies an Angle class II malocclusion, while a concave profile indicates an Angle class III relationship (Fig. 5.**7**).

There are several reasons why these concepts from orthognathic surgery are important for the rhinosurgeon:

1. With regard to the timing of profile-correcting rhinoplasty in adolescence, it should be borne in mind that jaw growth continues until about 16 years of age in girls and until about 18 years in boys.
2. Gnathic abnormalities lead to typical profile changes:
   - Mandibular prognathism: Protrusion of the pogonion
   - Retrognathia: Retrusion of the pogonion

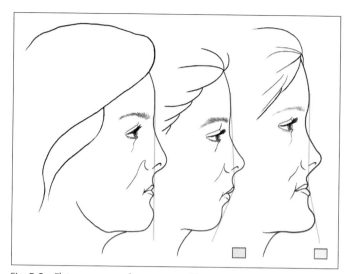

Fig. 5.**6**   Flat, convex, and concave profile types.

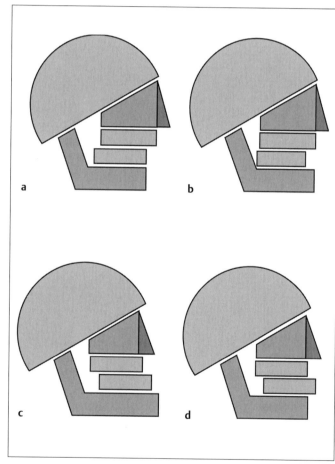

Fig. 5.**7 a, b**   Angle class II malocclusion. **c, d** Angle class III malocclusion. (**a**) Retrusion of the entire mandible. (**b**) Retrusion of the alveolar process of the mandible. (**c**) Protrusion of the entire mandible. (**d**) Protrusion of the alveolar process of the mandible. Normal relationship of the mandible and pogonion to the skull base (17).

- Maxillary prognathism: Protrusion of the subnasale and upper lip
3. The position of the nasal tip is influenced by the position of the jaws and midface. For example, an anterior sloping face can cause overprojection of the tip.

The Nasal Base

The shape of the nasal base is determined by the height ratio of the lobule to the columella, which is normally 1:3. The nares have an elliptical shape. The shape of the tip can be accurately assessed by viewing the nose from below. A *boxy tip* has a squared-off shape. A long-presumed interdomal ligament does not exist (21). The width of the nasal tip is determined by the shape of the alar cartilages, the skin, and the interdomal fat. The critical anatomical structures that define nasal shape are the nasal septum and the lateral and medial crura and footplates of the alar cartilages.

Bossing occurs when the transition from the dome area to the lateral alar cartilages is not harmonious. Often it takes several years for bossing to develop after rhinoplasty.

Palpation

Manual Examination Techniques

Visual inspection of the nose is followed by palpation. Before palpating the nose, the examiner should inform the patient that it is the only way to obtain essential information on the resilience and tension of critical nasal structures. Cartilages can be reoriented and preserved only if the surgeon has been able to assess the cartilage tension by palpation.

Visual examination and finger palpation are equally important in the nasal evaluation (Tardy, 19).

Palpation:
1. Palpate the junction of the cartilage and bony nasal dorsum in the keystone area. Rough spots, appositional bone growth following previous surgery, or an open roof can be appreciated in this way.
2a. Assess the *tip recoil* by pressing the nasal tip toward the anterior nasal spine with the index finger.
2b. Palpate over the anterior septal angle to assess the height and tension of the septal cartilage, especially in relation to the tip recoil.
3. The relationship of the bony nasal pyramid to the cartilaginous pyramid will affect surgical planning. Evaluate this by palpating over the nasal flank. Short nasal bones may be an indication for spreader grafts.
4. Palpate the structures of the nasal inlet to assess the shape and tension of the anterior septum, the size of the nasal spine, and the prominences of the premaxilla.
5. Bimanual palpation of the alar cartilage yields information on the shape, size, and consistency of the cartilage (Fig. 5.**8**).

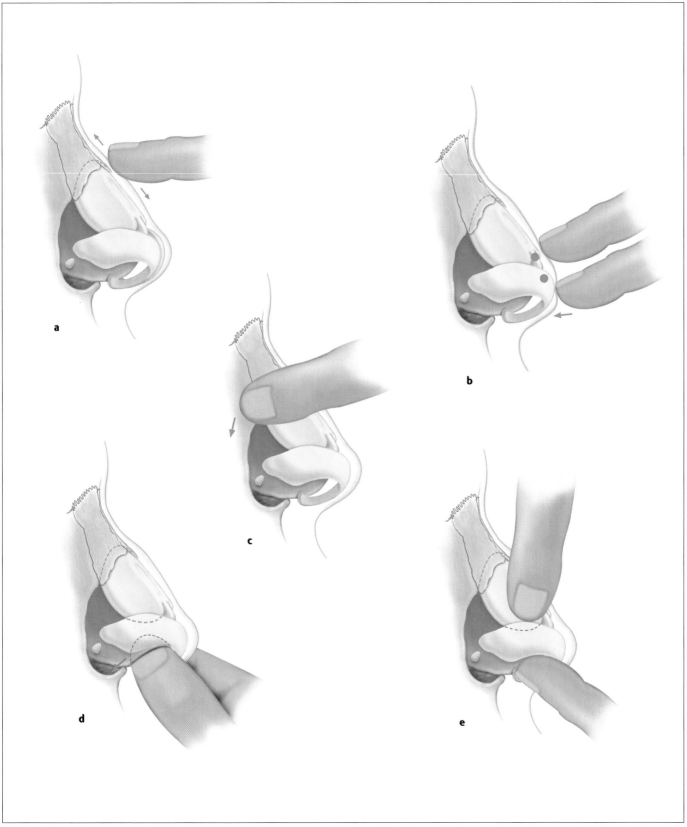

Fig. 5.**8a** Palpation of the bony and cartilaginous dorsum to explore elasticity, thickness and texture of the skin, irregularities, bony borders, open roof

b The tip recoil maneuver is an important indicator for tip support (arrow). The palpation of the anterior septal angle evaluates the size and tension of the anterior septum.

c Exploration of the length and strength of the bony nasal pramid, especially important is the relationship between the osseus and cartilaginous part.

d Palpation of the caudal septum, vestibules and nasal spine. The surgeon gains information about the tension, breadth and strength of the anterior septum, the size and shape of the nasal spine. Also information about the tension of the medial crura, the membranous septum and footplates is available.

e Bidigital evaluation of the shape, size and elasticity of the lower and upper cartilage, especially the cephalic and caudal edges.

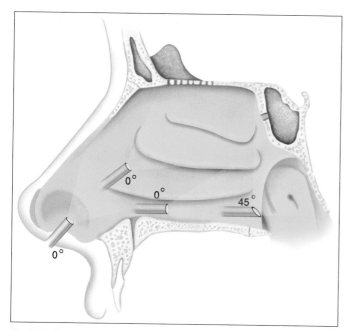

Fig. 5.**9** Systematic routine for nasal endoscopy.

Nasal Endoscopy

Nasal endoscopy should be a part of every nasal examination.

Evaluation of the mucosa. In allergic rhinitis, for example, hyperemia and increased vascular permeability develop in the mucosa as a result of local immune responses. The mucosa appears livid and edematous. In patients with a strong allergenic disposition, inflammatory redness of the mucosa is the dominant finding. The initially watery discharge becomes purulent when bacterial superinfection occurs. Polyps that develop in the ethmoid and project into the nose assume a pale, glassy appearance when the polyp stalk becomes constricted, occluding its blood supply.

Nasal endoscopy has an important application in recurrent and chronic inflammatory diseases of the paranasal sinuses. The endoscope can reveal the often subtle signs of a mucosal disease (e.g., rheological mucous changes, purulent tracks, edema) or anatomical variants in the shape of the lateral nasal wall (e.g., concha bullosa or paradoxical curvature of the middle turbinate).

Acute inflammatory exacerbations and especially suppurative diseases of the nasal mucosa are a contraindication for functional–esthetic rhinoplasty.

Endoscopy is also the best modality for evaluating noninflammatory diseases of the nose. Some lesions, such as polyps and papillomas, display pathognomonic features. There are other cases where polyps in the nose are not a pathogenetic entity but are a symptom of various diseases that can be identified by closer inspection.

Other diseases cannot be accurately classified by endoscopic examination (e.g., angiomatous tumors). When the 0° scope (4 mm) is used, endoscopy is useful for site-of-lesion determination in patients with obstructed nasal breathing.

Spurs, ridges, and displaced posttraumatic fragments, especially in the area of the posterior septum and perpendicular plate, can be evaluated and corrected as needed through an endoscopic approach (see Chapter 1, The Dual Character of Nasal Surgery).

The nasal valve can be assessed with a speculum without spreading open the vestibule. Inspiratory alar collapse can also be evaluated in this way.

Principles of Nasal Endoscopy

The patient can be examined in the sitting, semirecumbent, or supine position without premedication. If the mucosa is markedly swollen or vulnerable, it should be decongested and anesthetized with a tetracaine–epinephrine spray (10 drops epinephrine per 2 mL solution). In these cases we recommend inserting soft, moist pledgets (same solution) for 5 minutes prior to the examination. The pledgets should be placed under endoscopic control to avoid mucosal injuries. Even the smallest hemorrhages caused by careless endoscopic manipulation or instrumentation in the nose will seriously hamper the examination. The pledgets should be moist, not soggy, to avoid unnecessary wetting of the mucosa in the epipharynx, oropharynx, and hypopharynx.

- The basic instrument for nasal endoscopy is the 4-mm 0° wide-angle endoscope (Karl Storz, Tuttlingen).
- Endoscopy should always begin with the largest scope possible (4 mm), as this will provide maximum orientation within the nasal cavity.
- The primary use of a thinner scope (2.7 or 1 mm) is appropriate only as a second-line option, in small children, or if there is much deviation of the anterior septum.
- The endoscopic examination should always follow a systematic routine that covers specified regions.

Technique

The examination begins with the 0° endoscope. The nasal vestibule and nasal valve area are inspected first (Fig. 5.**9**).

By placing the endoscope at the entrance to the nasal cavity in front of the valve area, the examiner can assess the functional status of this region and check for collapse of the alar cartilages during normal and forced inspiration in a physiological position, without deforming the nares.

Next the endoscope is advanced into the nasal cavity, and the nasal floor is inspected. The scope can be carefully advanced between the septum and the body of the inferior turbinate toward the choana. In the presence of a vomerine ridge, which usually runs upward and backward, the posterior part of the nose is reached by advancing the scope strictly along the nasal floor.

The inferior turbinate has the same sagittal orientation as the pharyngeal orifice of the eustachian tube. The examiner inspects the nasopharynx, assessing the motility of the soft palate and the function of the pharyngeal tubal orifice. In children, the size and condition of the adenoids are evaluated.

Next the endoscope is partially withdrawn and redirected to inspect the middle turbinate. Endoscopy of this "window to the ethmoid" is of key importance for pathogenetic reasons. The middle turbinate is also the principal landmark for endoscopic operations (Fig. 5.**10**).

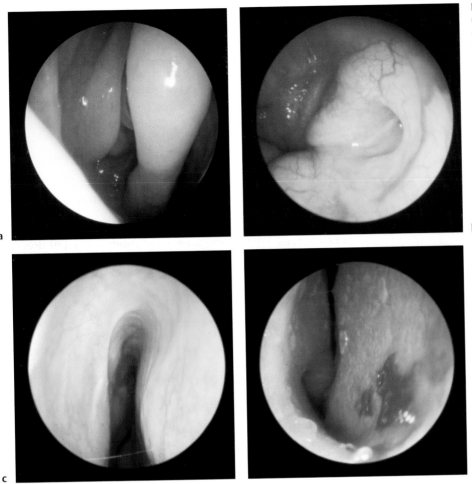

Fig. 5.10 Typical findings in nasal endoscopy. (**a**) View of the middle meatus with the 0° endoscope. (**b**) Mucosal polyps obstructing the middle meatus. (**c**) Papillomas. (**d**) View into the sphenoethmoid recess, showing the sphenoid sinus ostium. (All pictures 0°-telescopes, Karl Storz, Tuttlingen.)

Its medial lamina extends up to the cribriform plate and bears respiratory epithelium. In this way the upper part of the middle turbinate separates the cribriform plate from the ethmoid labyrinth located in the ethmoid part of the frontal bone.

The middle meatus of the nasal cavity is located between the middle and inferior turbinates. The middle turbinate is part of the ethmoid bone and also bounds the middle meatus medially. It inserts anterolateral to the cribriform plate and farther back on the lamina papyracea. Its basal lamina separates the mucus streams from the anterior and posterior ethmoids. The middle turbinate may be pneumatized by ethmoid cells and may reach considerable size (concha bullosa), leading to recurrent bouts of sinusitis.

The surface of the lateral nasal wall can be visualized by carefully displacing the middle turbinate medially with a narrow elevator. Anterior to the ethmoid bulla, which varies in size depending on its pneumatization, is the contour of the uncinate process. The inferior semilunar hiatus runs between the free posterior edge of the uncinate process and the anterior surface of the ethmoid bulla. It connects with the ethmoid infundibulum, which has a sagittal orientation. Continuous with the semilunar hiatus superiorly is the frontal recess.

The 30° endoscope is useful for locating the nasal orifice of the nasolacrimal duct. This orifice, usually elliptical in shape, can be found several millimeters behind the anterior attachment of the inferior turbinate.

The 30° scope is also useful for inspecting the sphenoethmoid recess, where the sphenoid sinus ostium is located. It is visualized by advancing the scope toward the choana, with the view angled upward, while keeping the barrel of the scope strictly on the nasal floor.

The entire nasopharynx can be inspected from below with the 45° or 70° scope. The olfactory groove, for example, can be examined to differentiate between a sensory or respiratory cause of hyposmia or anosmia.

Photographic Documentation

D. Jaeger and H. Behrbohm

A good general recommendation is to have a room, or at least a special area, set aside for taking high-quality, standardized clinical photographs. In the case of the nose, of course, the requirements of clinical and portrait photography overlap. With increasing experience in this area it will be recognized that photographs of the face capture much more than the actual clinical findings. The photographer should feel obligated, therefore, to exercise particular care.

Take a little extra time and help your subject overcome his/her natural inhibitions. Conversing with the patient during the photographic session will help to build trust and provide distraction. It does not matter whether the pictures are taken by a photographer, a dedicated assistant, or the surgeon, but the circle of photographers should be limited to experienced, committed colleagues. (The authors do all of their own clinical photography.)

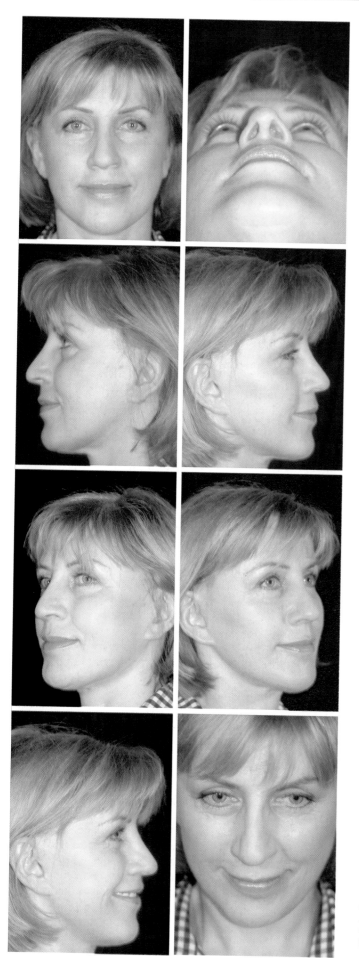

The camera lens should have a focal length sufficient to create some camera-to-subject distance. The flash should never be triggered "in the patient's face." Make sure to have a neutral backdrop and do not place the patient too close to it.

Generally the "golden section" principle should be applied in composing the picture. The field of view should be widened or narrowed to cover the essentials.

The goal of photodocumentation is the lifelike, distortion-free portrayal of nasal findings in standard photographic views taken before and after rhinoplasty. The following facial views are recommended:

- Frontal
- Right and left profile (with the canthomeatal plane horizontal)
- Right and left oblique (three-quarter profile)
- Basal view (projecting the nasal tip between the eyebrows)
- Nasal dorsum with the head tilted slightly forward
- Lateral smiling view (to show the effect of the mimetic musculature)
(Fig. 5.**11**)

Care and professionalism in taking pictures are definitely noticed by patients and can only enhance the surgeon's reputation.

Some important criteria are reviewed below.

Lighting

A small studio flash system is essential for obtaining reproducible lighting conditions that are unaffected by changes in natural light. The brightness of the flash unit should be fully adjustable. Umbrella reflectors produce a softer light. A bright, proportionately adjustable halogen modeling light lets the photographer check the lighting before triggering the flash.

Proper lighting helps to bring out the facial features. The *main light* defines the subject and should be placed within the photographic axis. Even slight changes in the vertical or horizontal angle of the light will affect the result. A *fill light* is placed on the opposite side of the camera from the main light. It fills in the shadows to provide more balanced contrast. The fill flash should have only half the brightness level of the main light. Collapsible reflectors or styrofoam panels can be used for added illumination (Fig. 5.**12**).

Focal Length of the Lens

The proper camera lens should be used to avoid documentation errors. An objective lens with a focal length of 100–130 mm is considered ideal for 35-mm photography. A single-lens reflex camera (SLR) is used to allow precise framing of the image. SLRs also have a built-in flash trigger, which is necessary for this type of work.

Image Scale

The image scale changes with the focal length of the objective lens and the camera-to-subject distance. Thus it influences the size of the image in relation to the subject.

Fig. 5.**11** Standard photographic views taken before and after nasal operations.

Framing the Image

Framing emphasizes the important image content. Choosing a favorable perspective further enhances the result.

Background

The background should have a neutral appearance. It is mainly for esthetic purposes. A black or blue backdrop will direct attention to the subject and is advantageous for light-colored hair.

Film Material

The choice of film material depends on the form in which the pictures will be filed. Slides are advantageous over negatives in that they can be accessed more quickly and are immediately available.

Films are designed for use with either daylight or artificial light. The color temperature of the flash requires the use of daylight film. Special portrait films are commercially available. These films are excellent for the accurate portrayal of skin color. The higher the film speed (ISO), the lower the image resolution. Because of this, high-speed films (400 ISO) are too grainy for clinical portrait photography. A 100 ISO film provides very fine detail and is recommended for clinical photography.

If a studio flash system is not available or affordable, the following tips should prove helpful:

- Use several high-intensity lights to illuminate the subject. Avoid multiple shadows.
- Place blue filters in front of the lights to reduce the yellow or use blue correction filters in front the lens.
- Use tracing paper to diffuse the flash.
- Placing orange paper in front of the flash will soften the skin color and make it appear more natural.
- Adjust the flash so that it does not strike the subject directly. Use half the normal flash intensity.

Informed Consent

The physician is obligated to present the patient with timely, comprehensive information before performing a functional–esthetic rhinoplastic procedure. The scope of this disclosure depends on the nature of the procedure, its necessity, and its urgency (12).

In the case of an esthetic operation, the patient should receive a particularly thorough explanation of the agreed goals and potential complications.

Bilateral olfactometry should be done prior to any surgical procedure on the nose (threshold test or the Cain identification test). The patient's self-assessment, history, and rhinoscopic findings should be documented (10).

Informed consent should be obtained at least 24 hours before the procedure. We recommend a staged disclosure in which the patient first receives written information in the form of a brochure and then meets with the physician for detailed counseling at a later date. In this meeting the physician provides verbal information and answers any questions

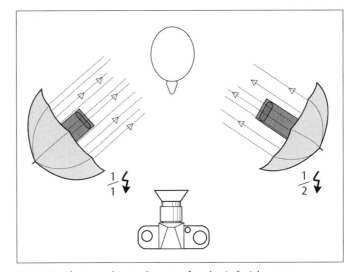

Fig. 5.**12**   Photographic studio setup for plastic facial surgery.

that the patient may have. The discussion should be carried out in layperson's language, avoiding medical jargon whenever possible. Drawings and diagrams are a helpful adjunct to informed consent in functional–esthetic rhinosurgery. All measures should be taken to eliminate misunderstandings. What is true of the language of the discussion is also true of its content: The physician must be clear and should avoid exaggerations and understatements. Written consent should be obtained.

From a legal standpoint, proof of informed consent is required. The best way to secure this is by having the patient sign a consent form which lists the principal risks of the procedure. A signature alone is not enough. The form must also state that the patient has been given full and complete information in terms that he/she can understand, and that this information has been given verbally by a physician (12).

This is an important point, because if the patient litigates, the physician must be able to document informed consent in detail. If he cannot do this, it will be assumed that the patient was not given information on the points that were not documented.

One should accurately document when the patient was given this detailed information, as well as the amount of time this took. With difficult patients, it is wise to summon a resident, physician's assistant, or nurse to act as a witness.

The physician must be able to prove informed consent. Because every surgical procedure is potentially unlawful, the surgeon must be able to document patient consent. This consent is valid only if the patient has received adequate, timely information prior to the procedure.

Personal Recommendations

During the office consultation, the patient has an opportunity to ask questions on the conduct of the operation, its risks, and possible complications. The surgeon should address these questions in detail. He/she should also be available for any further appointments that are needed to address unanswered questions or review certain details.

Upon request, patients should receive an information sheet that they can bring with them when on hospital admission, which may be scheduled weeks or months ahead.

On the day before the operation, the patient is again informed about all possible risks and complications.

While physicians have an obligation to fully inform the patient, they should do this without inducing needless uncertainty or anxiety. They should put the numerous possible risks into a realistic context by evaluating them with respect to the individual case. The tenor of the preoperative consultation should be optimistic and reassuring and ultimately should reinforce the informed decision for surgery.

Psychological Issues in Rhinoplasty

All symptoms and complaints have a psychosomatic aspect, but the relative proportions of the "psychic" and "somatic" elements of a disorder are highly variable. Esthetic surgery is always a form of psychosurgery. On the one hand, it can free the patient from the suffering and distress of a facial abnormality or deformity that is perceived as a stigma. In this way the surgery can contribute to a new feeling of self-worth and make the patient happy. But on the other hand, even a successful rhinoplasty that makes the patient more physically attractive may not solve his/her real problems. It may be, for example, that the patient is projecting problems of social interaction into an organic problem. This patient may expect that solving an esthetic problem will also solve conflicts that he believes are rooted in the physical condition. As a result of this, the patient may reject the successful result of a rhinoplasty because it has not solved the other problems. Common warning signs or possible contraindications to predominantly esthetic septorhinoplasties are listed below.

Potential Problem Patients

1. Be careful if you notice a disparity between a mild physical abnormality and a high degree of patient distress ("I can't stand to look at myself!"). If physical examination reveals only a subtle finding that does not definitely require surgical correction, this may mean that the patient has body dysmorphic disorder (BDD). BDD is present in 4.5–7% of persons who seek esthetic surgery (7, 18). Patients with this disorder are dissatisfied with the surgical result, lack insight, and are usually eager to have touch-up surgery after the first operation. A standardized scale can be used to assess these patients for BDD prior to the initial surgery. The following features are characteristic of BDD:
   - An obsessive preoccupation with an imagined defect or slight physical abnormality.
   - The preoccupation with the imagined defect causes significant distress or impairment in social, occupational, or other important areas in the person's life.
   - The preoccupation cannot be explained by some other mental disorder, such as whole body image dissatisfaction (as in anorexia nervosa).
   A score of 3 on all of these criteria (1 = no, 2 = may be, 3 = yes) warrants a diagnosis of BDD. A score of 2 on any of the criteria may be an indication of BDD. Psychiatric consultation is advised for these cases, and the patient is not considered a candidate for rhinoplasty.

2. There is no "simple" rhinoplasty. The more minor the anatomical problem, the greater the expectations that the surgeon must meet. Unrealistic expectations in a patient with perfectionist traits are a sign that surgery should be reconsidered.
3. Every operation, especially when elective, requires clear motivation and resolution on the part of the patient. Any uncertainties about the operation can be clarified through verbal discussion. It is not up to the surgeon to find a motivation for the operation. Unmotivated patients should not undergo surgery.
4. There are candidates for esthetic operations who go to doctor after doctor, shopping around for the best deal. Bargain hunters are poor candidates because they are reluctant to embark upon a trusting doctor–patient relationship and tend to renew their bargain hunt when the slightest problems arise. Also, these patients will try various ways to recoup their expenses after the operation (7).
5. The motivation for cosmetic rhinoplasty may be unclear in patients who are unkempt or seem disinterested in their appearance. These patients should first be told that their appearance can be improved by clothing, hair styling, makeup, or beauty consulting, and that surgery may not be necessary.
6. Be careful with patients who have already been operated elsewhere and come to you for a revision. It is always best when the same surgeon performs both the original operation and the revision. An even more difficult situation arises for the surgeon who "operates into" a lawsuit that is in progress.

Fortunately, the typical rhinoplasty patient is motivated, active, optimistic, and cooperative. The average degree of satisfaction with the surgical outcome varies depending on the patient's age and gender. For example, young women are pleased with their outcomes much more often than middle-aged males (9, 11). Surgeons are warned against the combination of factors known as SIMON: single, immature, male, over-expectant, narcissistic (19).

Preoperative Workup

Rhinological History

The patient is questioned specifically about a sensation of nasal obstruction (constant or variable) as well as olfactory impairment and facial pain. Is there prior history of cranial trauma? Is there evidence of perennial or seasonal allergy, analgesic intolerance, or asthma? Has the patient had otitis media or sinusitis?

Esthetic History

During the preoperative consultation, the physician acquires information on the wishes, motivation, and mental status of the rhinoplasty candidate. He obtains vital information about whether or not to operate. See page 90 for more details.

Evaluation of the External Nose

Inspection of the nose begins when the history is taken. Palpation should include the external and internal nose. Further details are presented in Analysis, Clinical Geometry above.

Endoscopic Examination

The goal of the endoscopic examination in a broad sense is to detect all endonasal disease. The capabilities and technique of nasal endoscopy are reviewed in the section Nasal Endoscopy above.

Diagnostic Imaging

A survey radiograph of the paranasal sinuses is sufficient for preoperative screening in patients who have no history of sinusitis. Otherwise, coronal computed tomography (CT) is standard.

Laboratory Tests

Detailed information can be found on pages 191 and 205.

Function Testing

Before any nasal surgery is performed, the nasal airflow (in cm^3/s) should be objectively determined by active anterior computerized rhinomanometry, and olfaction should be assessed with a threshold and identification test. If parallel signs of tympanic ventilation problems are noted, pure-tone audiometry and tympanometry should be performed.

Photographic Documentation

The face should be photographed in standardized positions under the reproducible conditions of a small studio. The photos are used for the preoperative documentation of findings and for postoperative comparison. See p. 99 for details.

Informed Consent

The patient is informed about all the risks of the operation and the desired goals. The information is presented verbally and must be documented in writing. The principles of informed consent are reviewed in the section Informed Consent Principles above.

Planning the Operation

The surgeon consults with the patient and obtains his/her input in planning the operation, taking into account all preoperative findings including the clinical photographs.

Preoperative planning is aided by the use of drawings, templates, or animated graphic computer programs.

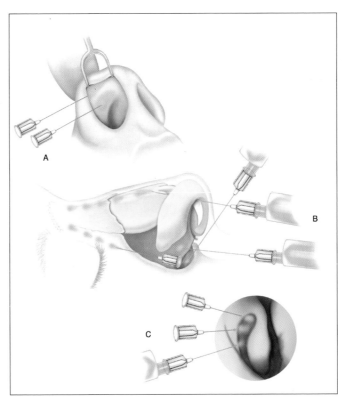

Fig. 5.**13**   Use of local anesthetics in rhinoplasty

Immediate Preoperative Preparations

Positioning

For septorhinoplasties and for endoscopic paranasal sinus operations, the patient is positioned supine with the head resting flat on the table. The surgeon should double-check the position, since any flexion or extension of the head will alter the inclination angle of the skull base. Gravity acts differently on the supine face than the upright face, and therefore the patient photographs (at least frontal and lateral) should be posted in the operating room along with CT scans and other images.

Local Anesthesia

The nasal mucosa is decongested 15 minutes before the operation with nose drops (xylometazoline hydrochloride). A local anesthetic (ultracaine with 1:100 000 or 1:50 000 epinephrine) is injected to induce local anesthesia, hypoemia, and hydrodissection. The agent should be injected at standard sites (see Fig. 5.**13**) beneath the superficial musculoaponeurotic system (SMAS) in the cartilaginous and bony nose and beneath the perichondrium of the septal cartilage.

The infiltration technique depends on the intended approach. The nasal dorsum is infiltrated in the supraperichondrial plane with a long, ultrathin needle inserted by the intercartilaginous route. Agent is injected over the periosteum

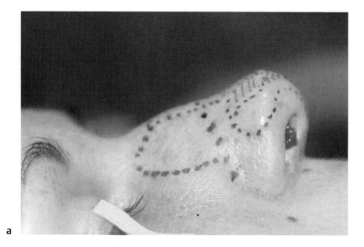

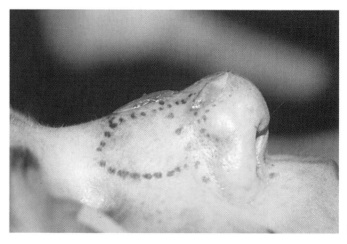

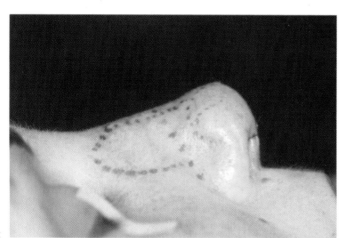

Fig. 5.**14** Preoperative markings indicate the proposed lines of incision, resection, osteotomies.

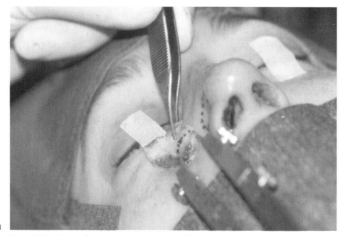

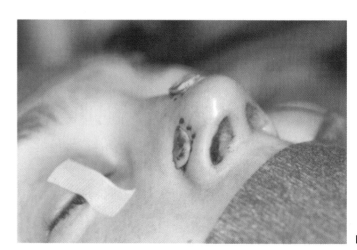

Fig. 5.**15** Use of a precision template for rhinoplasty.

and below the nasal mucosa (0.5–1 mucosal) along the lines for lateral osteotomies. For the cartilage-splitting approach, agent is injected beneath the vestibular skin until skin blanching is noted. A marginal incision in the alar cartilage requires only sparing infiltration along the cartilage rim. A small depot should always be placed over the nasal spine, premaxilla, and if necessary over the footplates of the medial crura. For skin incisions in the nasal base, agent is infiltrated along the intended lines of incision.

For the open approach, the anterior and lateral columella and the tissue between the domes are also infiltrated.

The septal mucosa is infiltrated with anesthetic solution in the subperichondrial plane. By placing carefully controlled pressure on the syringe, the surgeon can elevate the mucoperichondrium from the cartilage in the desired surgical plane (*hydraulic dissection*).

For endoscopic paranasal sinus surgery, the lateral nasal wall is infiltrated just in front of the head of the middle turbinate. The spread of the local anesthetic can be monitored by inspection with the 0° endoscope.

Marking the Operative Site

The proposed incisions should be marked on the nose before the operation is begun. A *rhinoplasty template* (Karl Storz, Tuttlingen) can be used for preoperative marking that is accurate to the millimeter.

Anesthetic Management in Rhinoplastic Operations

M. Goldstein

For operations that involve very pain-sensitive anatomical structures in the head and face, general anesthesia is the most effective way to reduce intraoperative stress responses. Combined with endotracheal intubation, it affords greater protection from the aspiration of secretions and blood compared with the combination of local anesthesia and analgosedation.

An essential component of anesthetic management is a detailed, confidence-building preoperative consultation with the patient.

On the day of the surgery, the patient is given oral midazolam for anxiolysis 45–60 minutes before the start of the operation.

The intravenous anesthetic agents propofol and remifentanil are used in combination as an alternative to inhalation anesthesia. *Total intravenous anesthesia* (TIVA) has a number of advantages over inhalation anesthesia:

- TIVA avoids all potential effects of halogenated hydrocarbons and nitrous oxide on the operating room personnel.
- There are no effects on gas-filled body cavities with the risk of pressure elevation due to changes in gas partial pressures.
- Continuous infusion rather than a bolus injection provides for a gentler, more comfortable induction of anesthesia.
- Both agents allow for excellent depth-of-anesthesia control ("on-off anesthesia"). In the case of remifentanil, it takes only a few minutes after administration is completed for the active level to fall by 50% (context-sensitive half-time), resulting in swifter anesthesia induction and shorter times to establish a new steady-state concentration after a change in infusion rate.
- The combined action of both agents on the respiratory center generally results in complete respiratory depression. This effect and the essential absence of intermittent motor activity obviate the need for repetitive doses of muscle relaxants.
- A marked reduction in the frequency of postoperative nausea and vomiting (PONV) compared with inhalation agents and nitrous oxide not only increases postoperative well-being but also reduces events (vomiting) that are associated with severe blood pressure elevation in the operative area. Oral feeding can be resumed immediately after recovery.
- Cognitive faculties are subject to very short recovery times.

The simplest method for the induction and maintenance of TIVA is the use of conventional syringe pumps, in which the dosage of propofol and remifentanil is adjusted for the patient's body weight and delivered at a specified rate in mL per unit time.

In *target-controlled infusion* (TCI), specially programmed syringe pumps are used to set and maintain the target concentration of the agents in the blood. After the anesthetist enters the desired blood level for inducing and maintaining the anesthesia, along with the patient's age and weight, the TCI perfusor calculates and injects the necessary dose of the agents. The tendency of propofol to accumulate is taken into account by reducing the administered volume with increasing duration of anesthesia. In this way TCI can avoid overdosing and reduce costs (22).

The combination of TCI with individual electroencephalogram (EEG) recording (e.g., using the processed EEG of the Narcotrend EEG monitor), setting Kugler stage D1–D2 as the targeted goal for the depth of anesthesia, leads to an accurate determination of the actual anesthetic requirement for any given patient (23, 24, 25, 26). Use of the processed EEG for monitoring and controlling the depth of anesthesia thus offers additional advantages:

- It avoids intraoperative wakefulness (probability of awareness: 0.2% = 1 case in 500 general anesthesias) (27).
- It shortens recovery times by avoiding undetected overdosing.

Due to the absence of analgesic hangover effects, TIVA with propofol and remifentanil requires the intraoperative initiation of pain therapy. Local anesthesia administered by the surgeon while the patient is still under general anesthesia, combined with systemically administered analgesics, will provide several hours of postoperative pain reduction or relief, which is then continued on the ward with an individual pain control regimen (26).

The resulting increase in subjective well-being will generally shorten the duration of postoperative immobilization.

Interactions among anesthetics, blood pressure response, and peripheral resistance on the one hand, combined with the intraoperative bleeding tendency that exists in plastic and otorhinolaryngological surgery, has prompted considerable research and discussion.

Propofol consistently lowers the blood pressure when administered at ordinary clinical doses. Several experimental studies attribute this effect to direct smooth-muscle relaxation in venous and arterial vessels (28, 29).

A direct smooth-muscle–mediated vasodilating action has not been confirmed at clinically relevant concentrations (30, 31), and low concentrations of propofol can even produce a vasoconstrictor effect (30).

The blood pressure response to propofol can also be interpreted as the result of different cardiovascular variables (32).

The inhibition of sympathetic-mediated vasoconstriction observed in several studies appears to be the most likely cause of the fall in blood pressure (33, 34).

To date there have been no high-quality comparative or controlled studies proving that the propofol-induced fall in blood pressure due to sympathetic inhibition has quantitative effects on intravenous hemorrhage.

References

1. Angle EH. *Die Okklusionsanomalien der Zähne.* 2nd ed. Berlin: Meusser: 1913.
2. Baud Ch. *Harmonie der Gesichtszüge.* La Chaux de Fonds: Clinique de la Tour: 1967.
3. Becker OJ. Rhinoplasty: Cultural, esthetic and psychological aspects. *Chicago Med.* 1961; 64:15.
4. Behrbohm H, Kaschke O, Nawka T. *Endoskopische Diagnostik und Therapie in der HNO.* Stuttgart: Gustav Fischer: 1997.
5. Behrbohm H. Septorhinoplastik–klinische Geometrie und virtuelle Op-Planung. *HNO-Nach.* 2001; 31:24–29.
6. Behrbohm H. Klinische Geometrie bei der Septorhinoplastik. *Mitteilungen. Norddeutsche Gesellschaft für ORL, Demeter.* 2002; 2:22–24.
7. Biemer E. Kommentar zu: Gestörte Körperwahrnehmung. *HNO akt.* 2001; 9:229–230.
8. Daley J. Introduction of an artistic point of view in regard to rhinoplastic diagnosis. *Arch.Otolaryngol.* 1945; 42:33.
9. Goin JM, Goin MK. *Changing the body: Psychological effects of plastic surgery.* Baltimore: Williams and Wilkins: 1981:121–143.
10. Gudziol H, Förster G. Zur Durchführung präoperativer Riechtests aus medikolegaler Sicht. *Laryngo-Rhino-Otol.* 2002; 81:586–590.
11. Hinderer VT. Dr. Vazquez Anon's last lesson. *Aesth Plast Surg.* 1978; 2:375–382.
12. Hirche W. *Arztrecht kompakt. Juristischer Ratgeber für die Arztpraxis.* München: MD-Verlag: 1994.
13. Lang J. *Klinische Anatomie der Nase, Nasenhöhle und Nebenhöhlen. Grundlagen für Diagnostik und Operation.* Stuttgart: Thieme: 1988.
14. Linfert A. *Von Polyklet zu Lysipp.* Dissertation, Freiburg: 1965
15. Naumann HH. Rhinologische Grundlagen und Indikationen für korrigierende plastische Eingriffe im Nasenbereich. In Gohrbrandt EJ, Gabka A, Berndorfer, eds. *Handbuch der plastischen Chirurgie, Vol. II.* Berlin: De Gryter: 1966:1–44.
16. Powell N, Humphreys B. *Proportions of the aesthetic face.* Stuttgart: Thieme:1984.
17. Rakosi T, Jonas J. *Kieferorthopädie. Diagnostik.* Stuttgart: Thieme: 1989.
18. Rohrich R. The who, what, when and why of cosmetic surgery: Do our patients need a preoperative psychiatric evaluation? *Plast. Reconstr. Surg.* 2000; 106:1605–1607.
19. Tardy ME. *Rhinoplasty: The art and the science. Vol. I.* Philadelphia: WB Saunders: 1997.
20. Wright MR. Management of patient dissatisfaction with results of cosmetic procedures. *Arch Otolaryngol Head Neck Surg.* 1980; 106:466–471.
21. Zhai LJ, Bruintjes Tj,D, Boschma Th, Huzing EH. The interdomal ligament does not exist. *Rhinology.* 1995; 33:135–137.
22. Bruhn J, Röpcke H, Bouillon T. Target-controlled Infusion (TCI): Die Verabreichung intravenöser Anästhetika mit computergesteuerten Spritzenpumpen. Anästhesiol Intensivmed. 2002; 43:547-557.
23. Schultz B, Grouven U, Schultz A. Automatic classification algorithms of the EEG monitor Narcotrend for routinely recorded EEG data from general anaesthesia: a validation study. Biomed Tech (Berl). 2002; 47:9-13.
24. Raymondos K, Piepenbrock S, Hausdörfer J, Panning B, Grouven U. Automatic EEG classification with Narcotrend into general stages of anaesthesia during remifentanil/propofol TIVA in elective inpatient surgery . Eur J Anaesthesiol. 2000; 17(Suppl. 19):22.
25. Kraus G, Mogendorf F, Bartlog M, Grouven U, Schultz B. Propofoldosierungen und Aufwachzeiten bei Carotis-OPs ohne und mit EEG-Monitoring (Narcotrend®). Anästhesiol Intensivmed 2000, 41:390.
26. Sandin RH, Enlund G, Samuelsson P, Lenmarken C. Awareness during anaesthesia: a prospective case study. Lancet. 2000; 355:707-711.
27. Goldstein M. TIVA mit Disoprivan® und Ultiva® in Kombination mit Konzepten der Schmerztherapie. Symposium "Anästhesie und perioperative Schmerztherapie". Park-Klinik Weissensee, Berlin. May 2000.
28. Bentley GN, Gent JP, Goodchild CS. Vascular effects of propofol: sm ooth muscle relaxation in isolated veins and arteries J Pharm Pharmaco l. 1989; 41:797-798.
29. Muzi M, Berens RA, Kampine JP, Ebert TJ. Venodilation contributes to propofol-mediated hypotension in humans. Anesth Analg. 1992; 74:877-883.
30. Nakamura K, Hatano Y, Hirakata H, Nishiwada M, Toda H, Mori K. Direct vasoconstrictor and vasodilator effects of propofol in isolated dog arteries. Br J Anaesth. 1992; 86):193-197.
31. Mimaroglu C, Utkan T, Kaya T, Kafali H, Sarioglu Y. Effects of propofol on vascular smooth muscle function in isolated rat aorta. Methods Find Exp Clin Pharmacol. 1994; 16:257-261.
32. Robinson BJ, Buyck HC, Galletly DC. Effect of propofol on heart rate, arterial pressure and digital plethysmograph variability. Br J Anaesth. 1994; 73):167-173.
33. Krassioukov AV, Gelb AW, Weaver LC. Action of propofol on centrals ympathetic mechanisms controlling blood pressure. Can J Anaesth. 1993; 40:761-769.
34. Robinson BJ, Ebert TJ, O'Brien TJ, Colinco MD, Muzi MD. Mechanisms whereby propofol mediates peripheral vasolidation in humans. Anesthesi ology. 1997; 86:64-72.

Principles of Modern Septoplasty

T. Hildebrandt

Contents

Introduction

The cartilaginous septum is the central structural element of the nose and has much the same function as a tent pole. It provides suspension for the upper lateral cartilages and anchors the anterior nose to the facial skeleton. Many nasal deformities are associated with septal problems and are interdependent in their pathogenesis. Functionally, the nasal septum is part of the aerodynamic mechanism of the nose. Abnormalities in the ventilation function of the nose are most frequently caused by septal deformities.

In the early 1900s, Killian and Freer developed the concept of the submucous septal resection. Unlike their predecessors, they stressed the need to preserve the mucosal layers and took into account the supportive function of the septal cartilage, feeling it was essential to preserve a dorsal and caudal cartilage strut for support. This is a relatively straightforward procedure that can achieve reasonably good short-term results in many patients. As such, it was still being used by many surgeons in the 1980s, even though Cottle, Fomon, and Metzenbaum had already laid the foundation for modern septoplasty several decades earlier. This modern approach is based on the principle of preserving or reconstructing cartilaginous and bony structures. Typical long-term complications such as saddle nose deformity or septal perforations are considerably less common when this principle is followed.

Rather than exploring all aspects of septal operations in detail, this chapter deals more with general principles that will help the surgeon to view the nasal septum within the context of complex rhinosurgery and take into account the long-term effects of specific procedures. Viewed in this manner, procedures on the nasal septum should actually not be considered as operations for beginners.

Indications

A successful concept of functional–esthetic rhinosurgery requires studied consideration of the nasal septum. The septum has special significance because it is involved in almost every rhinological problem to some degree.

Besides the mostly elective procedures, septal revision is a very common operation in patients who have sustained midfacial trauma.

The basic functional goal of septal surgery is to promote optimum nasal airflow while improving the aeration and drainage of the paranasal sinus system. Adjunctive septal procedures may also be necessary to provide sufficient access for treating diseases of the paranasal sinuses and pituitary.

The septum may also have a direct or indirect role in solving esthetic problems of the nose. For example, a saddle nose, tension nose, or crooked nose usually cannot be satisfactorily corrected without a septoplasty. At the same time, altering the septal cartilage can also affect the appearance of the nasal tip.

Strict criteria should be applied in selecting children for septal surgery. When atraumatic, structure-conserving techniques are used, the surgical correction of an obstructive deviated septum may be considered as early as four to six years of age. Whenever possible, major resections of the vomer should be avoided before 12 years of age (18).

Contraindications

Septal deviation in itself is not an indication for surgery. It is rare to find a perfectly straight septum, and ridges on the premaxilla are considered normal to some degree. Ideally, functional deficits should be detectable by objective measurements before they are considered an indication for surgery. But at the same time, surgery is not routinely indicated whenever an objective, septum-related functional deficit is found. It is not uncommon for surgeons to recommend a septal correction merely because of an incidental finding that is not associated with actual complaints. In some circumstances, the subjective discomfort of the patient can be as much of a concern in functional septal surgery as it is in esthetic rhinoplasty.

Preoperative Considerations

It should be established preoperatively whether the septoplasty is being done purely for functional improvement, is part of a complex operation with both functional and esthetic goals, or is a means for effecting purely esthetic changes in the shape of the nose. The intents of septoplasty can have various implications, such as the deliberate decision to leave a functionally significant septal deviation alone in selected patients. In some rhinoplasties that involve the broad mobilization of anatomical structures, the septum may provide a secure pillar that can prevent dynamic instability of the nasal skeleton. Consequently, the patient should understand that it may be necessary to accept a certain disparity in nasal breathing between the two sides of the nose—although a severe airway obstruction should not be allowed to persist. Similarly, the patient should be informed that undesired changes in the shape of the nose may occur that require immediate additional rhinoplasty or that become apparent only at follow-up. For this reason, it is advisable to obtain photographic documentation even for a "simple" septoplasty.

Septum and Turbinates

The goal of function-improving rhinoplasty should not be to transform the nasal airway into a clear cavity that allows maximum theoretical airflow through the nose. It is important to recognize that the septum, the turbinates, and the lateral nasal wall act in concert to create an efficient aerodynamic system. These structures are separated by a variable, cleftlike space that regulates the airflow velocity and ideally provides an optimum spatial and temporal balance of both laminar and turbulent flow. From a surgical standpoint as well, the septum and turbinates should be regarded as a unit. Before correcting the septum, it may be necessary in some cases for the surgeon to lateralize or "trim" the middle and/or inferior turbinates to create sufficient space on the concave side. Regardless of the specific method used, the medial mucosa should be left alone and the airfoil-like contour should remain largely intact. Septal and turbinate surgery should always be carefully coordinated. There is no justification for a general, "routine" turbinectomy (7).

Preoperative Analysis

Besides a detailed history, there are three basic steps for analyzing the preoperative septal findings and classifying them in a rhinological context:

Clinical Examination

The clinical examination should always include endoscopy of the nasal cavity. Endoscopy can reliably detect bony deviations or spurs located far back in the nose along with any preexisting posterior perforations. Endoscopy also makes it easier to determine whether a significant concha bullosa is present. Detailed inspection of the middle meatus and sphenoethmoid recess can provide evidence of chronic sinusitis. Classic anterior rhinoscopy is more useful for evaluating the septum-related component of nasal valve stenosis. Endoscopy and anterior rhinoscopy should be repeated after the mucosae have been decongested. Palpation of the entire nasal skeleton also adds essential information for preoperative planning.

It may be necessary to apply special preoperative care measures or administer perioperative cortisone therapy, depending on the condition of the mucosae.

Function Studies

Today the preoperative and postoperative use of rhinomanometry, supplemented if necessary by rhinoacoustic testing, has become a standard tool for objectifying the subjective assessment of nasal breathing by the doctor and patient and for obtaining quantitative information. Olfactometry is recommended before every septoplasty, chiefly for medicolegal reasons.

Imaging Studies

With clear-cut septal findings, a negative history, and no abnormalities by nasal endoscopy, plain radiographs of the paranasal sinuses are sufficient to exclude serious chronic sinusitis. Subtle changes in the ethmoid labyrinth, which are sometimes responsible for functional deficits, can be detected only by coronal computed tomography (CT). Coronal CT is also better for defining the lumen and extent of a concha bullosa that requires surgery, allowing for a more precise and less traumatic operating technique.

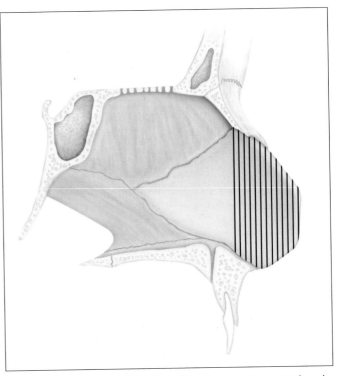

Fig. 6.**1**   The shaded caudal portion of the septal cartilage provides adequate support for the cartilaginous nasal dorsum.

Structural Principles of the Nasal Skeleton and their Surgical Significance

The Static Function of the Septum

The caudal portion of the septal cartilage, located past a line connecting the distal nasal bone to the anterior premaxilla, is responsible for providing support to the middle third of the nasal dorsum and the nasal tip (Fig. 6.**1**).

In terms of surgical anatomy, it is sufficient to subdivide the nasal septum into a caudal part and a cranial part. Although the septum is commonly subdivided into five portions, this has little practical relevance. An area of particular importance is the attachment of the septal cartilage and upper lateral cartilages to the bony nasal pyramid. This "K area," as called by Cottle, should not be unnecessarily weakened or destabilized at operation.

The static supporting function of the caudal septal cartilage is sensitive to disruption. This relates to intrinsic cartilaginous factors, on the one hand, and also to the way in which the cartilage is embedded in the surrounding structures. It is sometimes noted that even the slightest mobilization of the septal cartilage leads to a sudden, disproportionately strong decline in its supportive function. The situation is comparable to releasing the lock on a tightened spring. This phenomenon occurs mainly in conjunction with a weak K area, a relatively small nasal pyramid, and/or a very flexible septal cartilage that provides effective structural support only when it is stiffened by a certain degree of torsion.

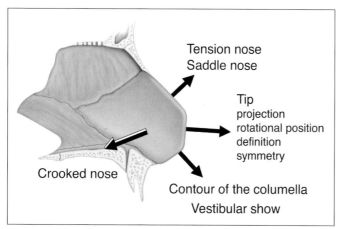

Fig. 6.**2**   Possible effects of the septal cartilage on the shape of the external nose.

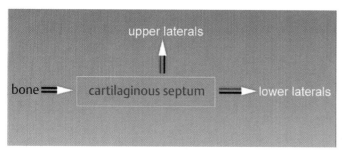

Fig. 6.**3**   Cascade of centrifugally arranged, superimposed extrinsic and intrinsic factors that shape the nasal skeleton. The septum as the central structural element "gets, has, and gives shape."

Superimposing Extrinsic and Intrinsic Morphological Features

Because of its central anatomical position, changes in the septal cartilage can have effects on the shape of the nose. The nasal septum helps to define the facial profile, contributes to axial deformities, and influences the esthetics of the nasal tip (Fig. 6.**2**). Very generally this relates to a deficiency or excess of cartilaginous substance within the sagittal plane or, in the case of the crooked nose, to deviation of the cartilaginous quadrangular plate from a sagittal alignment.

The structural analysis of nasal anatomy reveals a general principle whereby extrinsic and intrinsic factors interact in determining the shape of the internal and external nose. Starting from the bony components of the nasal skeleton, certain morphological features are transmitted in a centrifugal pattern, mainly via the quadrangular plate, to the cartilaginous nasal dorsum, the nasal tip, and the columella. The septal cartilage is held by its outer bony frame in a state of partial elastic deformation. This reversible elastic deformation is superimposed upon the intrinsic shape of the septal cartilage, and both of these in turn have an extrinsic effect on the distally located upper lateral and alar cartilages, which have their own intrinsic shape (Fig. 6.**3**).

Influence of the Septum on the Esthetics of the Nasal Tip

The esthetics of the nasal tip can be characterized reasonably well in terms of several criteria: projection, rotational position, definition, and symmetry. This simplified formula gives us a framework to systemize the desired or undesired effects of septal surgery on the appearance of the nasal tip. A useful tool in this regard is the Anderson tripod model to which the septum is added. Originally, Anderson used this model to show the interdependence of nasal tip projection and rotation, as in the resective surgery of the alar cartilages. If we include the septum in the model, it becomes clear how carefully coordinated septal and alar cartilage surgery must be, especially with regard to nasal tip rotation (Fig. 6.**4a–d**).

It is very often desirable in nasal tip surgery to produce cranial rotation of the tip. Measures on the lateral crura of the alar cartilages can be supplemented by a wedge excision to shorten the caudal septal margin (possibly including mucosa and portions of the membranous septum) and thus produce a synergistic rotation effect. Removing a basal cartilage strip can also produce tip rotation, provided the quadrangular plate has been separated from the perpendicular plate. This effect is associated with a loss of projection, however (Fig. 6.**4b**).

Overresection of the caudal septal margin, especially in a patient with very long alar lateral crura, and weakly developed medial crura can lead to retraction of the columella and unintended downward rotation of the nasal tip (Fig. 6.**4c**).

If there is too little work done on the lateral crura in relation to the resections on the septum to produce the desired cranial rotation, the angle between the lateral crura will be increased. This means a "blunting" of the nasal tip, or loss of tip definition. The rhomboid of the nasal tip is flattened and enlarged (Fig. 6.**4d**).

The extreme form of this case occurs if a saddle nose deformity develops. Depression in the middle third of the nasal dorsum is caused by a considerable loss of substance in the septal cartilage. The nasal tip loses projection, shows relative cranial rotation, and has an amorphous appearance (Fig. 6.**8**). The opposite effect is visible in the condition of a tension nose. The small angle between the lateral crura is partially due to a high septum.

The causes of the nasal tip asymmetry reside in the alar cartilages themselves and also in the effect of more proximal structures (see above). Bowing of the caudal septal cartilage is the most frequent extrinsic reason for distortion of the nasal tip.

Mechanical Uncoupling

The following practical conclusion can be drawn from the general structural principle of the nasal skeleton as a three-part, proximal-to-distal cascade of extrinsic and intrinsic shaping features: It is a good idea in septorhinoplasties to separate these three compartments in the proximal-to-distal direction, with preservation of the K area, before attempting to resect or reshape particular cartilage structures. This "mechanical uncoupling" is necessary so that the purely intrinsic shape characteristics of the septal cartilage, upper lateral cartilages, and alar cartilages can be clearly appreciated and operated

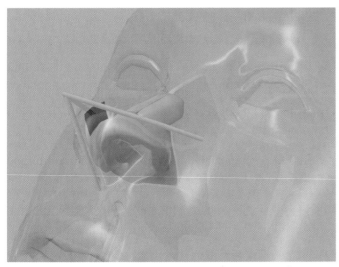

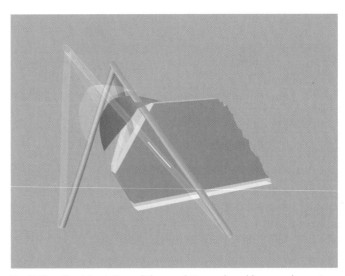

Fig. 6.**4**   The influence of altering the septal cartilage on the estetics of the nasal tip. **a** The tripod as a model for the alar cartilage complex in conjunction with the nasal septum. The rhomboid area between the supratip break point, the infratip break point, and the two tip-defining points describes the nasal tip area.

Fig. 6.**4b**   Cranial rotation of the nasal tip produced by complementary resections of the septum and lateral crura; unfortunately associated with a certain loss of projection.

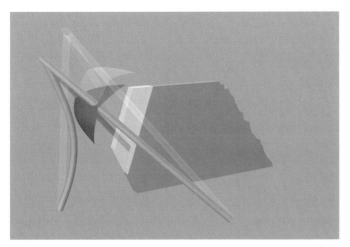

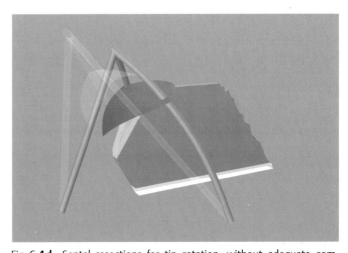

Fig. 6.**4c**   Overresection of the caudal septal margin can lead to downward rotation of the nasal tip, retraction of the columella, and significant loss of projection.

Fig. 6.**4d**   Septal resections for tip rotation, without adequate complementary correction of the alar cartilages, can reduce the definition of the nasal tip. This is illustrated in the figure by the flattened and enlarged tip area.

◁ Fig. 6.**5**   The typical, most frequent formation of bone and cartilage in septal deviations. The deformity of the perpendicular plate and vomer produce an extrinsic effect that also deforms the quadrangular plate. The cartilage may additionally show intrinsic deviation.

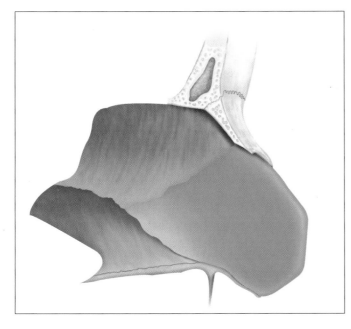

with good precision. The more complex the nasal deformities, the more important it is to strictly apply this operative strategy.

A common place phenomenon in septoplasty is a good example for the effectiveness of this surgical principle. Following complete separation of the basal and posterior osseocartilaginous junction, it is quite often to find an essentially straight, centrally positioned septal cartilage plate. Experience shows that a large percentage of septal deviations are caused almost entirely by a ridgelike fusion of the perpendicular plate and vomer. They are both laterally deviated toward the same side and deform the quadrangular plate. The cartilage may additionally show intrinsic deviation (Fig. 6.**5**).

In 1965 Gray also distinguished a purely cartilaginous septal deviation from the dominant osseocartilaginous type noted above. This nontraumatic septal deformity is believed to result from asymmetrical growth deformity processes in the fetal period and during puberty (Lang 1987, 25). Its prevalence in the general population might even be interpreted as an evolutionary selection advantage that reduces the risk of skull base impression caused by direct frontal trauma to the nose. The septal asymmetry possibly helps to redirect force vectors away from the skull base, reducing the risk of life-threatening injury.

Surgical Technique

A septoplasty generally consists of three steps:
1. Dissection and exposure
2. Mobilization and resection or correction
3. Reconstruction

Dissection and Exposure

The standard approach for septoplasty is the hemitransfixion incision. It preserves the attachment of the footplates to the caudal septal margin and provides good access to all portions of the cartilaginous and bony septum. The septum can also be exposed through posterior mucosal incisions, which are used mainly for endoscopic septal corrections that are done as an adjunct to paranasal sinus surgery. Septal operations that are combined with rhinoplasty are often performed through a transfixion incision. In open rhinoplasty, the mucosal layers can also be dissected from the upper lateral and alar cartilages. It is sometimes helpful to combine this approach by additional incisions for instance such as hemitransfixion or transfixion incision.

The surgeon should take the findings into account when creating the mucosal tunnels. The routine development of bilateral superior and inferior tunnels is not advised, but more extensive tunnels can be helpful for more complex deformities. The inferior tunnels are often easier to develop in a retrograde fashion. The maxillo–premaxillary approach described by Cottle (exposure of the spine and crest of the piriform aperture) is necessary in only a relatively few cases. The surgeon should pay attention to the incisive nerve when defining the lateral extent of the inferior tunnels. The key to an atraumatic dissection is to maintain a strict subperichondrial and subperiosteal plane of approach. Connective tissue fibers at the osseocartilaginous junction in the area of the premaxilla should be sharply divided. The same generally applies to scars in postoperative or posttraumatic cases.

In the great majority of cases, all or part of the mucosa can be left adherent to the cartilage on one side. In cases where the quadrangular plate is widely mobilized, this will effectively hold the cartilage plate in its original anatomical position and facilitate the reconstruction.

Many surgeons elevate the mucosa on the concave side first, because the mucosa on that side is under less tension when a marked deviation exists. If the mucosal dissection is started on the convex side, it may be easier to identify the apex more precisely, assess how much the deviated area contributes to structural support, and determine how much can be re-

sected if necessary. In cases with a very prominent or sharp-angled deviation, it is advisable to change to the opposite side with a vertical chondrotomy just in front of the deviation and then completely elevate the mucosa on the convex side after the cartilage has been mobilized.

Mobilization and Resection

Once the septum has been exposed through a suitable approach, the correction should be carried out in a posterior-to-anterior direction if possible, conforming to the structural principle of the nose explained above. The first step, then, is to correct the elastic deformation of the septal cartilage by its bony frame. Disconnecting the bony and cartilaginous portions of the septum is most effective and provides the best exposure when combined with temporary partial resection of the perpendicular plate and vomer. Sometimes, deviations of the vomer can be reduced in situ by fracturing. These measures should be limited geared toward the local findings and conform to the overall concept. At last, a "swinging door" is created by instrumental or manual disarticulation of the quadrangular plate from the premaxilla. This removes all tension from the cartilage, allowing the surgeon to make a definitive assessment of the intrinsic pathology. The sagittal extent of the cartilage plate can be modified as needed on its basal, caudal, and dorsal aspects. Also, significant deviations from the sagittal plane can be straightened.

From a didactic standpoint, it is helpful to distinguish between angular and curved cartilage deviations. Both can also lead to subluxation of the caudal septal margin. Angular deviations are often vertical and are correctible with a segmental resection, combined if necessary with suture reapproximation of the resection margins. Not infrequently, this type of deviation is accompanied by local areas of cartilage thickening. This makes it possible to remove cartilage tangentially without causing significant loss of continuity in the sagittal plane and without compromising the supportive function of the cartilage.

Large, curved deviations are more difficult to deal with surgically than angular deviations, especially when they also constrict the nasal valve.

Deep cartilage incisions that are made on the concave side in the direction in which the deviation is oriented can in some cases reduce or even reverse the bowing tendency of the cartilage. This allows the intrinsic tensile forces in the tissue to establish a new equilibrium (12). It should be added that this also reduces the mechanical strength of the cartilage. If necessary, the bending effect can be reinforced with a through-and-through mattress suture according the tension-band principle.

When the mucosa is left intact on one side, the convexity of the cartilaginous septum can be reduced over a circumscribed area by outlining one or more cartilage islands with chondrotomies and moving them closer to the midline. This technique can be particularly helpful in cases where a curved septal deviation has caused nasal valve stenosis. In some cases these cartilage areas can also be morselized and straightened in situ after the mucosa has been elevated on both sides.

If the bowing extends into the nasal dorsum, it is advisable to separate the upper lateral cartilages from the septum in order to achieve an adequate correction. A meticulous reconstruction of the cartilaginous nasal dorsum should be carried out.

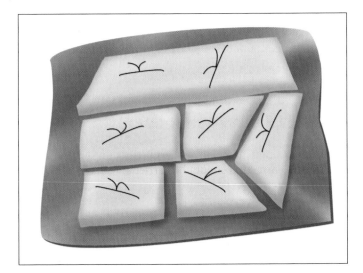

Fig. 6.**6**   Compound graft for septal reconstruction consisting of a PDS foil and cartilage grafts sutured onto it.

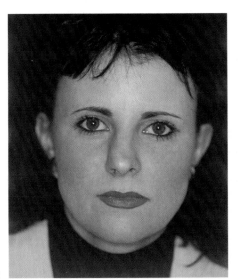

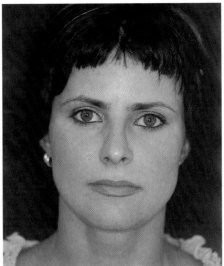

a

b

Fig. 6.**7 a–d**   Osseocartilaginous deviation as a result of early childhood trauma with a tension septum and overprojected nasal tip. The condition was corrected by an open septorhinoplasty.

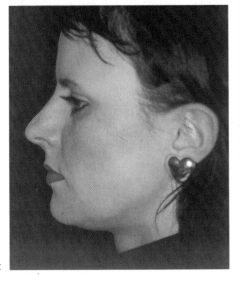

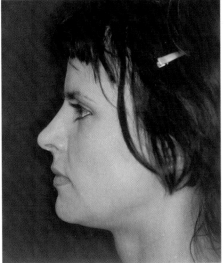

c

d

Reconstruction

With very complex or extreme septal cartilage deformities, it is best in some cases to resect all of the cartilage and construct a neoseptum. The so-called compound graft has yielded good re-

sults in such cases (9). A sheet of polydioxanone suture (PDS) can serve as a scaffold for several small, autologous cartilage grafts. This provides a sturdy construction whose size can be adjusted as needed after the grafts are in place (Fig. 6.**6**). Even very large septal cartilage defects (due to trauma or previous surgery) can be reconstructed with this technique, for example

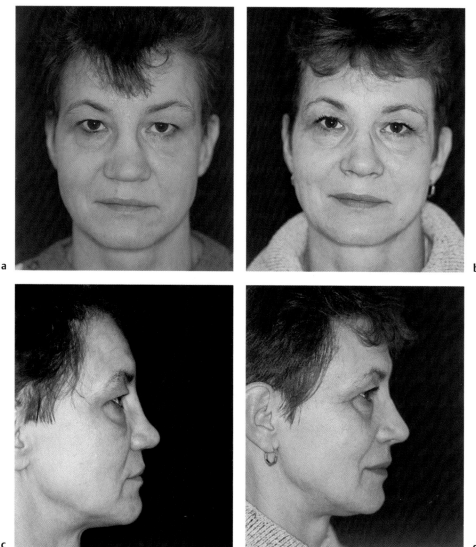

a

b

c

d

Fig. 6.**8 a–d**   Postoperative saddle nose. Septal reconstruction with a compound graft.

by using auricular cartilage. Thus, costal cartilage harvesting is often avoidable.

At the end of every septoplasty, the surgeon must make certain that all supportive cartilage structures are in a secure position. This may require the use of a spine suture in some cases. While performing the operation, the surgeon should constantly gear his actions toward the preservation or controlled modification of the supporting function of the septum. Repeated intraoperative palpation of the entire nose is the only way to gain an accurate impression in this regard.

Any defects that remain in the bony septum should be repaired in mosaic fashion with suitable pieces of bone and/or cartilage. This will prevent the development of mucosal atrophy. The flexibility of the repaired area, similar to that of a chain link, allows for good adaptation of the postoperative packing.

If only small, slitlike mucosal perforations have occurred during the operation, there is no urgent need to suture them. They can even provide useful drainage, provided they are not located at corresponding sites. Silicone endoprostheses (e.g., Doyle splints) are particularly advantageous for temporary postoperative packing or splinting. They provide mechanical strength, reduce edema formation, and create a moist milieu that promotes mucosal regeneration. Generally these splints are well tolerated and can be left in place for several days if necessary.

References

1. Aiach G. *Atlas of rhinoplasty: Open and endonasal approaches*. St. Louis: Quality Medical Publishing, Inc.: 1996.
2. Anderson JR. A reasoned approach to nasal base surgery. *Arch Otolaryngol.* 1984; 110:349–358.
3. Anderson JR. The dynamics of rhinoplasty. In *Proceedings of the Ninth International Congress in Otolaryngology.* Amsterdam: Experta Medica: 1969:206.
4. Anderson JR. Ries WR, *Rhinoplasty Emphasizing the External Approach.* Stuttgart-New York: Thieme; 1986.
5. Behrbohm H, Hildebrandt T, Kaschke O. *Funktionell-Ästhetische Chirurgie der Nase.* Tuttlingen: Endopress: 2001.
6. Behrbohm H, Hildebrandt T, Kaschke O, Jahnke V. Funktionell-ästhetische Chirurgie der Nase—Ziele, präoperative Diagnostik, Operationsplanung. *HNO aktuell.* 2000; 8:129–137.
7. Behrbohm H., Kaschke O, Nawka T. *Endoskopische Diagnostik und Therapie in der HNO.* Stuttgart: Fischer: 1997.

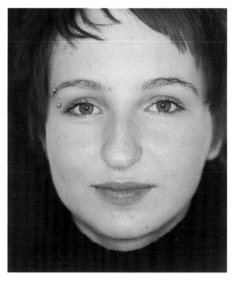
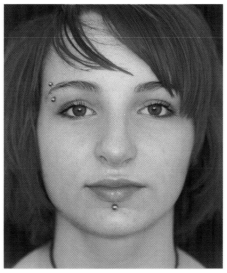

a   b

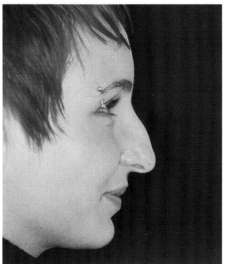
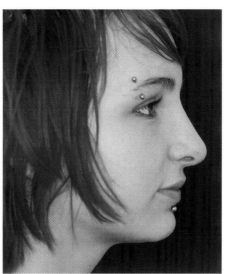

c   d

Fig. 6.**9 a–d** Long, humped nose. Managed by complementary correction of the septum and alar cartilage complex through an open approach.

8. Bönisch M, Mink A. Heilungsprozess des Knorpels in Verbindung mit PDS-Folie. *HNO*. 2000; 10:743–746.

9. Bönisch M, Mink A. Septumrekonstruktion mit PDS-Folie. *HNO*. 1999; 47:546–550.

10. Cottle MH, et al. The "maxilla-premaxilla" approach to extensive nasal septum surgery. *Arch Otolaryngol*. 1958; 68:301.

11. Cottle MH, Loring RM. Surgery of the nasal septum. New operating procedures and indications. *Ann Otol (St. Louis)*. 1948; 57:707.

12. Fry HJ. Interlocked stress in human septal cartilage. *Br J Plast Surg*. 1966; 18:276.

13. Fry HJ. Nasal skeletal trauma and the nasal septal cartilage . *Br J Plast Surg*. 1967; 20:146.

14. Gray L. The deviated nasal septum-I-Aetiology. *J Laryng*. 1965a; 79:567–575.

15. Gubisch W. Das schwierige Septum. *HNO*. 1998; 36:286–289.

16. Hildebrandt T, Behrbohm H. Functional aesthetic surgery of the nose—the influence of the septum on the aesthetics of the nasal tip. CD-ROM KS 533; Karl-Storz MediaSercice: 2001.

17. Hildebrandt T, Behrbohm H, Jahnke V, Kaschke O. Neue Aspekte der Septumplastik bei Nasenkorrekturen. *HNO aktuell*. 2000; 8:161–170.

18. Kastenbauer E R, Masing H. Chirurgie der inneren Nase—Versorgung von Nasenverletzungen. In Naumann HH, Helms J, Herberhold RA, Jahrsdoerfer ER, Kastenbauer ER, Panje WR, Tardy ME, *Kopf- und Hals-Chirurgie* Vol.1, Part I. Stuttgart-New York: Thieme; 1995:361–446.

19. Killian G. Die submuköse Fensterresektion der Nasenscheidewand. *Arch Laryng Rhin* (Berlin). 1904; 16:326

20. Lang J. Klinische Anatomie der Nase, Nasenhöhle und Nebenhöhlen. *Aktuelle Oto-Rhino-Laryngologie*. Stuttgart-New York: Thieme: 1988: Vol.11.

21. Masing H, Rettinger G. Eingriffe an der Nase. In Theissing J, *Mund-, Hals- und Nasenoperationen*. Stuttgart-New York: Thieme: 1988:49–114.

22. Metzenbaum M. Replacement of the lower end of the dislocated septal cartilage versus submucous resection of the dislocated end of the septal cartilage. *Arch Otolaryngol*. 1929; 9:282.

23. Middelwerd M J. Septoplasty and turbinate surgery. In: Nolst Trenité G J. *Rhinoplasty—A practical guide to functional and aesthetic surgery of the nose*. Amsterdam-New York: Kugler: 1992:37–43.

24. Nolst Trenité GJ. *Rhinoplasty—A practical guide to functional and aesthetic surgery of the nose*. Amsterdam-New York: Kugler: 1992.

25. Takahashi R. The evolution of the nasal septum and the formation of septal deformity. *Rhinology*. 1988; Suppl. 6.

26. Tardy ME. *Rhinoplasty: The art and the science*. Philadelphia: WB Saunders: 1997.

27. Walter C. *Plastisch-chirurgische Eingriffe im Kopf-Hals-Bereich*. Stuttgart-New York: Thieme: 1997.

Open Structure Rhinoplasty

D. W. Kim and D. M. Toriumi

Contents

Introduction

The primary objective of rhinoplasty is to create predictable changes in nasal contour while maximizing nasal function. Reproducible, consistent outcomes in rhinoplasty come with the surgeon's ability to create a stable nasal structure and predict the effects of scar contracture on this structure. In complex cases, endonasal approaches may not provide the exposure needed to execute complex grafting. The external approach allows maximal exposure of the cartilaginous nasal structures, bony vault, and septum. The surgeon is thus able to directly visualize the repositioning, alteration, and augmentation of the nasal structures.

Joseph and Gillies both reported cases utilizing an open approach to rhinoplasty in the early part of the 20th century. Over the ensuing decades, the technique evolved to include a transcolumellar incision which extended onto the vestibular skin allowing for wider exposure. In North America, the approach has steadily gained in popularity since its introduction by Padovan in 1970. Early criticism of the visible columellar scar has been addressed by numerous reports of favorable results with scar camouflage.

One must remember that external rhinoplasty is only a means to access the underlying nasal structures. Once exposure is achieved, there are a multitude of maneuvers that may be executed depending on the patient's individual anatomy. A description of the external approach itself and the maneuvers commonly performed during structural rhinoplasty are presented in the following.

Indications

While there are no absolute indications to external rhinoplasty, there are certain problems which are best corrected through techniques requiring wide exposure. In general these methods involve extensive rearrangement of existing structures or addition of structural grafts. Indications include:
1. Significant tip deformity with an asymmetric, ptotic, overprojected/underprojected, bulbous, or buckled tip structure.
2. Secondary rhinoplasty—previously disrupted structural supports may need to be reconstituted or replaced.
3. Non-Caucasian rhinoplasty—may require significant increases in projection and support of inherently weak alar cartilages.
4. Cleft lip nasal deformity.
5. Crooked nose—may require precise repositioning of upper or lower lateral cartilages (LLC) or extensive septal correction or reconstruction.
6. Major nasal reconstruction.
7. Unclear diagnosis—in cases in which the surgeon is uncertain as to the anatomical cause of the deformity, the external approach allows for accurate diagnosis prior to structural modification.

Contraindications

A relative contraindication to the external approach for rhinoplasty is the presence of severely damaged or thinned skin. Such conditions may occur following multiple previous operations, particularly in thin skinned individuals. The presence of acquired cutaneous telangiectasias, purple or blue discoloration of the nasal skin with cold temperature, and visible irregularities are signs of such a condition. In these cases, an endonasal approach with limited soft-tissue elevation may reduce the risk of further cutaneous compromise.

Alternative Techniques

Although there are no absolute contraindications to the external approach during rhinoplasty, an endonasal approach may be a reasonable alternative in cases in which minimal changes are required.

Nondelivery approaches have the advantage of preserving all major tip support mechanisms of the nose. Access may be gained through a cartilage-splitting or retrograde approach. The main disadvantage of these approaches is the limited exposure of the tip cartilages. While the delivery approach provides greater exposure than nondelivery approaches, it does so at the cost of compromising tip support. Specifically, the intercartilaginous incision disrupts the attachment of the upper lateral cartilages (ULCs) and LLCs. Although the lower lateral crura are widely exposed with this method, the chondrocutaneous flap is delivered in a nonanatomical orientation, creating potential difficulty for the inexperienced surgeon.

Preoperative Considerations

In all rhinoplasty, a clear understanding must be reached between surgeon and patient regarding the perceived nasal deformities, surgical plan, and expected outcomes. The relationship between nasal airway function and appearance must be emphasized.

It is imperative that the patient understand that the postoperative period is a prolonged and dynamic process. Initially, the patient must anticipate a significant amount of swelling which will slowly subside. Over the ensuing months and years, ongoing resolution of edema and contraction of the soft-tissue envelope will create more definition to the nose. The patient must therefore be prepared to wait for several months for a significant improvement from surgery. This is especially true for thick skinned individuals, revision patients requiring extensive manipulations, or patients with only subtle problems. The patient should be aware that the incision on the columella will be visible for several weeks and will fade with time.

Photographic documentation is essential before and after surgery. Full face frontal, oblique, lateral images, and close-up base views are essential. Images should be obtained with dual flash sources angled 45° toward the patient. An additional frontal view taken with a single flash placed in front of and above the patient allows for shadowing which highlights the dorsal line. A blue screen or wall is ideal for establishing contrast between the patient and background. Standard 35 mm or digital photography are both viable options; at the time of writing, however, slides produced from a high-quality 35 mm camera provide better resolution and color than even the most advanced digital cameras. As technology advances, digital photography may eventually match or surpass traditional methods.

Computer image modification programs are commercially available and are becoming increasingly popular for consultation of cosmetic surgery patients. In rhinoplasty, these programs allow the consultant to alter a downloaded image on a computer screen in order to display the possible postoperative appearance of the nose. Such technology can facilitate a mutual understanding between patient and surgeon regarding surgical goals and expectations. As many patients enter the process with vague or unrealistic wishes or with an esthetic sense that conflicts with that of the surgeon, such programs may help to focus the patient's expectations toward a defined and reasonable goal.

Special Surgical Requirements

The patient should be advised to stop all blood thinning agents such as aspirin, ibuprofen, and vitamin E for at least two weeks prior to surgery. The individual should be in relatively good health and free of active nasal infection at the time of surgery. Any concerning medical condition should be cleared by the patient's primary care physician or appropriate consulting specialist.

It is the preference of the senior author to perform the operation under general anesthesic in order to protect the airway from dependent blood drainage. A single dose of i.v. cephalexin is given prior to the start of the case. If ear cartilage is to be harvested, an antipseudomonal agent such as ciprofloxacin is administered.

A standard rhinoplasty set should be available. The following is a list of essential instruments—the preference of the senior author is indicated in italics:
- #11 and #15 blade scalpels
- Assorted fine skin hooks
- Fine dissecting scissors—*Converse*
- Fine needle holders—*Webster and Castroviejo*
- Fine forceps—*Toothed adson and Bishop-Harmen*
- Tissue forceps—*Brown-Adson*
- Freer elevator
- Retractors—*Converse*
- Suture—*5.0 and 6.0 polydioxanone suture (PDS) for stabilization of cartilaginous grafts; 5.0 clear nylon for permanent suture modification to the shape of native cartilage; 4.0 plain gut on a straight septal needle for closure of septal flaps; 5.0 chromic for closure of vestibular skin incisions; 6.0 PDS for subcutaneous closure of columellar incision; and 7.0 nylon for columellar skin closure.*

Preoperative Analysis

The surgeon must note the thickness and sebaceous quality of the nasal skin–soft-tissue envelope (SSTE). In darker skinned individuals with thick skin, incisions may take longer to heal with increased potential for a visible scar. In addition, the underlying structural framework of the nose must push into the thick soft-tissue envelope in order for form to project through. Moreover, a significant tissue void in such patients will result in exuberant scar formation and poor definition, particularly in the tip and supra-tip areas. Thus the postoperative soft-tissue pollybeak may be prevented by avoiding overreduction of the structural framework of the thick skinned nose and opting instead to achieve balance by augmentation to areas of relative deficiency (Fig. 7.1). In thin skinned patients, there is more tolerance for leaving a small amount of dead space as a greater degree of soft-tissue contracture will allow for "truer" redraping. This advantage in thin skinned noses is counterbalanced by the added risk of contour irregularities becoming visible or palpable. Care must therefore be taken in ensuring that all existing bony and cartilaginous structures, grafts, and implants are precisely positioned and smoothly contoured (1).

It is crucial to obtain a clear idea of the patient's nasal airflow. Many patients present to the rhinoplasty surgeon with functional complaints, while others display variant anatomy which predisposes to postsurgical obstruction. Assessment should be undertaken prior to and after decongestion in order to differentiate between inflammatory and anatomical causes of obstruction. The surgeon must note the external stigmata of an obstructed nose or one that is prone to develop postoperative problems. These characteristics include thin SSTE, a narrow middle vault, short nasal bones, supra-alar pinching, narrow nasal base, a prominent supra-alar crease, narrow nostrils, and thin lateral nasal walls. Intranasal exam may reveal a narrow internal valve angle, dynamic lateral wall collapse, septal deviation, and inferior turbinate hypertrophy. All of these factors must be considered in formulating a surgical plan which will preserve a functional airway.

Cosmetic nasal analysis begins with a global assessment of the most apparent deformities. Often one or two areas are immediately noticeable to the observer. These may include a crooked dorsum, a large dorsal prominence, a bulbous tip, a dependent or foreshortened tip, or a wide base. It is useful to conceptualize a nose in terms of such traits so that priority can be given to these deformities during surgery. In rhinoplasty, each subunit of the nose affects the appearance of the other subunits. Thus, in order to create a natural well-proportioned appearance, the surgeon modifies a given subunit based on the status of adjacent structures. Knowing that one aspect of the nose is particularly problematical allows the surgeon to focus on it and modify the rest of the nose around those corrections. For example, in a patient with a long nose and ptotic tip, the surgeon may wish to establish tip projection and rotation first, and then set the dorsal height appropriate to the new tip position.

Analysis should then continue with a systematic assessment of each view of the nose. While analysis of the patient is done in the office setting, quality preoperative photographs allow for more detailed study at a later time. On the frontal view, symmetry and width should be assessed in each of the

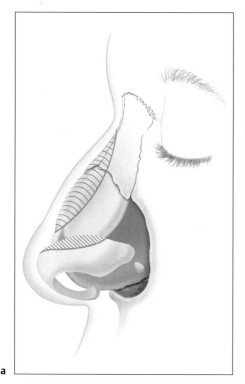

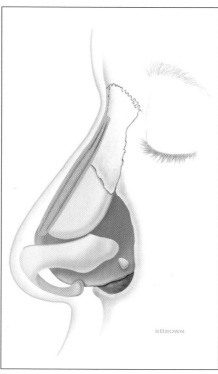

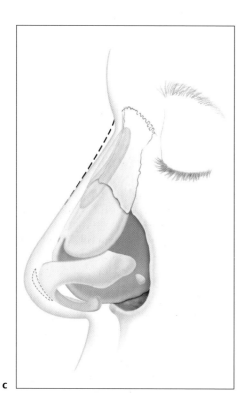

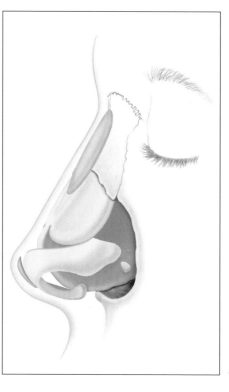

Fig. 7.1 Polybeak deformity due to overreduction of nasal dorsum. (**a**) A patient with thick skin needs to undergo expansion of structure into the thick skin. Excess reduction can result in a polybeak deformity. (**b**) Dorsal profile is overreduced, leaving excess SSTE and polybeak deformity. The problem in these patients is the excess, thick nasal tip skin. Reduction of tip projection and loss of dorsal height acts to accentuate the deformity. (**c**) Treatment of the polybeak deformity may require enlarging the nose by placing a dorsal graft and increasing nasal tip projection. (**d**) Expansion of the thick nasal skin can improve the tip-supratip relationship and balance the nose.

vertical thirds of the nose. The brow–tip esthetic lines should follow a gentle, unbroken curve following the relative normal variation of nasal width: slightly wider cephalad at the brow/nasal root transition, narrower in the middle vault, and wider again at the tip. If the brow–tip esthetic lines are irregular or asymmetrical, the anatomical cause of the problem should be noted. Bony and cartilaginous vault irregularities are easily discernable with a single light source placed above the patient to enhance shadowing. The general tip shape should be determined from the frontal and base views (e.g., bulbous, deviated,

wide, amorphous, asymmetrical). The base view also provides information about the shape and size of the columella, alar base, nostrils, and lobule. In general, the frontal and base views should reveal a triangular shape of the nose in which the nasal base (interface of nose and face) is wider than the tip and dorsal line. The triangularity of the tip depends on the presence of an unbroken line from the nasal tip-defining points to the lateral alar margin. Poor structural support in this area will manifest as alar pinching or concavity of the alar margins on frontal and base views. In cases of variant anatomy in which the base is excessively narrow or the tip too wide, the correct relationship must be restored.

On the lateral view, the nasofrontal angle should be approximately 120°. This angle is measured at the nasal starting point and is determined by the height of the radix and the angle of the forehead. A deep nasofrontal angle creates an illusion of a shorter nose, independent of the actual vertical position of the nasal starting point. Conversely, a shallow angle creates an appearance of a longer nose. The dorsum is assessed for smoothness, convexity or concavity, and presence of a supratip break. In the lower third, the overall projection and rotation of the nasal tip must be assessed. Using Goode's method, the nasal tip projection as defined from the alar crease to the tip-defining point, should be just over half the length of the nose. The nasolabial angle in men should be between 90° and 95° and in women between 95° and 105°. This angle can be affected by variations in the size and shape of the upper lip and premaxillary bone. Therefore, the nasolabial angle does not always reflect the degree of tip rotation. The alar–columellar relationship and degree of infratip break should also be noted (2, 3, 5).

Surgical Technique

Incisions—Nuances and Technique

Up to 10 cc of local anesthetic with 1:100 000 epinephrine is placed intranasally in the submucoperichondrial plane on both sides of the septum, nasal floor, and inferior turbinate. This larger volume generally will not cause significant hemodynamic disturbances in a healthy patient. The anesthetic is useful in providing vasoconstriction and hydrodissection. The external nasal SSTE is infiltrated with a smaller volume in order to prevent distortion of the baseline shape. The areas injected include the columella, the intradomal area to the nasal spine, the tip and supratip, and the dorsum and side walls. It is useful to mark the salient anatomy and abnormalities with a pen prior to injection.

The marginal incisions may be scored lightly with a 15 blade while everting the alar rims with a wide skin hook to provide direct visualization. The incision should be designed at the caudal margin of the lateral crura. The cephalic border of the nasal vibrissae is an inconstant landmark that may help in localizing the caudal edge of the lateral crura. Palpation of the cartilage with the back of the scalpel is a more reliable localizing technique. The transcolumellar incision is then made with an 11 blade at the level of the midcolumella in an inverted V orientation. The apex of the V should form an angle approaching 90° (Fig. 7.2). Creating an overly acute angle will increase the chance of skin ischemia and breakdown at the apex. The incision should be connected to the columellar extension of the marginal incisions that follow the caudal margin of the medial crura and lie 2 mm posterior to the lateral border of the columella. Particularly in thin skinned patients and in patients with prominent medial and intermediate crura, these incisions must be placed superficially in order to avoid cutting the underlying cartilage.

Elevation of the soft-tissue envelope is then performed in a supraperichondrial plane. The columellar incision is first opened with Converse scissors. The tips of the scissors should

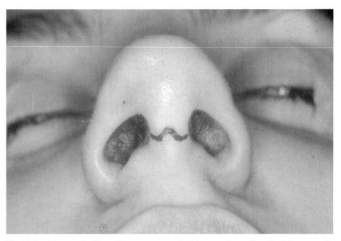

Fig. 7.**2** External rhinoplasty approach. Transcolumellar incision made midway between the top of the nostril and base of the nose.

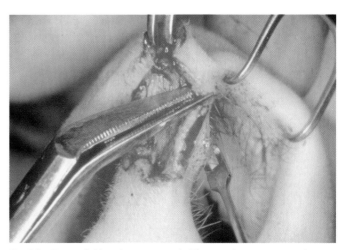

Fig. 7.**3** External rhinoplasty approach. Three-point countertraction can aid in delivery of the lower lateral cartilages into the operative field.

be used to establish a tunnel beneath the transverse columellar incision, bridging the two vertical incisions. The scissors should be used as a palpation instrument in this maneuver in order to avoid damaging the underlying medial crura. The scissors may then be gently opened in order to widen the tunnel and to better demarcate the transverse incision. The transverse incision may then be safely completed as the soft-tissue envelope should be elevated from the cartilage at this point. Often there are small columellar arteries at the inferior skin flap that may need to be controlled with a fine tip bipolar cautery.

Elevation of the soft-tissue envelope then proceeds cephalad toward the domes. Three-point retraction greatly aids in the development of the correct plane of dissection. A fine double-prong skin hook retracts the superior flap of the columella cephalically, another fine skin hook is placed at the undersurface of the medial crus in order to retract the intermediate crus and dome inferolaterally, and a third wide double-prong skin hook is placed at the alar rim margin to expose the marginal incision (Fig. 7.3). Dissection is performed with Converse scissors in a plane immediately superficial to the perichondrium. The scissors should be slightly angled downward toward the cartilage and the plane developed with fine cuts using the tips of the scissors rather than through a spreading motion. A cotton-tip applicator may be used as a blunt dissec-

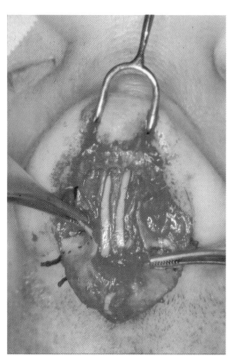

Fig. 7.**4** Spreader grafts applied between the upper lateral cartilages and dorsal margin of the septum. Note how the spreader grafts extend from the osseocartilaginous junction to the anterior septal angle.

tor to further develop the plane. As the dissection plane is developed cephalad, the vestibular skin is incised flush with the caudal border of the lateral crura (previously scored). The second fine double-prong skin hook may be advanced laterally on the lateral crus as dissection continues cephalad and laterally. Dissection should be taken to the lateral 25 % of the lateral crus in order to gain enough exposure for work in the upper two thirds of the nose. Dissection too far laterally may result in destabilizing the ligamentous lateral support of the LLCs.

Once both lateral crura are exposed, dissection may be continued cephalad over the middle vault. Dissection below the muscle is critical to avoid thinning the overlying skin soft tissue envelope.

Dissection of the soft-tissue envelope over the upper third should be elevated in a subperiostial plane. Starting at the rhinion, a Joseph elevator is used to incise the periosteum. Dissection proceeds cephalad in this plane. The size of the subperiostial pocket depends on the planned surgical maneuvers. If significant reduction or rasping of the bony dorsum is needed, a wider area of dissection may be required. If elevation of the radix is planned, a narrow pocket may be preferred for better fixation of the radix graft (1, 3).

Middle Vault

The middle vault has significant functional and cosmetic implications for the nose. Functionally, the internal nasal valve area is partly dependent on the relationship of the ULC and the dorsal septum. Excessive narrowing of the angle between these structures will lead to obstruction at the internal valve. Previous surgery causing destabilization of this area will result in inferomedial collapse of the ULC into the airway. In particular, patients with short nasal bones and long ULCs are at risk of lateral collapse. Cosmetically, the width and symmetry of the

front view of the nose depends on symmetrical reconstruction of the ULC and septum.

Spreader grafts are long rectangular cartilaginous grafts placed between the dorsal cartilaginous septum and ULC. These grafts are useful for correcting functional and cosmetic problems related to a narrow or asymmetrical middle vault. In addition, these grafts should be used in primary rhinoplasty to prevent middle vault collapse in high-risk patients. In particular, when reduction of a cartilaginous dorsal hump leads to excision of the horizontal articulation of the dorsal septum and ULCs, spreader grafts will stabilize the middle vault and help restore appropriate horizontal width.

The dimensions of spreader grafts will vary depending on specific needs and anatomy, but range from 6–12 mm in length, 3–5 mm in height, and 2–4 mm in thickness. More than one graft may be needed depending on available grafting material and the deformities. In general the thicker aspect of the spreader graft is beveled and then positioned cephalad at the rhinion in order to create the normal appearance of slightly increased width in this area. The grafts may be placed from a dorsal approach after the ULCs are freed from the septum. Mucoperichondrial flaps must first be elevated from the junction of the ULC and septum in order to prevent injury to the mucosal lining and subsequent cicatrix. Two 5.0 PDS mattress sutures placed through the ULC, spreaders, and septum should be used for stabilization. The caudal ULC should be pulled caudally during the suture stabilization in order to straighten any redundancy or curvature. The dorsal profile of the spreader grafts, ULC, and septum should be coplanar and smooth. In situ trimming of the grafts may be needed to ensure an even dorsal surface (Fig. 7.**4**).

An alternative method of placing spreader grafts is through a tight subperichondrial tunnel at the junction of the ULC and dorsal septum. In this method, elevation of the septal flaps must not include the dorsal aspect of the quadrilateral cartilage. A mucoperichondrial incision is made high on the septum just caudal to the junction of the ULC and septum. A narrow dissection instrument, such as a Freer elevator, is then used to create a long, tight pocket just beneath the dorsal junction between the ULC and septum. Snug placement of a spreader graft into this tunnel will cantilever the ULC away from the dorsal septum, effecting additional widening of the internal nasal valve, as compared to placing spreaders through an open dorsal approach. In the latter, the ULC is lateralized, but the absolute angle between the septum and ULC does not change. The precise pocket spreader graft creates lateralization and mild flaring of the ULC, leading to increased width and angulation. This effect is achieved because of the bulk of the spreader graft placed below the intact connection between the dorsal margin of the septum and the ULC. This translates to additional airway improvement. This method should be considered in patients with severe obstruction referable to the internal valve. A drawback to this method is the additional width that is incurred. Careful patient selection is therefore required (3,4).

Other methods to modify middle vault width have been described in the literature and include flaring sutures, suspension sutures, and butterfly grafts (6). In our experience, these methods are less predictable and/or less durable than properly placed spreader grafts.

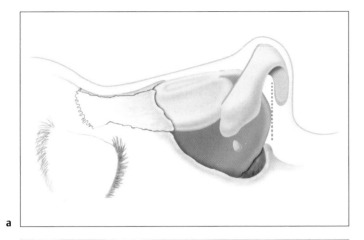

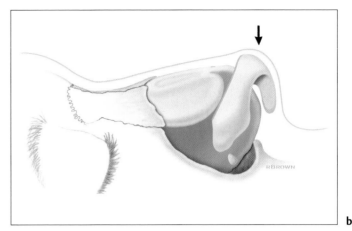

a   b

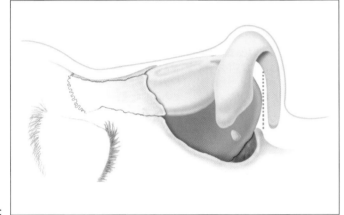

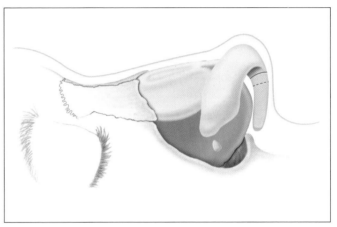

c   d

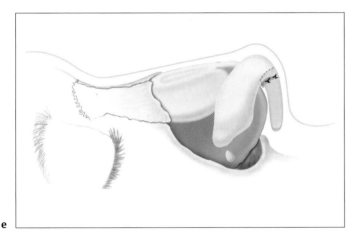

Fig. 7.**5**   Tripod principle of tip projection. (**a, b**) Tip projection can be decreased in a patient with shorter, less supportive medial crura by performing a full transfixion incision. (**c**) A full transfixion incision in a patient with long, strong medial crura will not be an effective means of decreasing tip projection as the medial crura will resist deprojection. (**d,e**) Shortening the medial crura is an effective means of decreasing tip projection in patients with long, strong medial crura. This can be accomplished by dividing and overlapping the overly long medial crura.

e

Tip–Base Stabilization

Refinement of the nasal tip is one of the most difficult aspects of rhinoplasty. The external approach allows direct visualization of the underlying variant anatomy which may cause tip deformities. The main variables that are addressed are tip shape and position. Typically, modifications to the inherent shape of the tip are performed through a combination of conservative excision, suture modification, and structural grafting of the LLCs. The specific maneuvers performed vary tremendously, depending on the size, shape, position, and strength of the existing LLCs and caudal septum (1).

Equally important is establishing the appropriate tip position. The projection and rotation of the nasal tip may be con-

ceptualized through Anderson's tripod paradigm. The two lateral crura and the conjoined medial crura create the three limbs of the tripod. Other factors notwithstanding, shortening the medial crura will counterrotate and deproject the tip; lengthening the medial crura will rotate and project; shortening the lateral crura will rotate and deproject; and lengthening the lateral crura will counterrotate and project (Figs. 7.**5**–7.**7**). Certain maneuvers will lead to immediate changes to the tripod architecture. These maneuvers may be performed through a combination of *repositioning techniques* such as suture retropositioning the medial crura onto the caudal septum in order to decrease projection and rotation; *modification of structural shape* such as dome suturing to increase projection (variable effect on rotation); *structural grafting* such as tip

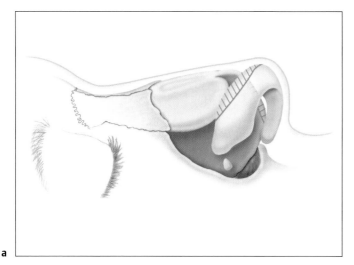

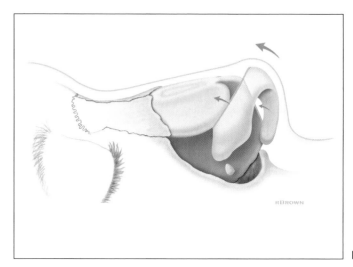

a

b

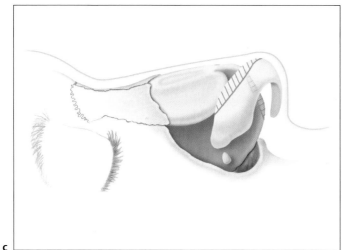

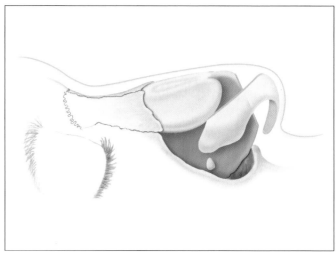

c

d

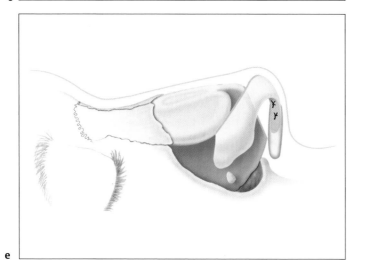

e

Fig. 7.**6**   Tripod principle of tip rotation. (**a, b**) In the patient with strong medial crura, the combination of cephalic trim of the lateral crura and removing an inverted triangle of cartilage from the caudal margin of the nasal septum will result in tip rotation. (**c, d**) Cephalic trim and removal of an inverted triangle of cartilage from the caudal septum in a patient with short, weak medial crura will likely result in tip ptosis rather than tip rotation. (**e**) Placement of a columellar strut and dome sutures will aid in supporting weak medial crura and increase the likelihood of tip rotation.

grafting to increase projection; or *overlapping* techniques such as lateral crural overlay in order to deproject and increase rotation (Fig. 7.**8**). It is preferable to avoid excessive reduction, excision, or weakening of tip structures. Details of refinement to tip shape and position are discussed elsewhere (1, 2, 7).

Often overlooked in rhinoplasty are the dynamic changes that the tip will undergo long after surgery. The combination of the long-term effects of scar contracture, gravity, and mimetic

forces stresses the structural integrity of the nasal tip. Anderson's paradigm is valid only if one understands that the entire tripod is a mobile and compressible structure. The concept of tip support is well-established. The major support mechanisms are the integrity of the LLCs, and the ligamentous attachments between the LLC and the ULC and between the LLC and the septum. Surgical destabilization of these structures often occurs during rhinoplasty. Cartilage excision, morselization,

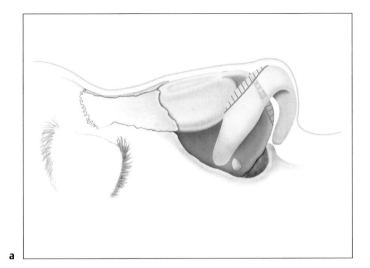

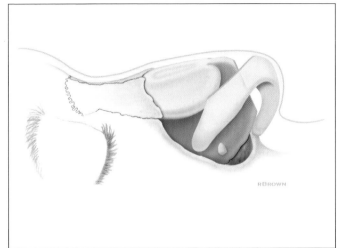

a

b

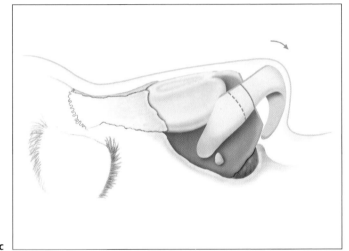

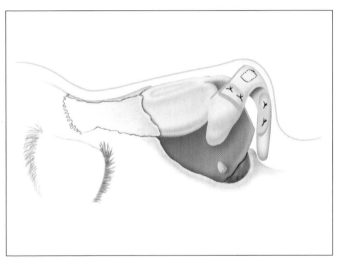

c

d

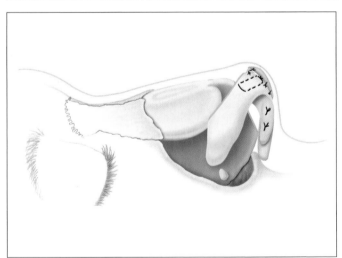

e

Fig. 7.**7** Tripod principle for tip ptosis. (**a, b**) Performing cephalic trim and caudal septal resection in a patient with overly long lateral crura will not result in tip rotation. In many cases, tip ptosis may worsen. (**c, d**) Shortening the overly long lateral crura can effectively rotate the nasal tip. This can be accomplished by dividing and overlapping the overly long lateral crura using the lateral crural overlay technique. Placement of a columellar strut and dome sutures will aid in increasing tip rotation. (**e**) If additional tip projection is desired, a tip graft and buttress graft can be used in combination with dome sutures.

and cross-hatching will weaken the inherent structural support of the tip architecture. Separating the medial crura from the septum and the ULC from the LLC compromise the main ligamentous tip supports. Unless the tip is soundly resupported at the time of surgery, a high risk of postoperative loss of tip projection and tip ptosis is incurred. For these reasons, stabilization of the nasal base is essential in order to achieve durable results in tip modification.

The method chosen to stabilize the nasal base depends on the particular anatomy and surgical goals. Typically, any given method of base stabilization may be adjusted to effect subtle changes in tip projection and rotation as well. The techniques most commonly employed by the senior author include fixation of the medial crura onto the caudal septum, caudal extension graft, suture fixated columellar strut, or extended columellar strut. In each of these techniques, a stable midline

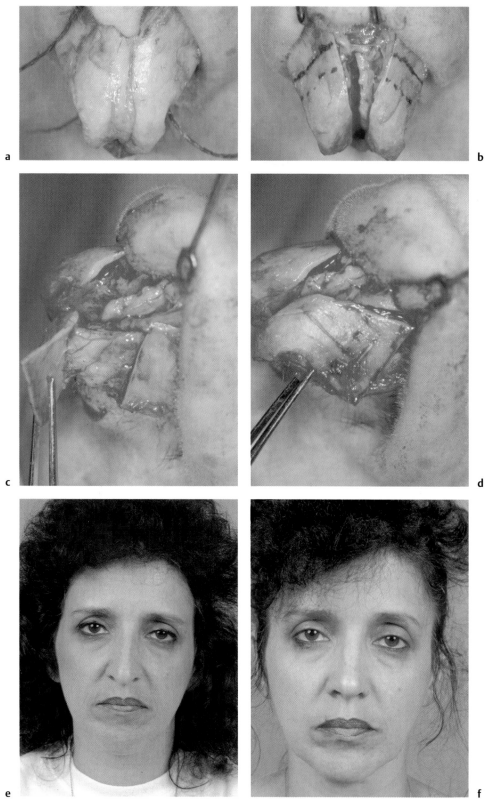

Fig. 7.8 g–l ▷

Fig. 7.**8**   Patient with a dependant nasal tip. Using the lateral crural overlay technique results in shortening of the lateral crura and increased tip rotation. The medial crura were also sutured to the caudal septum to support the nasal base. (**a**) Overly long lateral crura creating dependant nasal tip. (**b**) Lateral crura marked in preparation for lateral crural overlay. (**c**) Lateral crura divided lateral to the domes and cartilage elevated off underlying vestibular skin. (**d**) Lateral crura are overlapped and resutured with 6–0 PDS suture. Preoperative views: **e, g, i, k**. Postoperative views: **f, h, j, l**.

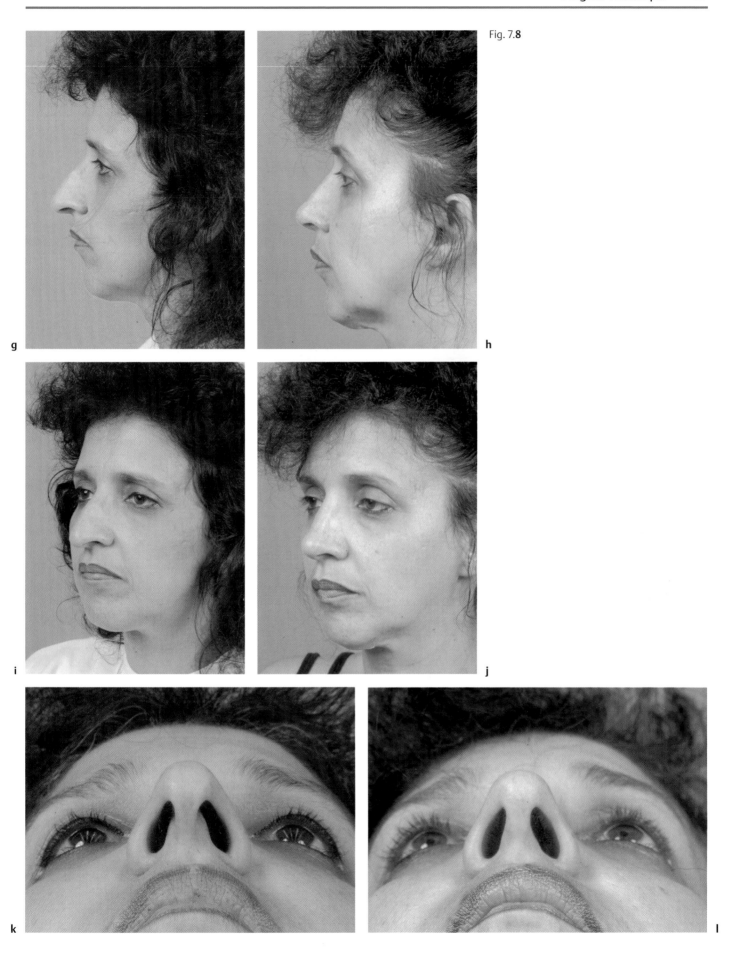

Fig. 7.**8**

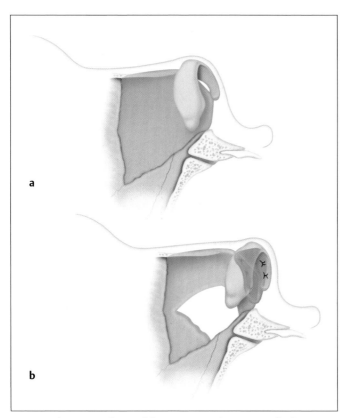

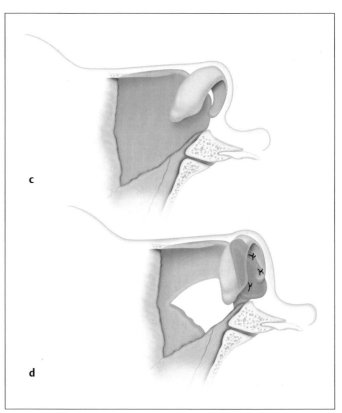

Fig. 7.**9**   Placement of a caudal extension graft is one method to resupport the nasal base. The shape and orientation of the graft may be altered to effect changes in tip shape and position. (**a, b**) A graft with a more projecting anterior margin will allow one to lengthen and counterrotate the nose. (**c, d**) A graft with a longer posterior margin will allow one to augment the nasolabial angle and create an illusion of increased rotation.

cartilaginous structure is employed to add support to the nasal base and tip. The tripod is effectively stabilized to this structure and may be differentially positioned relative to it in order to create subtle alterations of tip position. Major changes in tip projection and rotation require other techniques.

The medial crura may be suture stabilized onto the caudal septum in patients with a relatively long midline caudal septum. Such patients may present with a hanging columella, tension nose deformity, or overprojected tip and usually require trimming of the caudal septum. If the medial crura are sutured to a normally positioned caudal septum, then retraction of the columella may be created. The medial crura are separated and dissected free of the caudal septum. Bilateral mucoperichondrial flaps are raised on the septum so that mucosal redundancy created by tip repositioning may be distributed cephalically. The medial crura are fixated with horizontal mattress sutures in a tongue-in-groove manner. An initial fixation suture may be placed full thickness through the medial crura, caudal septum, and vestibular skin of the membranous septum with a straight needle and rapidly absorbing suture such as chromic or plain gut. Once the desired positioning is achieved, 5.0 PDS suture may be used to reinforce the fixation between the inner surface of the medial crura and septum. The septal flaps must be redistributed evenly and tightly to the midline with several passes of a 5.0 plain gut suture on a straight needle.

The caudal extension graft relies on the same principle as the previous technique. The difference is that the caudal septum is effectively lengthened with a cartilage graft so that the medial crura may be readily sutured to it. Patients with a relative caudal septal deficiency may present with columellar retraction and an underprojected, overrotated tip. This technique is often employed in secondary rhinoplasty after previous excessive shortening of the septum. The graft should overlap the existing caudal septum and be suture stabilized with at least two horizontal mattress sutures. The caudal aspect of the graft should be in the midline so that the medial crura may be stabilized in a midline position. Both the caudal septal stabilization technique and the caudal extension graft allow for changes in projection, rotation, nasolabial angle, and columellar show by variably positioning the medial crura onto the septum or caudal extension graft. The latter technique has the potential for a greater degree of tip alteration as the shape and orientation of the effective caudal septal margin may be altered. For instance, if the caudal extension graft is longer anteriorly toward the tip, counterrotation may be achieved (Fig. 7.**9 a, b**). If the graft is longer posteriorly near the nasal spine, the nasolabial angle may be opened with a resultant appearance of increased tip rotation (Fig. 7.**9 c, d**). These techniques rely on the stability of the septum to stabilize the tip. Therefore, the caudal septum itself must be structurally intact and securely attached to the nasal spine and maxillary crest in order to ensure durable stabilization.

The columellar strut is a reliable technique which may be used to stabilize the nasal base. This technique is useful in cases in which major tip alterations are not needed. The strut should be rectangular and may vary from 5–12 mm in length, 3–6 mm in width, and 1–3 mm thick. The strut is placed in a pocket between the medial crura and sutured to the medial crura in a horizontal mattress fashion. Because the strut does not extend to the nasal spine, it cannot push the tip beyond its existing projection. Thus, while the floating columellar strut will provide some support to the medial crura, such struts may not be adequate for patients with a deficient nasal base.

As a columellar strut extends closer to the nasal spine, a theoretical increase in tip support is gained. The strut, however, must be strong enough to withstand the downward tension of the tip, particularly if it is designed to push the tip beyond its current projection. This is the concept of the extended columellar strut. This technique aims to create a significant increase in projection in patients with a major deficiency of tip support. The non-Caucasian patient and the patient with a congenital nasal deformity often exhibit this scenario. Other anatomical findings indicative of a patient with a deficient nasal base include a ptotic or underprojected nasal tip, and the nasolabial angle may be overly acute. The graft is typically harvested from costal cartilage in order to impart sufficient strength to the nasal base and tip. The strut is suture fixated to the periostium of the nasal spine. A notch in the undersurface of the strut may be made to articulate with the spine and prevent migration from the midline. Alternatively, the graft may be incorporated with a separate premaxillary graft in a tongue-in-groove manner. This may be necessary in patients with an exceptional degree of premaxillary deficiency. As in the other techniques, the medial crura are sutured to the extended columellar strut to achieve the desired projection.

Once the nasal base is stabilized, we prefer to use dome binding sutures to set the width of the domes. Dome sutures will also provide an increase in tip projection and rotation (Fig. 7.**10**). Once the width of the domes is set, the distance between the domes can be set with an interdomal suture. This suture goes through both intermediate crura and should not be tied too tight otherwise the columellar lobular angle can be effaced. If a cleft remains between the domes, a small piece of crushed cartilage can be placed between the domes. In cases in which the alar margins are bowed outward or the tip is bulbous, the lateral crura may be convex. Convex or bulbous lateral crura can be improved with dome sutures. Additionally, straightening curved lateral crura may create the appearance of a less bulbous tip. Lateral crural struts are useful grafts in such cases. These flat cartilage grafts are placed between the undersurface of the lateral crura and the vestibular skin. The vestibular skin should be carefully elevated from the lateral crura from cephalad to caudal. The caudal attachment of the lateral crus and skin should remain intact to prevent caudal migration of the graft. The graft should extend from just lateral to the domes to the lateral aspect of the lateral crura. The lateral cural strut graft may be stabilized with a full thickness chromic suture, but should be finally secured to the LLC with a 5.0 clear nylon suture. In patients with thick nasal tip skin we frequently use a sutured-in-place tip graft to provide additional projection and tip contour. Tip grafts frequently measure 10–12 mm in length, 5–7 mm in width, and 2–4 mm in thickness. Tip grafts are sutured to the caudal margin of the medial crura (Fig. 7.**11**). Tip grafts should not be used in patients with thin skin as these grafts may become visible over time (1).

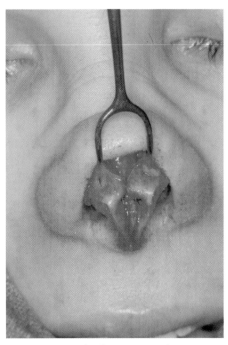

Fig. 7.**10** Dome-binding sutures. These sutures are placed through the domes and decrease tip bulbosity and can increase tip projection. An interdomal suture can be used to set interdomal width or a tip graft can be sutured to the medial crura.

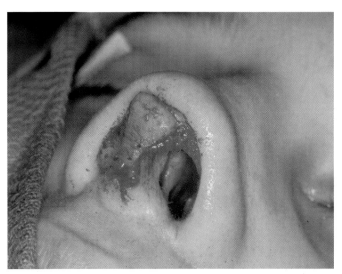

Fig. 7.**11** Sutured-in-place tip graft. Note how the tip graft projects a couple of millimeters above the exiting domes. Four to six 6–0 PDS sutures are used to fix the tip graft to the medial and intermediate crura.

Secondary Rhinoplasty

Several special considerations must be made for secondary rhinoplasty. The external approach is an excellent method to gain exposure of the cartilaginous structures as dense scar often impedes dissection. In such cases the direct visualization provided by the external approach may be needed in addition to the tactile feedback upon which endonasal dissection depends. In cases with severe scar formation, even with

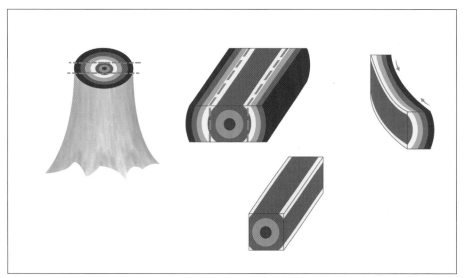

Fig. 7.**12** Carving of costal cartilage grafts must be performed in a symmetrical fashion. An effort should be made to obtain the graft from the center of a straight segment of rib. Eccentrically carved grafts will become subject to asymmetrical forces of contracture and have a tendency to warp over time. This concept is illustrated by analogy with a tree trunk with concentric rings. If one carves from the periphery of the trunk, the wood will warp toward the periphery. If one carves a graft from the center of the rings, forces of contracture will be symmetrical and the wood will not warp. (**a**) A tree trunk has many circumferential rings that create fibrous regions of the tree. (**b**) If a segment of wood is cut from the tree trunk, opposing fibrous structures can be seen. (**c**) If the segment is carved asymmetrically, warping can be expected to occur. (**d**) If the wood is carved symmetrically from the center of the trunk, warping is much less likely.

direct visualization, it may be difficult to differentiate scar from cartilage. As in primary cases, three-point retraction while applying downward pressure with the tips of a pair of Converse scissors will aid in finding and maintaining the correct plane. The surgeon should always protect the integrity of the SSTE.

A common reason patients seek secondary rhinoplasty is for the correction of postoperative nasal obstruction. In such cases, previous surgery has led to overreduction, destabilization, and/or collapse of normal nasal support structures. The most common causes of postrhinoplasty obstruction are lateral wall collapse, middle vault collapse, and persistent or inadequately treated septal deformities. Certain cosmetic stigmata are associated with these functional deficits. These include a narrow middle vault, an inverted V deformity at the cartilaginous–bony junction of the dorsum, supra-alar pinching, and alar pinching. Prevention of these deformities during primary rhinoplasty is a far better option than secondary correction. Avoidance of overresection of the LLCs, stabilization of the base and tip, and reconstitution of the middle vault are key steps in avoiding such complications (1).

One difficulty of secondary rhinoplasty is the lack of septal cartilage available for grafting material. In these cases it is often necessary to harvest cartilage from one or both ears. A vertical skin incision is made approximately 1 cm in front of the postauricular sulcus on the posterior conchal bowl. The skin and perichondrium is then elevated from the posterior concha with Converse scissors. Retraction with a small skin hook and blunt dissection with a cotton-tipped applicator aids in this process. Care should be taken to leave the peripheral vertical component of the concha intact so that no change in shape of the ear occurs. The harvested segment may extend toward the canal meatus, but the emenentia corresponding to

the root of the helix should not be excised. The resulting piece is usually kidney shaped and will vary from 2–4 cm in largest dimension. The skin flaps should be judiciously cauterized to prevent thermal injury. Closure with a few subcutaneous 5.0 PDS sutures followed by a running 5.0 fast-absorbing gut should be placed. A bolster in the anterior conchal bowl may be fashioned from a dental roll and sutured through the ear with a 3.0 nylon suture (3).

In cases when ear cartilage is also insufficient or exceptionally strong grafting material is needed, costal cartilage may be harvested. Typically, the cartilage is taken from rib VII, VIII, or IX. A 3–5 cm incision is placed over the medial aspect of the rib. The muscle is separated in the direction of its fibers to access the rib surface. Subperichondrial dissection around the rib is performed with an elevator. It is important to retain a subperichondrial dissection on the deep surface of the rib in order to avoid injury to the pleura. Under direct visualization, the graft is freed from the surrounding perichondrium and the desired segment sharply excised. A malleable retractor may be placed deep to rib to protect the pleura. A needle may be inserted into areas of the rib in which it is unclear whether bone or cartilage is present. Closure should be performed in a layered fashion after hemostasis is achieved (3).

When carving costal cartilage, it is crucial that the surgeon obtain the grafts from the center of a relatively straight segment of rib cartilage. The cartilaginous matrix is circumferentially oriented much like the cross section of a tree trunk. An oblique longitudinal cut will result in asymmetrical forces of contracture and result in warping toward the periphery of the graft. A graft obtained through symmetrical trimming from the periphery toward the center of the rib will result in a graft with equal circumferential forces of contracture and thus a decreased chance of warping (Fig. 7.**12**).

The presence of damaged or incomplete nasal cartilage poses one of the biggest challenges during secondary rhinoplasty. Components of the structural framework of the nose must often be strengthened or completely reconstructed in order to restore appearance and function. Common problem areas in secondary rhinoplasty include the nasal tip, the lateral nasal wall, the alar margin, and the middle vault.

Postoperative tip weakness may occur if the nasal base is inadequately supported during primary rhinoplasty. In some cases, this manifests as a ptotic, underprojected tip with an acute nasolabial angle. In other cases, concurrent maneuvers such as caudal septal resection or scarring from lateral crural excision may create forces which counteract tip ptosis and result in a tip with normal or excessive rotation, but is none the less poorly supported. The corrective technique depends upon the status of the alar cartilages. Often, the LLCs have been weakened and have lost inherent structural strength. The base must be restabilized through one of the techniques outlined above. In cases of previous caudal septal resection, medial crural stabilization with a caudal extension graft will achieve base stabilization as well as setting tip position. In cases of severe loss of tip support and projection, a costal cartilage extended columellar strut may be indicated.

Tip shape is determined by the size, shape, and orientation of the cartilage of the intermediate and lateral crura. Asymmetries, bossae, bulbosity, and other abnormalities may result from previous surgery. In many cases, the cartilage is so damaged that reorientation of existing structures cannot create adequate tip support. Particularly in thick skinned patients, a robust tip structure must project into the soft-tissue flap to transmit shape through the skin. In such cases, a shield-shaped tip graft may be used to this end. The graft is sutured to the intermediate and medial crura. The dimensions of the shield graft depend on the desired augmentation to the infratip lobule and tip. These structures may be altered without changing the nasal base. The leading edge of the shield graft may project beyond the domes by as much as 8 mm when a significant increase in projection is needed. A buttress or cap graft may be placed cephalad to the leading edge of the graft in order to support the graft and camouflage the transition to the supratip. Lateral crural grafts are placed on the existing lateral crura and sutured to the lateral edge of the shield graft when the tip graft projects more than 3 mm above the existing domes. These also provide additional support and camouflage to the shield graft. Lateral crural grafts also bolster lateral alar support in cases in which the native lateral crura have been weakened or removed.

Lateral nasal wall narrowing and collapse is often the consequence of excessive cephalic trim of the lateral crura. Patients with a long narrow nose and a preexisting prominent supra-alar crease are susceptible to this complication. Examination of such patients may reveal pinching in the supra-alar area with dynamic collapse during inspiration. Correction of this problem requires strengthening the lateral nasal wall and may be performed with alar batten grafts. These grafts are curved cartilaginous supports placed into the area of maximal lateral wall weakness (Fig. 7.**13**). Through the external approach, the grafts are placed into tight pockets which overlap and extend lateral to the lateral crura. The curvature of the graft should be oriented to lateralize the supra-alar area with the concave surface medial. The lateral aspect of the graft is usually caudal to the lateral crura, depending on the area of

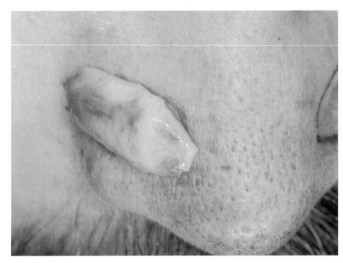

Fig. 7.**13**   Alar batten graft for lateral wall weakness. Alar batten grafts are placed into precise pockets lateral to the lateral crura along the supra-alar crease.

maximal pinching. In severe cases, the grafts may extend all the way to the piriform aperture in order to add support. In cases in which lateral recurvature of the native lateral crura impinges on the nostril width, the lateral crura may be sutured to the alar batten grafts for lateral stabilization. Internal vestibular stents may be placed in the postoperative period to prevent postoperative medialization of the lateral wall. These stents may be constructed with pliable plastic stents and may be kept in the nasal vestibules at night-time for a period of three to 12 weeks, depending on the severity of the initial problem (1, 8, 9).

Like other complications, secondary deformities of the alar rim may result from overresection or weakening of the alar cartilages. Aggressive cephalic trim may cause cephalic retraction of the alar rim margin and excessive columellar show. Weakening at the alar margin will lead to notching and collapse, most evident by a loss of the favorable triangular base view. Alar rim grafts may be used to correct this type of deficiency. These are narrow cartilaginous grafts which are placed into precise pockets along the alar rim just caudal to the marginal incision (Fig. 7.**14**). They measure 2–3 mm in thickness and width and 5–8 mm in length. Softer material, such as cartilage harvested from the ear or from cephalic trim of the LLC, is preferable. The medial aspect of these grafts may be gently bruised to aid in camouflage. They may be stabilized to the surrounding soft tissue or to the lateral aspect of a shield graft with 6.0 PDS suture. These grafts will improve upon the concave or "knock-kneed" appearance of the rim on base view and create a more triangular appearance to the basal view (Fig. 7.**15**). Severe cases of alar retraction may require the use of composite grafts of ear cartilage and skin placed into the marginal incisions to reposition the alar margins in a more caudal position (Fig. 7.**16**).

Inferomedial collapse of the ULC with associated internal valve collapse, a pinched mid-dorsum, and an inverted V deformity are consequences of destabilization of the horizontal segment of the middle vault. As in primary rhinoplasty, the application of spreader grafts is a valuable tool in restoring middle vault support and symmetry. The same principles apply as in primary rhinoplasty. However, in revision cases, a greater

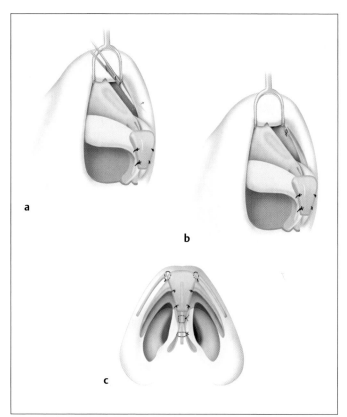

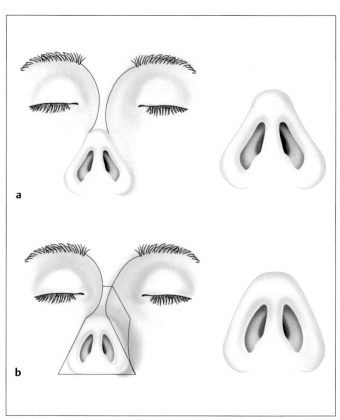

Fig. 7.**14**   Alar rim grafts are placed into pockets along the alar rims. (**a, b**) These soft, thin grafts are placed into pockets along the caudal aspect of the marginal incision and extend toward the tip in order to support the alar margin. They may serve to correct mild alar pinching, alar retraction, and can help re-establish a smooth transition from the nasal tip to the base. (**c**) These grafts may be sutured to the lateral aspect of a tip graft in order to aid in the camouflage and transition of tip structures. Creating a continuous line of support from the tip graft to alar rim significantly decreases the chances of postoperative visibility of the tip graft.

Fig. 7.**15**   When the transition between the tip and nasal base along the alar margin is pinched, irregular, or retracted, there is loss of normal triangularity even if there is appropriate tip width and base width. Placement of alar rim grafts can restore this unbroken transition, re-establishing a natural triangular appearance on basal view and contributing to a normal hour-glass shape on frontal view. (**a**) Pinched appearance to nasal tip. (**b**) Normal tip shape with smooth transition from tip to nasal base.

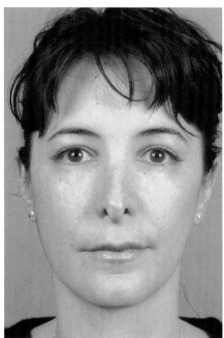

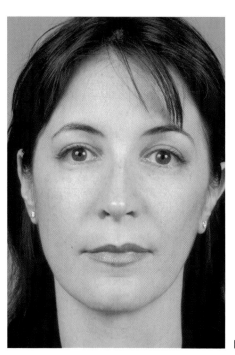

Fig. 7.**16**   Secondary rhinoplasty. Patient with pinched middle vault and nasal tip and severe alar retraction. Tip graft was used in combination with lateral crural grafts to reconstruct the nasal tip. Alar batten grafts were used to stabilize the lateral walls of the nose and correct the airway obstruction. Composite grafts were used to correct the alar retraction. Preoperative views: **a, c, e, g**. Postoperative views: **b, d, f, h**.

a

b

Fig. 7.**16 c–h** ▷

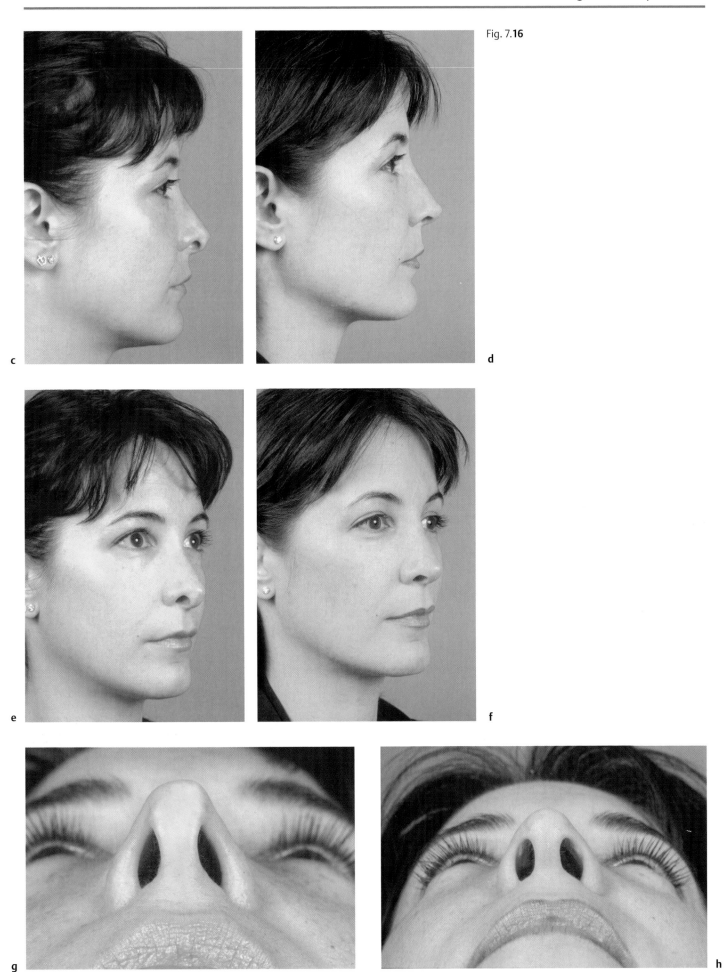

Fig. 7.**16**

c

d

e

f

g

h

degree of collapse or asymmetry may be present. The surgeon must therefore be prepared to insert wider or more numerous spreader grafts than in standard primary rhinoplasty.

The osseous vault may demonstrate an assortment of problems related to previous rhinoplasty. Most common are slight asymmetries or irregularities due to unequal osteotomies or inadequate repositioning. A bony open roof may result if previous dorsal hump reduction was performed without lateral osteotomies and medialization of the nasal bones. Treatment of the above problems requires mobilizing the bones through osteotomies, repositioning them into the proper position, and smoothing the dorsal contour as needed. If the dorsum has been excessively lowered, a dorsal onlay graft or a radix grafts may be required. A difficult problem is the case of excessively narrowed nasal bones. Treatment in this case requires osteotomies followed by outfracture of the nasal bones. As the bones will have a tendency to medialize back into their previous position, internal nasal stents may be placed high in the nasal airway to maintain the bones in the proper lateral position (10).

Closure

A single 6.0 PDS subcutaneous suture may be placed in the midline of the columellar incision in order to alleviate tension at the skin closure. A slight degree of eversion should be achieved with placement of this suture. The columellar skin should be closed with several interrupted 7.0 nylon sutures in a vertical mattress fashion. The two sutures just off midline should be angled from medial on the lower flap to lateral on the upper flap in order to better align the skin edges. The edges should be evenly opposed and everted after closure. This will allow for optimal healing over time. The vestibular skin incisions may be closed with interrupted 6.0 chromic sutures. Care should be taken not to distort the alar margin position with the closure of the marginal incision. Bacitracin-soaked Telfa packs are placed in the inferior nasal airway bilaterally to decrease bleeding and the nasal dorsum is supported with tape and an Aquaplast themoplastic cast. If inferior turbinate work has been done concurrently, small plastic splints are sutured to the septum to prevent synechiae between the septal incision and turbinates.

Key Technical Points

1. A limited volume of local anesthetic should be used in order to prevent distortion of the anatomy.
2. A transcolumellar incision in an inverted V orientation at the level of the midcolumella is connected to bilateral marginal incisions.
3. Use of three-point retraction and sharp dissection will allow development of a plane immediately superficial to the perichondrium at the domes, lateral crura, and middle vault.
4. Septal cartilage is approached in a subperichondrial plane through an intranasal hemitransfixion, or Killian incision, or through an external approach with dissection between the medial crura.
5. The upper vault is exposed in a subperiostial plane with a narrow pocket preserved for possible graft placement.

6. The horizontal junction of the ULC and dorsal septum must be stable and symmetrical. Placement of spreader grafts may aid in restoring support to this area and setting middle vault width.
7. The nasal tip shape and position depend on surgical manipulations to the LLCs. Durable effects depend on stabilization of the nasal base in order to support the tip against forces of scar contracture, gravity, and facial musculature. The main techniques for base stabilization include securing the medial crura onto the caudal septum, caudal extension graft, sutured-in-place columellar strut, and extended columellar strut.
8. Secondary rhinoplasty often aims to correct the functional and cosmetic sequellae of the weakened or deficient structural framework of the nose. Corrective surgery must restore the support structures of the nasal tip, lateral nasal wall, alar margin, and middle vault. The dependable techniques for these problems include shield grafts, alar batten grafts, alar rim grafts, lateral crural struts, and spreader grafts.
9. The columellar incision should be closed with fine sutures and maximal eversion.

Postoperative Care

In most cases, the patient is discharged home a few hours after surgery. Elderly patients or patients with medical conditions which may increase the risks of early complications may be admitted for overnight observation. Antibiotics are given for at least 10 days postoperatively. A first-generation cephalosporin is used for simple primary cases in order to cover skin and intranasal flora. In complex secondary cases, particularly if ear cartilage is harvested, a quinolone such as ciprofloxacin or levofloxacin is used in order to add antipseudomonal coverage. Vicodin is given for pain control, but the patient is encouraged to change to acetominophen once discomfort begins to subside. The patient is also instructed to clean the nasal lining with hydrogen peroxide on a cotton-tipped applicator and apply Bacitracin ointment over the incisions. The patient is instructed to avoid salt in his/her diet, exertion, and overheating, all of which may induce increased edema.

The patient should return on the first postoperative day for a general check. If significant bleeding has not occurred since surgery, the nasal packing may be removed. If turbinate surgery was performed, the packing may remain for an additional day. The sutures, tape, cast, and ear bolsters are removed between the fifth and seventh postoperative day. The patient should be reminded at this time that significant swelling is expected at this early stage. The internal septal splints are removed two to three weeks after surgery. These should remain longer in cases in which the integrity of the septal flaps is tenuous.

After this point, frequency of follow-up depends on the complexity of the surgery and the individual postoperative course. On average, patients are seen three times within the first month, five to ten more times over the next 12 months, and at least yearly after that. These repeat visits are critical so that the nose may be closely monitored as edema resolves and the SSTE contracts. Over time, slight asymmetries may become apparent at the tip, supratip, or dorsum. If the fullness is compressible, it may be caused by unequal resolution of edema. An area in which more dissection or manipulation was performed may be swollen to a greater degree and duration. If the area of fullness is firmer, it may correspond to a cartilage graft which may have shifted. In either case, the patient may use repeated digital exercises over the area in an attempt to reduce the prominence. The pad of the forefinger or thumb is firmly placed over the palpable fullness several times a day for 5–10 minutes. This will lead to faster resolution of edema in the area and/or gradual shifting of a cartilage graft into a more appropriate position.

Local steroid injection is another technique to improve areas of soft-tissue fullness that are slow to resolve. This technique may help alleviate slight asymmetries that are not fully corrected by digital exercises. Injections will also expedite the resolution of tip and supratip fullness—a process that is particularly extended in the thick skinned patient. Steroid injections may expedite this process. Care should be taken not to inject deep into the dermis more than once every 3 months.

Some irregularities or asymmetries due to cartilage grafts may be refractory to digital exercises. In these cases, a corrective office procedure may be performed under local anesthesic. A 16-gauge needle is placed transcutaneously to access the cartilage graft in question and used to shave the graft into the desired shape. The excised portions of cartilage are selectively crushed and distributed under the skin. A conservative approach should be taken for this procedure in order not to risk overreducing the graft. Additional procedures may be performed so that the desired result may be obtained in a stepwise fashion. If significant imperfections persist despite these efforts, a revision procedure may be required. Usually such a procedure, if needed, is fairly minor and may simply require adjusting the position or shape of a graft. Often, these procedures may be performed under local anesthetic.

Frequent follow-up is crucial in order to detect these abnormalities as early as possible and to correct them through the methods described. Long-term visits are important as the nose continues to change for many years after surgery. Photographs should be taken throughout the postoperative course in order to follow these changes. Only through repeated follow-ups, study of photographs, correlation to operative worksheets, and ongoing analysis will the rhinoplasty surgeon learn from previous mistakes and gain better surgical results.

Complications

Bleeding is the earliest common postoperative complication following rhinoplasty. The placement of packing will help to prevent bleeding, but does not guarantee against it. Larger packs should be used in cases in which intraoperative blood loss was greater than normal. For patients with questionable hemostasis, the packing should remain for an additional one to two days beyond the standard 24 hours. At this period, the packing should be extracted partially to assess for bleeding around it before completely removing it. If slow oozing persists after pack removal, topical decongestants may be sprayed intranasally. Often, the vasoconstrictive effect will control such a problem. More severe bleeding may require replacing the packing material for another few days.

Rarely, bleeding continues beyond several days after surgery. In such cases, a careful intranasal examination with a rigid endoscope and suction may be required to identify the source of bleeding. Chemical cautery and repeat packing may address the problem. In some cases, an exam and electrocautery or suture control is required under anesthesia. In these cases, it may be an exposed vessel on the inferior turbinate or septum or granulation tissue around the septal splint which may be the source of the bleeding.

Postoperative infection is rare and is characterized by increased pain, swelling, and erythema. It must be determined if the patient has been compliant with the antibiotic regimen. If not, the appropriate antibiotics should be resumed. Nausea and dysphagia are two common reasons for failing to take oral medications. Antiemetics, liquid medicines, or i. v. administration of the antibiotics may therefore be needed. If infection has occurred despite taking antibiotics, a broader spectrum agent may be considered. If infection progresses despite these measures or if fluctuance develops, the intranasal incisions may need to be opened to allow drainage and irrigation beneath the SSTE. The presence of infection is compounded in the presence of multiple grafts or alloplastic materials.

Long-term complications related to collapse of nasal structures and contracture of the SSTE may manifest as lateral wall pinching, collapse of the middle vault, alar retraction, and tip ptosis. As stated previously, these complications are avoidable through stabilization of these structures and avoidance of overresection during primary surgery. These types of problems may not become apparent for several years after surgery. If severe, revision surgery to reconstruct the deficient areas may be required.

References

1. Toriumi DM. Structure approach in rhinoplasty. *Facial Plastic Clinics of North America.* 2000; 8:515–537.
2. Tardy ME. *Rhinoplasty: The art and science.* Philadelphia, W.B. Saunders: 1997.
3. Toriumi DM, Becker DG. *Rhinoplasty dissection manual.* Philadelphia: Lippincott: 1999.
4. Toriumi DM. Management of the middle nasal vault. *Op Tech Plast Reconst Surg* 1995; 2:16–30.
5. Orten SS, Hilger PA. Facial analysis of the rhinoplasty patient. In: Papel ID, ed. *Facial Plastic and Reconstructive Surgery*, 2nd ed. New York: Thieme Medical Publishers, Inc: 2002; 361–368.
6. Park SS. Treatment of the internal nasal valve. *Facial Plastic Clinics of North America.* 1999; 7:333–346.
7. Tardy ME, Walter MA, Patt BS. The overprojecting nose: anatomic component analysis and repair. *Facial Plastic Surgery.* 1993; 9:306–316.
8. Chand MS, Toriumi DM. Treatment of the external nasal valve. *Facial Plastic Clinics of North America.* 1999; 7:347–356.
9. Toriumi DM, Josen J, Weinberger M, Tardy ME. Use of alar batten grafts for correction of nasal valve collapse. *Arch Otolaryngol Head Neck Surg.* 1997; 123:802–8.
10. Toriumi DM, Hecht DA. Skeletal modifications in rhinoplasty. *Facial Plastic Clinics of North America.* 2000; 8:413–432.

Suggested Reading

Tardy ME. *Rhinoplasty: The art and science.* Philadelphia: W.B. Saunders: 1997.
Toriumi DM, Becker DG. *Rhinoplasty dissection manual.* Philadelphia: Lippincott: 1999.

Endonasal Tip Approaches and Techniques

S. W. Perkins

Contents

Introduction

Often, the most challenging part of rhinoplasty is modifying and refining the nasal tip. Endonasal delivery flap techniques have an extensive and successful history. This chapter will focus on the beauty, versatility, and the simplicity of endonasal tip surgery.

Achieving tip definition has evolved since Joseph introduced cosmetic rhinoplasty in the late 1800s. This evolution is described well by Tebbetts (1). Initially, nasal tip shaping techniques were destructive, consisting mostly of incising and resecting cartilage. Often the tip was approached in either a retrograde or a cartilage-splitting fashion. The limited visibility of these approaches lowered the threshold for possible asymmetry or other deformity. These early destructive techniques resulted in consistent loss of tip support and increased the risk of secondary deformities.

Then came the era of open structure rhinoplasty with the routine use of tip grafts. This increased the number of variables in the surgical maneuvers and long-term healing results where modifying and sculpting the normal anatomical structures could produce the same or better results. We now have evolved into an era of nondestructive tip-shaping techniques. These methods allow achievement of the desired esthetic appearance while maintaining or recreating projection and functional tip support. This assures excellent results not just at one year, but also at five years, 10 years, and more.

Our approach is based on the creation of the double-dome unit as described by McCollough and English (2). In addition, individual treatment of each dome to create the correct contour is further described. Long-term success using these techniques has been well described (3). We will first describe our basic surgical technique, followed by specific nasal tip deformities and steps utilized to correct these.

Indications

The ideal patient for these techniques has been described by Tardy et al. (4). The ideal patient has a slightly bifid or broad tip with dual dome highlights. Thin skin and sparse subcutaneous tissue allow for more refined results from these endonasal techniques. The alar cartilages themselves must be firm and strong. Finally, the alar sidewalls should be thin and delicate, yet resist collapse and recurvature. Most patients do not have these ideal features. Yet by using the endonasal approach and a progressive method with each tip, excellent esthetic results can still be achieved.

Contraindications

There are certain conditions in our experience that favor the use of the external columellar approach. It is often difficult to deliver, in a safe and adequate manner, alar cartilages in a patient with scar tissue in the lobule from previous surgery or trauma. Middle nasal vault deformities, in our experience, are more easily corrected through the external columellar approach. Patients with marked asymmetry in the nasal tip, with thin skin and bossa, may require camouflage tip grafting sutured in place. Also, marked twisting of the columella with significant discrepancies between the two medial crura may necessitate the external approach. Other indications for the external columellar approach are extremely soft alar cartilages with no inherent support as well as marked overprojection, overrotation, underprojection, and underrotation of the lobule.

Preoperative Considerations

All patients are initially seen in consultation with their selected surgeon. The consultation room is designed to put the patient at ease while still maintaining a professional environment. The nasal analysis begins with the patient on a comfortable bar stool in front of a three-way mirror with the physician directly behind him/her. Together they analyze the nose with the physician gently guiding the discussion. The three-way mirror offers a more three-dimensional conversation.

An in-depth nasal history is taken during the consultation. Inquiries include any previous nasal trauma or surgery, difficulties breathing through the nose, any history of sinus disease or allergies, and current nasal medications. The physician reviews a more extensive overall history form, completed by the patient prior to consultation, at this time. Intranasal exam is also performed at this time to detect deformities of the septum, enlargement of the turbinates, or other intranasal pathology. A preprinted nose form helps to ensure a complete evaluation (Fig. 8.**1 a, b**).

The procedure should be thoroughly discussed at this time and goals summarized with the patient. The physician reviews with the patient what to expect on the day of surgery, including the length of surgery, anesthesia, recovery, and discharge. Initial postoperative care and restrictions regarding certain activities are also discussed. Finally, the limitations of the surgery as well as possible complications are given as part of obtaining informed consent.

The consultation is then continued in the photography suite, where computer imaging is utilized to illustrate the physician's goals for surgery. This allows for confirmation that both the patient and the surgeon agree on the desired goals to be achieved. Following this a full set of nasal images are taken for preoperative documentation.

The last phase of the consultation is spent with the scheduling nurse, where questions can be answered in what often is a more comfortable setting for the patient. Fees are reviewed with the patient and signed copies of the procedures and fees are given to the patient. Any necessary lab work is arranged at this time.

Prior to surgery, all patients receive folders with detailed instructions on surgery, prescriptions, and a booklet reviewing postoperative healing and expectations. All patients start an oral antibiotic the day prior to surgery, most often either oral Keflex or Zithromax, and continue this for five days.

Fig. 8.**1 a, b**   Preprinted nasal history and physical evaluation form (side 1 and side 2).

PERKINS HAMILTON FACIAL PLASTIC SURGERY, P.C.

NASAL HISTORY AND PHYSICAL

Patient:_____

_____ History of trauma to nose: _____

_____ Previous surgery: _____
_____ Difficulty breathing:_____
_____ Patient Desires: **Improved tip: Smaller** ☐   **More defined** ☐
         Improved dorsum: Straighter ☐   **Narrower** ☐   **Hump removed** ☐

COSMETIC ABNORMALITIES

_____ Deviated nasal bones	_____ Dorsal hump
_____ Fractured nasal bones	_____ Traumatic dorsal hump
_____ C-shaped deformity R _____ L _____	_____ Dorsal saddling
_____ Irregular nasal bones	_____ Angulated R_____ L_____
_____ Nasal bones holding septum off center	_____ Dorsal curved septum only R_____ L_____
_____ Too short	_____ Dorsal ridge R_____ L_____
_____ Too long: Whole lobule ☐ Infra tip lobule ☐	_____ Avulsed/Depressed ULC's
_____ Projection: Over ☐ Under ☐	_____ Acute/deep N-F angle
_____ Soft lobular cartilages	_____ Obtuse N-F angle
_____ Rotation: Over ☐ Under ☐	_____ Poor tip support

TIP

_____ Supratip fullness:
     Soft tissue ☐
     Cartilage ☐
_____ Bulbous tip   _____ Asymmetric tip
_____ Broad tip
_____ Bifid tip
_____ Amorphous tip
_____ Infantile tip

LLC's asymmetric	R _____	L _____
Concave LLC	R _____	L _____
Bossa	R _____	L _____
Retracted ala	R _____	L _____
Nostrils wide: Horizontal	R _____	L _____
Asymmetrical	R _____	L _____
Wide alae	R _____	L _____
Alar base flare	R _____	L _____
Unusual cartilage bump	R _____	L _____

COLUMELLA

_____ Crooked   R _____ L _____
_____ Show: Elong. septum:
_____ Hanging
_____ Retracted
_____ Short ☐   Long ☐
_____ Twisted
_____ Short infra tip lobule

_____ MC Buckle   R _____ L _____
_____ Medial crural shift caudally   R _____ L _____
_____ Acute Nasolabial angle _____ %
    (60 - 65 - 70 - 75 - 80 - 85 - 90 - 95 - 100 - 105)
_____ Bifid

DORSUM

_____ Dorsal hump   Cartilage _____ Bone _____
_____ Dorsal irregularities   Cartilage _____ Bone _____
_____ Dorsal saddle   Cartilage _____ Bone _____
_____ Dorsum wide
_____ Open roof deformity   Central ☐   Right ☐   Left ☐
_____ Thick skin
_____ Thin skin
_____ Skin irregularities
_____ Weak chin

Doctor:_____   Date: ___/___/___   NASHISFUNC

Fig. 8.**1 b** ▷

Preoperative Analysis

It is critical to determine the exact tip deformities before creating a surgical plan. What is the esthetic problem of the tip and what is one attempting to achieve? This begins with a detailed examination during the consultation period. Standardized forms are helpful for assuring a complete examination as well as simplifying documentation (Fig. 8.**1 a, b**). The tip shape should be described, for example, as bulbous, twisted, or infantile. Both the degree of rotation and the extent of projection should be evaluated. It is critical to assess skin thickness and this issue alone may dictate approach and/or procedure to be performed. Palpation is helpful in determining the nature, volume, strength, and resiliency of the lobular cartilages as well as in evaluating tip support. Finally, it is important to note columellar abnormalities and their relation to the alar cartilages.

Fig. 8.**1 b**

PERKINS HAMILTON FACIAL PLASTIC SURGERY, P.C.

NASAL HISTORY AND PHYSICAL

Patient:_____

———— History of trauma to nose:_____
_____

———— Previous surgery:_____
———— Difficulty breathing: R ☐   L ☐   Bilateral ☐   Snoring——— Mouth breathing———
———— Patient desires: Straighter nose ☐   Improved breathing ☐
———— Sinus disease
———— Medications tried:_____   _____   _____   _____

FUNCTIONAL ABNORMALITIES

———— Deviated nasal bones
———— Fractured nasal bones
———— C-shaped deformity   R ☐   L ☐
———— Irregular nasal bones
———— Nasal bones holding
        septum off center

———— Traumatic dorsal hump
———— Dorsal saddling:
        Cartilage ☐ Bone ☐ Both ☐
———— Angulated   R ☐   L ☐
———— Dorsal ridge   R ☐   L ☐

Pyramid	**Drawing**	Septum
R	L R	L

———— Septum deviated   R ☐   L ☐
———— Spurs   R ☐   L ☐
———— Caudal end deflected   R ☐   L ☐
        blocking vestibule
———— Floor obstruction   R ☐   L ☐

———— Intranasal synnechia(e) R ☐   L ☐
———— Inferior turbinate
        hypertrophy   R ☐   L ☐
———— Middle turbinate hypertrophy
        or concha bullosa   R ☐   L ☐
———— Septal ulcer   R ☐   L ☐
———— Septal varices   R ☐   L ☐
———— Septal perforation:
           Size:_____
           Location:_____

———— Nasal valve collapse   R ☐   L ☐
        Internal ———— Alar
———— Middle vault narrowing
        or collapse   R ☐   L ☐
———— Loss of tip support
———— Collapsed lobule with
        valve collapse   R ☐   L ☐
———— Avulsed / depressed
        ULC's   R ☐   L ☐
———— Soft lobular cartilages

———— Nasal polyposis: R ☐ L ☐
———— Retraction of columella
———— Acute nasolabial angle
———— Premaxillary deficiency: R ☐ L ☐ Complete ☐
———— Cleft lip nasal deformity: R ☐ L ☐ Bilateral ☐

% Airway obstruction

R_____   L_____

(60 - 65 - 70 - 75 - 80 - 85 -
90 - 95 - 100 - 105)

NOTES:_____
_____
_____
_____

Doctor:_____   Date: ___/___/___

Surgical Technique

One and a half hours prior to surgery, patients are given oral Valium, phenergan. Reglan, and decadron, as well as Afrin nasal spray. In the operating room, deep sedation, typically utilizing i. v. propofol, is utilized prior to beginning local anesthesia. First pledgets soaked in 10% cocaine are placed intranasally. After adequate time for decongestion, infiltration is started with 2% Xylocaine with 1:50 000 epinephrine. No more than 7–8 cc is injected with minimal volume distortion.

The delivery approach is begun by making either a complete transfixion or high septal transfixion incision, depending on tip projection (Fig. 8.**2**). Curved, sharp scissors are then used to dissect up over the anterior superior angle and expose the upper lateral cartilages. Next, intercartilaginous and marginal incisions are made in a standard fashion (Fig. 8.**3**). Thin Metzenbaum scissors are then used to separate the overlying skin from the underlying lower lateral cartilages, nasal domes, and infratip lobule (intermediate crura). Finally, the alar cartilages are delivered with a single hook and supported with Metzenbaum scissors (Fig. 8.**4**). In this fashion each dome is assessed and recontoured individually.

The first step in achieving improved tip definition is the removal of fibrofatty tissue between the domes. This allows greater approximation of the two alar domes. An intact or complete strip can be performed next by excising the cephalic

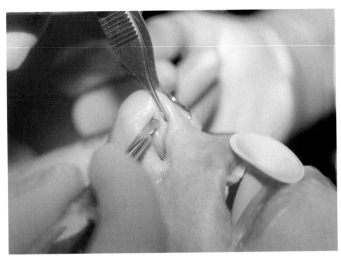

Fig. 8.**2**   Complete high septal transfixion incision.

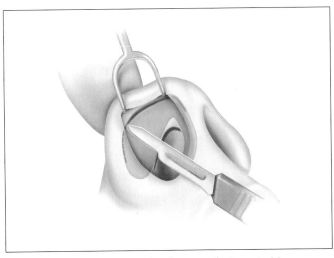

Fig. 8.**3**   Illustration of marginal and intercartilaginous incisions.

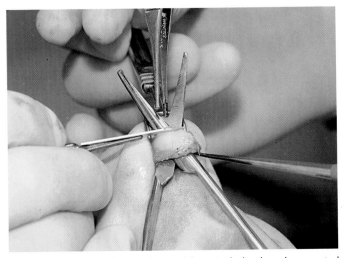

Fig. 8.**4**   Delivery of alar cartilages with a single hook and supported with Metzenbaum scissors.

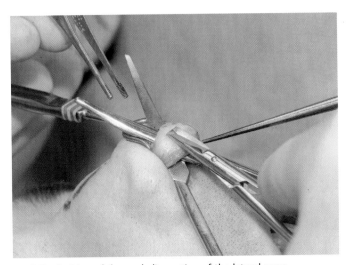

Fig. 8.**5**   Excision of the cephalic portion of the lateral crura.

portion of the lateral crura (Fig. 8.**5**). This achieves both volume reduction as well as improved supratip definition. It is essential to preserve a piece of cartilage at least 7–9 mm wide. In a few select cases, this may be all that is required and the cartilages may be replaced in situ. In most cases, however, other techniques are required to achieve satisfactory tip definition and symmetry.

The ideal alar configuration has been described as being when the domal segment is convex, the adjacent lateral crura is slightly concave, and the overlying soft tissue is thin (5). Occasionally, careful "pinching" of the individual dome cartilages can mold the cartilage into the ideal shape. Most often, however, individual dome treatment with suture is required. Prior to placing the single dome suture, the vestibular skin is separated from the undersurface of the domal cartilage (Fig. 8.**6**). A 5–0 absorbable synthetic polyglycolic acid (Dexon) mattress suture is placed at the junction of the lateral and medial crura. The knot is tightened to the point where the proper amount of domal definition is achieved (Fig. 8.**7**).

If the individual domes remain asymmetrical or improved supratip definition is desired, individual dome trimming can be performed. This involves "beveling" the cephalic portion of the single dome unit (Fig. 8.**8 a, b**).

With achievement of symmetrical, esthetically pleasing individual domes, the entire tip is reevaluated. Utilization of the endonasal approach allows this continual critiquing. A double-dome or transdomal mattress suture is next used to bring the individually defined domes together and stabilize these into one unit.

Stabilization is the key to maintenance of long-term results.

The suture is placed horizontally through the lateral and medial crura of both domes. We typically utilize a 5–0 clear polypropylene (Prolene) suture. The desired amount of lobular narrowing can be achieved by altering the tension of the stitch. With the domes replaced, the amount of narrowing can be seen as one tightens the knot (Fig. 8.**9**). It is important to avoid cinching down the suture and creating a unitip appearance.

The tip is then reevaluated. At this point the decision is made whether or not more aggressive steps will be required to achieve the desired tip esthetics. This could include steps such as lateral crural flap, dome division or the Lipsett maneuver. Marked disparity in length between the two medial crura is best corrected with the Lipsett procedure. With this technique the lengthier medial crura is delivered and dissected free from its attachments. An appropriate length of crura is resected to achieve equality in length between the medial crura. The two

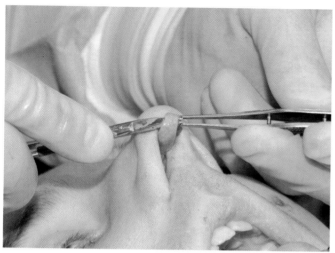

Fig. 8.**6** Separation of vestibular skin from the undersurface of the domal cartilage.

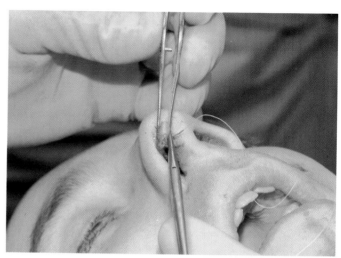

Fig. 8.**7** Mattress suture placed at the junction of lateral and medial crura.

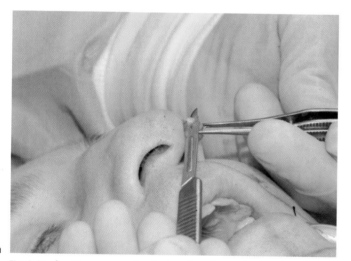

a

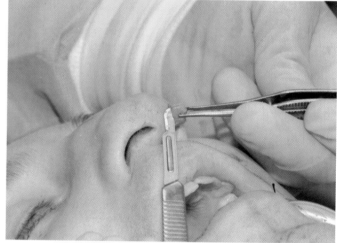

b

Fig. 8.**8 a, b** Dome narrowing by beveling the cephalic portion of the single dome unit.

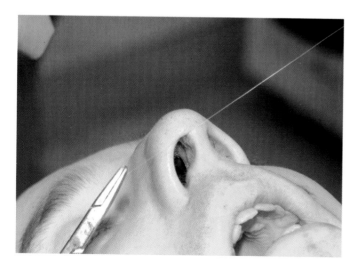

Fig. 8.**9** Narrowing of domes by tightening a 5–0 clear prolene suture knot.

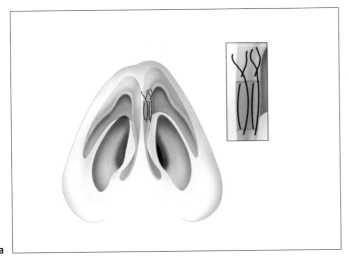

a

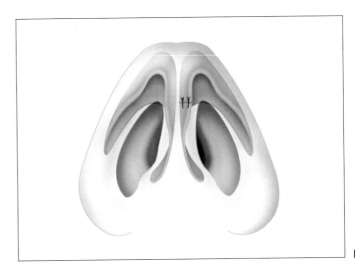

b

Fig. 8.**10 a, b**   Illustration of Lipsett maneuver.

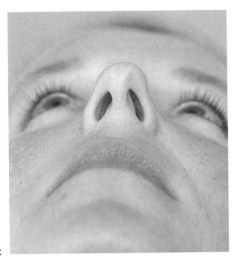

c

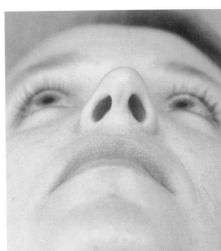

d

Fig. 8.**10 c, d**   Preoperative and postoperative basal view showing results of a unilateral, left Lipsett procedure.

resected ends are then reapproximated with 6–0 monocryl (Fig. 8.**10 a-d**).

Removing or replacing the double-dome mattress sutures and addressing the anterior–posterior or caudal–cephalic placement of a suture in relation to the other dome may address minor asymmetries.

Dome division is utilized for a variety of situations when the above more conservative techniques have not been successful. Dome division can allow for more tip narrowing, which is especially required in those with thick skin. Dome division can also be used to achieve upward rotation and increase or decrease tip projection. Finally, correction of tip asymmetries may be more easily addressed with dome division.

Dome division can be performed medial to the dome, lateral to the dome, or at the dome (Fig. 8.**11 a, b**).

Conservative upward rotation of the tip is typically achieved by resection of an inverted triangle of caudal septum with corresponding vestibular skin and using a columellar strut to assist in "pushing" the lobule cephalically. If further rotation is required following this, the lateral crural flap technique can be employed. This can involve a full incision of the lateral crura or simply a cephalic wedge excision (Fig. 8.**12 a, b**). The lateral crura can be overlapped and sutured to shorten their length and create upward rotation.

Following achievement of a symmetrical and well-defined tip, attention is then turned to the septum, the dorsum, and, lastly, osteotomies. A columellar strut fashioned from septal cartilage is placed between the medial crura and anterior to the nasal spine prior to osteotomies. Intranasal incisions are closed with 5–0 catgut. In closing the marginal incisions, it is important to avoid the lateral crura when suturing. Retraction

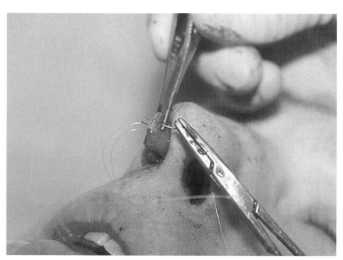

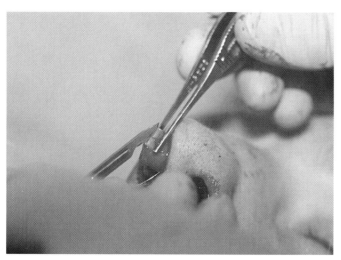

a   b

Fig. 8.**11 a, b**   Dome division can be performed medial to the dome, lateral to the dome, or at the dome.

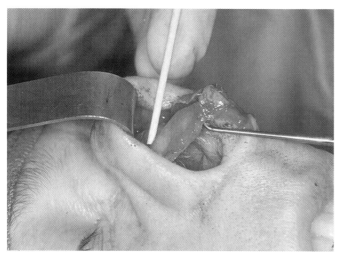

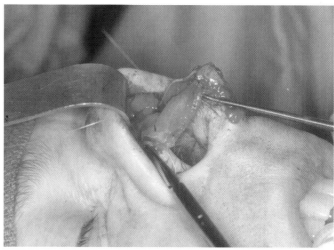

Fig. 8.**12 a**   Cephalic "wedge" excised at the lateral aspect of the lateral crus.

Fig. 8.**12 b**   Lateral crural flap. Complete transection, overlap, and suture of the lateral aspect of the lateral crus.

of the lateral crura could lead to possible alar collapse and nostril asymmetries.

Case Studies

Broad/Wide Tip

Tips that demonstrate minimal deformity and minimally excess width can be addressed in the most conservative fashion. Single-dome suture treatment is often not required in these patients if the alar dome cartilages are delicate, thin, or soft. A conservative cephalic trim followed by a double-dome suture alone can often achieve the desire result (Fig. 8.**13 a, b**).

Bulbous/Boxy Tip

The bulbous tip requires individual treatment of the domes. This is most often addressed with a conservative cephalic trim and an individual single-dome mattress suture. Reconstitution of the double-dome unit with a 5–0 clear prolene completes tip refinement (Fig. 8.**14 a-d**).

Bifid Tip

The bifid tip often requires both single-dome and double-dome mattress treatment of the tip complex. Occasionally, suture approximation of the tip alone will eliminate the bifidity. Most often, however, placement of either a nonsutured tip graft or a columellar filler graft is required (Fig. 8.**15 a-d**).

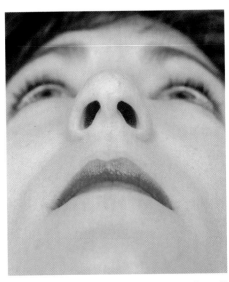

Fig. 8.**13 a**   Preoperative basal view of a broad/ wide nasal tip.

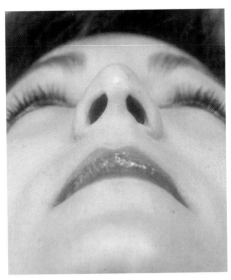

Fig. 8.**13 b**   Postoperative basal view of a conservative cephalic trim followed by double-dome suture.

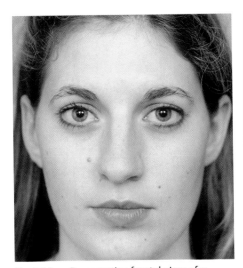

Fig. 8.**14 a**   Preoperative frontal view of a bulbous/boxy tip.

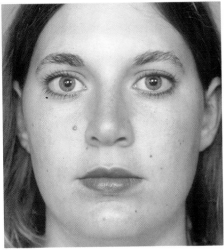

Fig. 8.**14 b**   Postoperative frontal view of tip refinement of a bulbous/boxy tip.

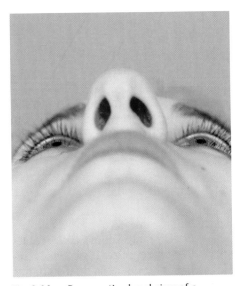

Fig. 8.**14 c**   Preoperative basal view of a bulbous/boxy tip.

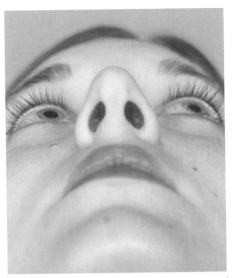

Fig. 8.**14 d**   Postoperatve basal view of tip refinement of a bulbous/boxy tip.

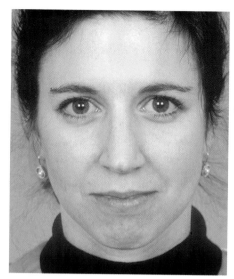

Fig. 8.**15a** Preoperative frontal view of a bifid tip.

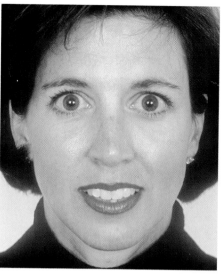

Fig. 8.**15b** Postoperative frontal view of tip complex after treatment of a bifid tip.

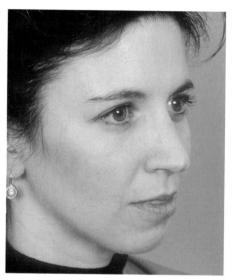

Fig. 8.**15c** Preoperative oblique view of a bifid tip.

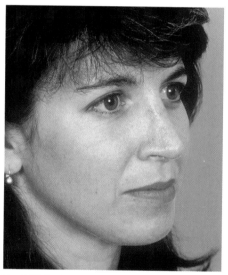

Fig. 8.**15d** Postoperative oblique view of tip complex after graft placement for treatment of a bifid tip.

Trapezoid Tip

The trapezoid tip deformity is due to divergent intermediate crura (Fig. 8.**16a-d**). Cartilage splitting or transcartilaginous cephalic margin resection is unwise in these patients as both can often lead to the late development of bossae. The alar cartilages have to be reoriented more caudally, or lateral alar batten grafts or possibly even alar struts must be added. This can be necessary if the lateral alar sidewalls are weak and tend to collapse or recurve inward when the domes are brought together.

Reconstitution of the interdomal ligament—single-dome and double-dome suture techniques—is required for correction. Tip grafting of the infratip lobule is also often necessary. Oftentimes even when the above aggressive techniques are employed, an esthetic tip cannot be achieved. In these more difficult cases, dome division is indicated to narrow the tip and straighten the lateral ala.

Asymmetrical Tip

A variety of techniques can be utilized to correct the asymmetrical tip, depending on the degree and the exact deformity. Minor deformities may be corrected with double-dome suture techniques alone. If asymmetry is due primarily to a disparity in medial crura length, the Lipsett procedure may be employed. For marked asymmetry between the domes, dome division is utilized (Fig. 8.**17a, b**). Typically the overprojecting dome is truncated and the double-dome unit is reconstituted. When the entire nose is overprojected, bilateral dome truncation may be performed.

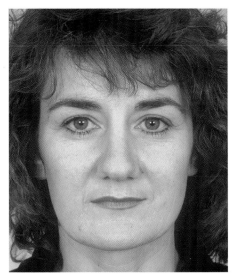

Fig. 8.**16 a**   Preoperative frontal view of a trapezoid tip deformity.

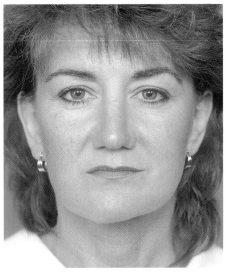

Fig. 8.**16 b**   Postoperative frontal view of a trapezoid tip deformity.

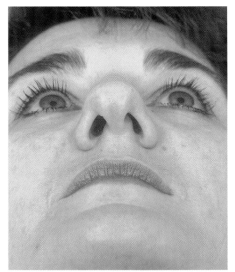

Fig. 8.**16 c**   Preoperative basal view of a trapezoid tip deformity.

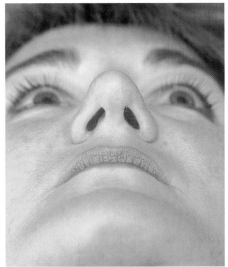

Fig. 8.**16 d**   Postoperative basal view of a trapezoid tip deformity.

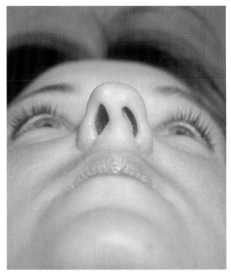

Fig. 8.**17 a**   Preoperative basal view of marked asymmetry between the domes, for which dome division is utilized.

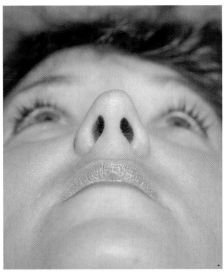

Fig. 8.**17 b**   Postoperative basal view of marked asymmetry between the domes, for which dome division is utilized.

Postoperative Care

A small, rolled piece of absorbable oxidized regenerated cellulose (Surgicel) is placed inside the nose within the vestibule of each newly constructed dome to add stability and prevent hematoma. One quarter circle shaped telfa pads are placed just inside the nose for absorbtion of drainage during the first night and are removed the following morning. A drip pad is also utilized the first 24 hours. Tan surgical tape (Micropore) along with an alloy metal splint is used for the external dressing that is removed at one week. Patient instructions include no strenuous activity for two weeks, no heavy lifting for three weeks, and avoidance of glasses on the nose for six weeks. Patients are closely followed for the entire first year. Revision surgery is considered only following a full twelve months of healing. Annual follow-up is strongly encouraged following the first postoperative year.

Complications

Bossa Formation

Knuckling of the lower lateral cartilages with healing can occur. Typically this is due to weakening of the lateral crura secondary to either overresection or cartilage-splitting techniques. Patients with thin skin, strong cartilages, and nasal tip bifidity are at the highest risk for this. Bossae can be treated by resecting the deformed cartilage through a marginal incision. Further camouflage can be provided by either morselized cartilage or fascia.

Alar Retraction

Retraction of ala is usually due to either overresection of the lateral crura or excess resection of vestibular mucosa. Improper suture placement during closure of the marginal incision can also retract the alar rim. Preservation of a complete strip of 8 mm or more in patients with a thin alar rim will help to prevent retraction.

Alar retraction can be corrected by taking a composite graft from the cymba concha of the ear (6). A marginal incision is made in the area of retraction and a small pocket is corrected. The graft is then sutured into place, in effect pushing down the alar rim.

Tip Asymmetry

Postoperative asymmetry of the tip can be due to a variety of causes. Most often it is due to uneven placement of the double-dome stitch. Healing forces can alter what was symmetrical initially during the postoperative period. Minor asymmetries not noted before surgery may become more obvious with a more overall symmetrical nose. Preoperative identification of tip asymmetries and meticulous technique can help to prevent their occurrence.

Improper Projection

Intercartilaginous as well as transfixion incisions do lead to decreased tip support as well as decreased projection. This is usually counterbalanced by the increased strength of the medial crura with creation of the double-dome unit. Struts provide further strength and projection.

Most commonly, due to the inherent strength achieved with the double-dome unit, overprojection is the more common minor complication. Preoperative planning and continual intraoperative assessment will help to avoid either overprojection or underprojection.

Summary

The advantages that open rhinoplasty offers with increased exposure come with many downsides. The external incision itself can be a source of noticeable scarring, alar notching, or even trap door deformity. Patients are required to make a special visit for removal of the columellar sutures at five days postoperatively. This is both an inconvenience as well as a somewhat painful experience. Finally, resolution of tip edema is significantly prolonged with the external approach. For all of these reasons, our first choice is to utilize endonasal techniques whenever possible.

Endonasal double-dome techniques are based on the philosophy of utilization of the normal anatomical structures of the nasal tip (lobule). The merits of these techniques are many. Results of individual steps can continuously be reevaluated. Most of these incremental steps are reversible. Often, use of grafts can be avoided as well as the possibility of secondary deformities that come with them. The disadvantages of these techniques include the need for greater surgical finesse in delivering and suturing the alar cartilages. Also, techniques for the correction of certain deformities may be better addressed through the external columellar approach. Nevertheless, for most primary cosmetic tip rhinoplasties, the beauty and expedient nature of the endonasal delivery flap approach with double-dome techniques provides consistent, long-term results and few complications.

References

1. Tebbetts JB. Rethinking the logic and techniques of primary tip rhinoplasty: a perspective of the evolution of surgery of the nasal tip (review). *Clin Plast. Surg.* 1996; 23:245–253.
2. McCollough EG, English JL. A new twist in nasal tip surgery: an alternative to the Goldman tip for the wide or bulbous lobule. *Arch Otolaryngol.* 1985; 111:524–529.
3. Perkins SW, Hamilton MM, MacDonald K. A successful 15-year experience in double-dome tip surgery via the endonasal approach. *Arch. Fac. Plastic Surg.* 2001; 3:157–164.
4. Tardy ME jr, Pratt BS, Walter MA. Transdomal suture refinement of the nasal tip: long-term outcomes. *Facial Plast. Surg.* 1993; 9:275–284.
5. Daniel RK. Rhinoplasty: creating an aesthetic tip: a preliminary report. *Plast. Reconstr. Surg.* 1987; 80:775–783.
6. Tardy ME. Toriumi DM, Alar retraction: A composite correction. *Fac. Plast. Surg.* 1989; 6 (2):101–107.

Suggested Reading

Tardy ME. *Rhinoplasty: The art and the science.* Philadelphia: WB Saunders: 1997.

Alar Reduction and Sculpture

R. Thomas and M. E. Tardy, Jr.

Contents

Introduction

Modification of the alar base and lobule anatomy during rhinoplasty by various forms of alar reduction, repositioning, reorientation, or sculpturing assists in balancing the final appearance of the nose. Esthetic narrowing of the nasal skeleton and tip must, in selected patients, be balanced by concomitant reduction refinement of the alar base (usually as the final step in the operation), else the nose appears "bottom-heavy" and disproportionate. Classically, a vertical line dropped from each inner canthus alongside the nose should define the lateral limits of the alae for an ideal normal appearance on frontal view (Fig. 9.1). Wider or more flaring alae suggest consideration for alar base reduction techniques (Fig. 9.2). These, like nasal tip sculpture techniques, are best executed in a graduated fashion, planned entirely upon the individual anatomy encountered and the esthetic appearance desired. In most retropositioning tip techniques employed to correct the overprojected nose, lateral flaring of the alar sidewalls results, inviting alar reduction in both width and overall alar sidewall length.

Weir is credited with the first published reference to alar base narrowing (1). Thus alar base narrowing is traditionally referred to by surgeons as the "Weir procedure"; we prefer the term "alar base reduction," since the exact procedure recommended by Weir is indistinct. His seminal article fails to illustrate the exact technique recommended. Others throughout the twentieth century, however, have refined precise indications for and techniques of alar base reduction and narrowing during rhinoplasty.

Indications

The exact alar reduction technique chosen will be dependent upon the individual anatomy encountered, the esthetic outcome desired, and the need to camouflage resultant epithelial scars. Alar modifications are rather consistently required to balance the nasal anatomy in certain ethnic anatomical types (i.e., Black, Asian, Oriental, and Mestizo noses), while the need to perform alar reduction in the more typical Caucasian nose is less frequent. None the less, alar base modifications are indicated when alar flaring, bulbosity, or excessive width of the nasal base are present, or when retropositioning of excessive tip projection results in a displeasing postoperative alar flare on the operating table. An excessively wide nostril floor dimension may also dictate the need for alar sill or nostril floor modifications. If preoperative asymmetry exists (as in the cleft lip/nose complex anomaly), alar modification should be considered.

Alar surgical modifications are usually most accurately performed as one of the final steps in esthetic rhinoplasty, after

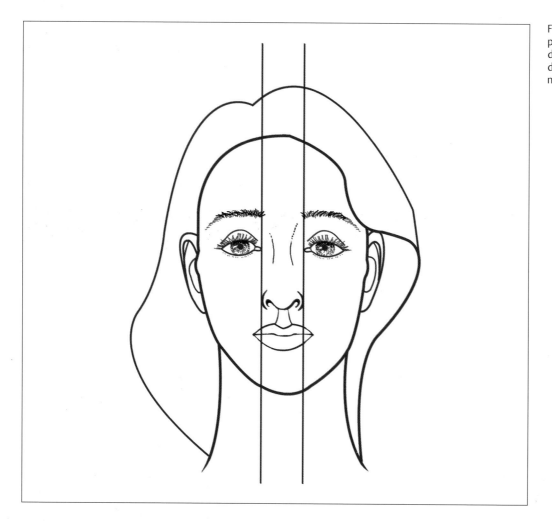

Fig. 9.1   In faces with normal proportions, an imaginary line dropped from the inner canthi defines the normal width of the nasal alar base.

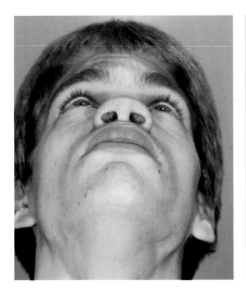 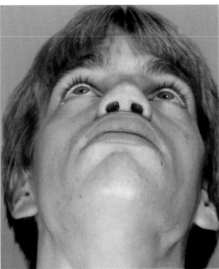

Fig. 9.2   (left) Unusually wide nasal base, significantly narrowed with a sliding alar flap procedure combined with improvement of tip projection (right).

all major and adjunctive procedures have been completed. At this time the general appearance of the surgically modified tip may be assessed, and the indicated method of alar sculpturing may be selected and carried out. If any doubt exists about nasal proportions, it is best to defer alar reduction until a later date, when postoperative nasal-tip healing is more exact, and more accurate evaluation of the modified, healing nasal anatomy becomes clear.

Alar reduction of any type must be carried out in a *conservative* and *symmetrical* manner, *lest one deformity be substituted for another.* Even subtle or minimal asymmetries or overreductions may create a major deformity where only a minor balance abnormality preexisted. If overaggressive resection of the alar base occurs, correction is difficult at best. In addition, it is important that the surgeon bring all his skills into play in the effort to minimize and camouflage the resultant alar scars, which can draw unwanted attention to an otherwise excellent rhinoplasty outcome.

In revision rhinoplasty, alar abase reduction or modification is indicated if a widened or asymmetrical alar base exists. Similarly, poor or visible scars resultant from primary alar base reduction deserve improvement and camouflage.

Contraindications

Only relative contraindications exist for alar base reduction surgery. Infantile nostrils, even in patients with a widened alar base disproportion, should not be rendered to an unacceptably smaller dimension by alar reduction. Overly small nostril openings resultant from previous surgery should not be made unacceptably small by attempts to camouflage unsightly alar lobule or nostril sill scars.

Alar reduction of major magnitude should be contemplated with caution when revision open rhinoplasty is carried out. Compromised blood supply to the tip has been reported in a few patients in this category.

Alternative Techniques

Internal buried alar cinch suture techniques can narrow the alar base modestly, but generally at the expense of alar base tissue distortion and possible asymmetry. Moreover, long-term continuous tension created by permanent suture cinching is always subject to eventual suture tear-out and failure. Precision surgical alar excision and repair remains the more acceptable surgical choice.

Preoperative Considerations

Thorough informed consent is essential before alar reduction is contemplated. Patients must understand that bilateral alar–facial junction scars will be present (although generally nicely camouflaged). If available, preoperative computer imaging can assist in confirming for the patient the benefit of surgical alar base reduction. Standard four-view rhinoplasty photographic documentation is essential, with an optional close-up basal view helpful.

Special Surgical Requirements

1. 5–0 fast-absorbing catgut suture
2. 5–0 polydioxane (PDA) suture
3. Needlepoint microcautery
4. Histacryl Blue or Dermabond tissue glue
5. 15c Bard-Parker knife blade
6. Surgical measuring calipers

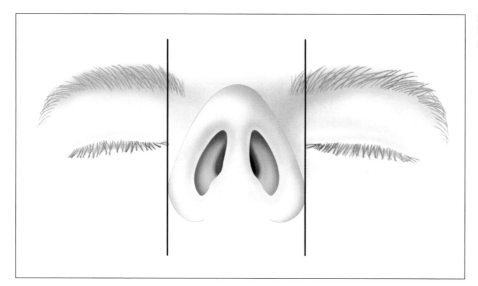

Fig. 9.**3**   The normal alar base width defined by lines dropped from the inner canthi to the alar–facial junctions bilaterally.

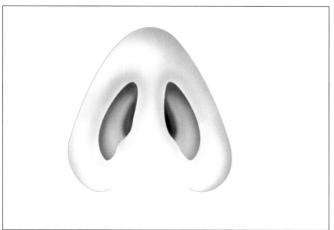

Fig. 9.**4**   Normal triangularity of the nasal base, with the preferred terminology applied to each anatomical element.

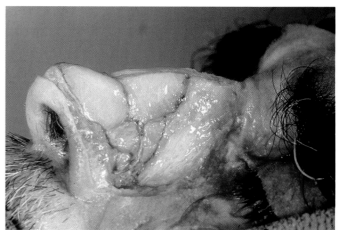

Fig. 9.**5**   The alar lobule is devoid of cartilage, being composed of highly vascular fibroareolar tissue, muscle, and fat.

Preoperative Analysis

Nothing equals the importance of extremely accurate and precise analysis and diagnosis in planning alar reduction surgery. The frontal and base views play the most important role in preoperative evaluation. A vertical line dropped from each inner canthus helps to define the esthetic appropriateness of alar base anatomy (Fig. 9.**1**). On base view, the same vertical lines from the inner canthus define the correct alar–facial junction relationship (Fig. 9.**3**). If the alar lobules fall outside (lateral to) this vertical line, alar base reduction is indicated to avoid a postoperative "bottom-heavy" nasal appearance.

The preferred terminology, desirable ideal normal anatomy, and preferred esthetic relationships of the alae and nostrils to the face and nose are depicted in Figure 9.**4**. In general, the alar lobule is composed of fibrofatty areolar tissues covered by epithelium both internally and externally (Fig. 9.**5**). Completely devoid of alar or sesamoid cartilage, the alae assume markedly different shapes, sizes, and configurations in different ethnic groups and even within similar ethnic groups (Fig. 9.**6**) (2). In the typical Caucasian patient, the alar sidewalls

serve as minor or adjunctive supportive mechanisms for the nasal tip, but if thin, delicate, and somewhat anatomically frail, may contribute nothing to tip support and are in danger of potential eventual collapse if an overabundance of supportive alar cartilage is resected during tip sculpturing.

The site and position of insertion of the alae into the face influence nasal proportions and esthetics dramatically. A more cephalic location of the alar–facial junction may create a high, arched appearance to the alae, exposing an excessive and undesirable amount of columella; when this anatomical variant is even more profound, a snarl-like appearance may result. More caudal insertions of the alae into the face produce the appearance of a disproportionately large and bulbous alar lobule, resulting in alar "hooding," and inadequate exposure of the esthetically appropriate amount of columellar anatomy. More commonly, less profound variations of anatomy between these two extremes exist, and are among the easiest to correct.

Thick, fat sidewalls detract from the overall delicacy and balance of the nose. Although not always amenable to total correction, defatting and thinning through skin incisions at the nostril border (or if possible just internal to the alar margin), may be justified to improve appearance and balance of the nasal base.

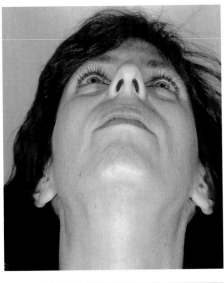

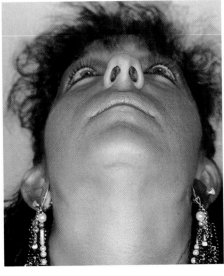

a

b

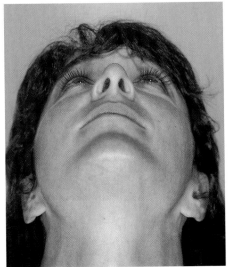

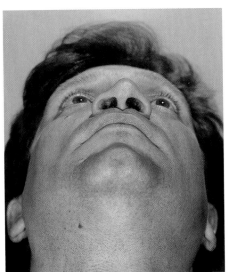

c

d

Fig. 9.**6 a–d** Alar base anatomy is highly diverse, varying in size, shape, inclination, and curvature of the alar sidewalls. The manner by which the alar sidewalls insert into the face, columella, or upper lip demonstrates extreme variability as well.

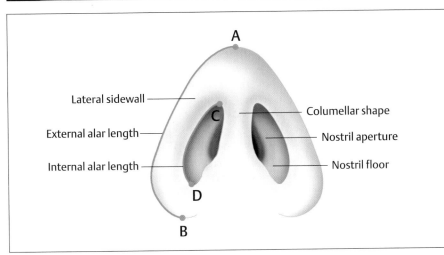

Fig. 9.**7** Analysis of the anatomy of the alar base should take into account:
- The internal length of the alar sidewall (C–D)
- The external length of the alar sidewall (A–B)
- The width and shape of the nostril floor and sill
- The shape and size of the nostril aperture
- The anatomy of the columella and related medial crural footplates, including both the length of the medial crurs and lateral flare of the footplates
- The overall length of the lateral alar sidewalls, determined by the site of insertion of the alae into the face.

The ideal alar lobule should not stand alone as a distinctive individual component of the nasal anatomy, but should blend the remainder of the nose into the face gracefully and without disharmony.

The site of incisions and the amount, degree, and geometry of alar reductions depend upon a host of anatomical variations predetermined before and during surgery (3). Although the surgeon's esthetic judgement will ultimately determine the site and degree of resection, a more precise surgical approach may be determined if several anatomical guidelines are assessed and integrated into the surgical plan. *Conservative* surgical alar reduction is mandatory to avoid overreduction and asymmetry, conditions almost impossible to correct satisfactorily.

To determine the planned approach and the site and geometry of incisions and excisions, the following anatomical factors are carefully evaluated (Fig. 9.**7**) (3):

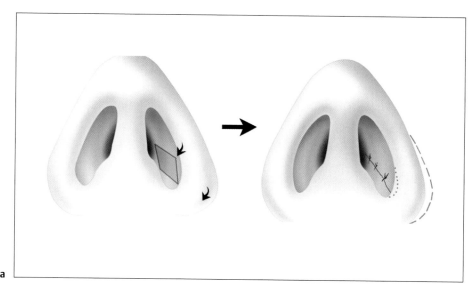

Fig. 9.8 (a) Subtle alar base narrowing by removing a diamond- or crescent-shaped segment at the junction of the floor of the nose with the alar sidewall. (b) Before narrowing. (c) After narrowing refinement.

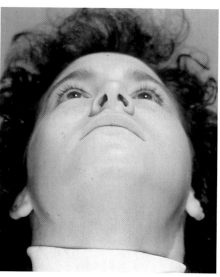

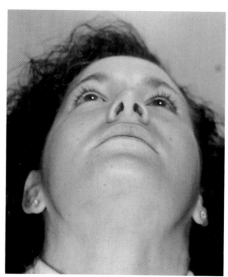

1. The *internal* (medial) length, shape, thickness, and lateral flare of the alar margin (C–D).
2. The *external* (lateral) length, shape, thickness, and lateral flare of the alar margin (A–B).
3. The width and shape of the *nostril floor and sill*.
4. The shape of the *nostril aperture*.
5. The shape (anatomy) of the *columella* and related medial crural footplates, including both the length of the medial crura and lateral flare of the medial crural footplates.
6. The length of the *lateral sidewalls of the nose*, determined by the site of insertion of the alae to the face

Graduated Surgical Techniques

The decision to perform alar base reduction during rhinoplasty is best made prior to surgery, when surgical edema infiltration anesthesia have not temporarily distorted the true anatomy (4). Once a decision is reached about which of the above anatomical factors are in need of modification, a *graduated* surgi-

cal scheme is employed to achieve the desired esthetic outcome. Based upon the anatomy encountered, alar excision and sculpture will range from minimal to major, depending upon the anatomy encountered (5). Like much of rhinoplasty, alar reduction represents a *compromise* operation, in which greater reductions exact the penalty of a larger and perhaps potentially more visible scar.

Internal Nostril Floor Reduction

In patients who require only minimal narrowing of the alar base dimensions, excision of a small wedge of epithelium and soft tissue from the nostril floor only will reduce the slight alar flare by reducing the dimension of the internal (medial) border of the alar sidewall. Although the outward curve of the sidewall is slightly altered, no medial repositioning or the alar–facial junction is created. The scar is effectively hidden within the nostril floor and the sill is not violated. Subtle, conservative but effective improvements are possible with this approach (Fig. 9.**8**).

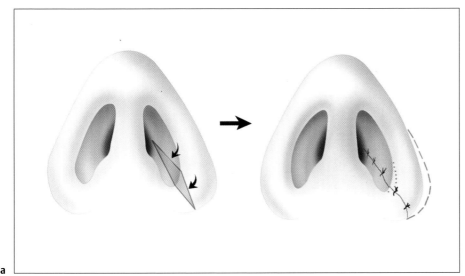

Fig. 9.**9** (**a**) A wedge removed of the alar base which is carried across the nostril sill into the alar sidewall. (**b**) Before narrowing. (**c**) Improved appearance after this type of subtle alar base narrowing.

a

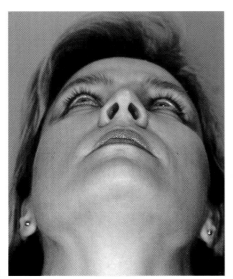

b

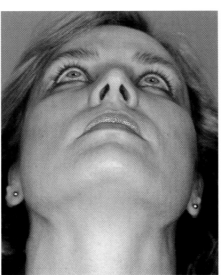

c

Wedge Excision Nostril Floor and Sill

Further reduction of alar flare is accomplished by carrying the incision across the sill into the alar–facial junction. Reduction of lateral flare as well as slight reduction of the bulk is effected (Fig. 9.**9**).

Alar Wedge Excision

If the alar development is excessive and bulbous, excision of a wedge of ala just above the alar–facial junction will reduce the overall bulkiness of the alar anatomy (Fig. 9.**10**). Some medial repositioning of the alae will be effected with this maneuver. Reduction of the overall length of the alar sidewalls occurs when generous wedges are excised, ideal in the overall reduction of the overprojecting tip.

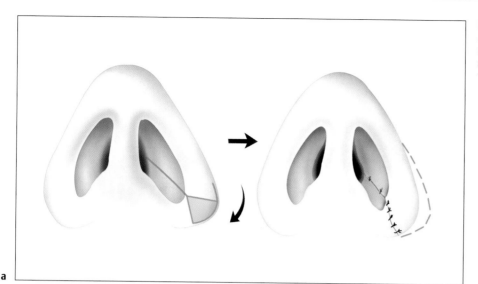

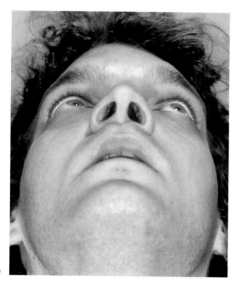

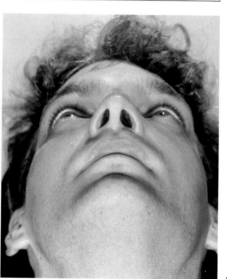

Fig. 9.**10**   (**a**) Excision of a major wedge of the alar sidewall to effect a more profound medial rotation of the alar sidewall, significantly narrowing the alar base. (**b**) Before narrowing with this technique. (**c**) Result obtained.

a

b

c

Alar Flap

Minimal alar reduction and slight medial repositioning of the alar–facial junction with excellent scar camouflage is accomplished with the approach described by Sheen (9) (Fig. 9.**11**). In this approach the incision remains on the alar surface and does not traverse the nostril sill, thus avoiding a potential "notched" appearance of the sill. Only very modest changes are possible with this technique.

Sliding Alar Flap

Maximal alar reduction with medial repositioning is effected with a generous incision in the alar–facial junction with various degrees of alar excision (Fig. 9.**12**). Reducton of the volume, curve, and flare of both the internal and external alar margins will result from this procedure, the extent of each being dependent upon the angulation of the alar incision. A back-cut placed 2 mm above the alar–facial junction allows the

alar flap to slide medially, narrowing the alar base significantly (6).

Of equal importance to the planning of the indicated technique for alar sculpturing is the precision plastic repair of the resultant scar (7). The ultimate appearance of far too many alar junction scars is compromised by imprecise opposition of the cut edges, resulting in level discrepancies and notches, which cast shadows, and thus diminish scar camouflage. Abundant sebaceous glands at the alar–facial junction in many patients tend to compromise precise healing.

Skin sutures placed across the junction often lead to permanent suture marks, typical of any incision which traverses an epithelial concavity (3).

The key to ideal scar camouflage of alar and nostril sill scars lies in *exacting everting approximation* of the cut edges with fast-absorbing catgut sutures, supplemented by tissue glue. Although bleeding from small alar vessels usually diminishes as the abundant small alar vessels retract and clamp down soon after alar incisions, exacting hemostasis may be hastened with needlepoint microcautery. If the tissue gap is

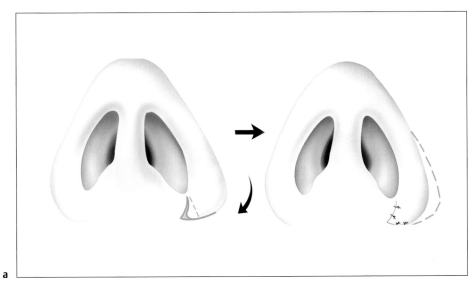

Fig. 9.**11** (**a**) Method developed by Sheen (9) to create modest medial translation of the lateral alar sidewall without compromising the alar sill. (**b**) Before and (**c**) result obtained after this subtle type of alar base narrowing.

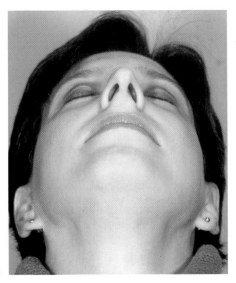

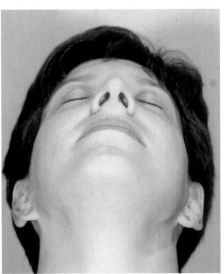

large (as in major sliding alar flaps), buried interrupted sutures of 5–0 polydioxanone suture material (PDS) are initially placed subcutaneously to accurately oppose the wound edges and relieve tension on the delicate catgut sutures. External suture marks may thus be largely eliminated with this sequence of steps. Nonabsorbable sutures are always best avoided, since suture marks almost inevitably result. Effective camouflage at alar–facial junction may be facilitated by positioning incisions 1–2 mm above the alar–facial crease (Fig. 9.**13**), avoiding the thick sebaceous glands located in this junction. The 1–2 mm cuff of skin remaining above the exact alar–facial crease facilitates exact edge-to-edge closure; magnification is helpful in achieving precise closure. This simple but critical approach to incision siting almost completely eliminates visible scars, suture marks, and widened visible sebaceous gland openings. Tissue glue reinforces the gentle suture closure (Fig. 9.**14**). At approximately five to seven days the tissue glue generally spontaneously falls away, carrying any suture remnant with it. Tedious suture removal is thus avoided.

Key Technical Points

1. Exacting preoperative analysis is critical to planning the extent and type of excision.
2. Precise, gentle suturing with gently tied fast-absorbing catgut suture negates possible suture marks.
3. Siting the scar 1.5–2 mm on the alar lobule side of the alar–facial junction improves ultimate scar camouflage.
4. Symmetrical excision and repair is essential (unless preoperative asymmetry exists).
5. Slight eversion of the opposed skin edges is desirable, although this is more difficult on the fibrofatty alar lobule than in skin elsewhere.
6. Avoiding incisions across the nostril sill (when made possible by existing anatomy) avoids potential notching of this delicate landmark.

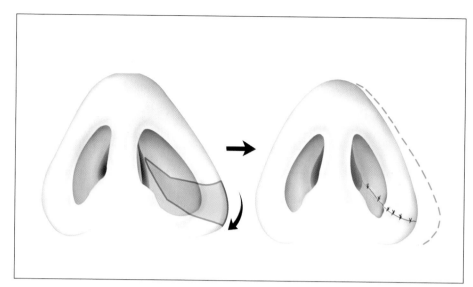

Fig. 9.**12** (**a**) A major sliding alar flap technique employed when a significant degree of medial translation of the alar sidewall is required.
(**b**) Before and (**c**) after larger sliding alar flap procedure.

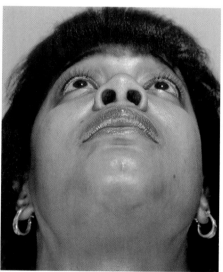
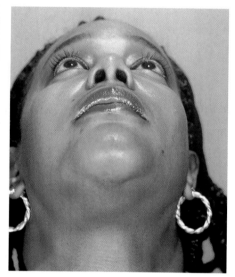

Postoperative Care

The patient should avoid rubbing or manipulating the alar base for two weeks.

1. If not already fallen away, the tissue glue seal may be gently teased away at five to seven days.
2. A Neomycin–steroid ophthalmic ointment is applied to the healing incisions for two weeks.
3. Photographs are taken at one week, one month, three months, 12 months, and regularly at intervals for as long as the patient is willing to return. (Long-term follow-up and critical evaluation constitutes the most important factor in self-education and feedback to the rhinoplasty surgeon).

Complications

Complications, which are uncommon, include:
- Visible alar scars
- Asymmetrical alar resection
- Notching of alar sill
- Overreduction with nostril distortion and overnarrowing
- Infection
- Wound separation and avulsion

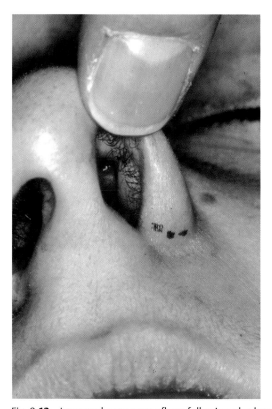

Fig. 9.**13** Improved scar camouflage following alar base narrowing re-section procedures is facilitated by leaving a cuff of 1–2 mm of epithelium above the alar–facial junction. This maneuver avoids the need for sutures to be placed across the concavity of the alar–facial junction, where abundant sebaceous glands are located.

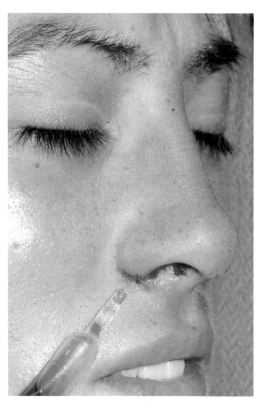

Fig. 9.**14** After gentle suturing of the cut edges of the alar excision, tissue glue is applied to seal the wound, resulting in immediate cessation of any bleeding, and generally leading to improved scar camouflage.

Conclusions

If the alar base appears disproportionate or inordinately wide before or at the conclusion of rhinoplasty, alar base reduction and narrowing should be considered. Judgements regarding the siting of alar reduction incisions and the geometry of alar excisions must be based upon the existent anatomy. The magnitude and extent of alar reductions are determined based on an assessment of the internal (medial) length and the flare of the alar margin, the external (lateral) length and flare of the alar margin, the width and shape of the nostril floor and sill, the shape of the nostril aperture, the anatomy of the columella, and the overall length of the lateral alar sidewalls.

The surgeon should assess which of the above factors must be surgically modified, and then formulate a progressive graduated formulation for alar base reduction, calculated to achieve a balanced, symmetrical alar base appearance with minimal scar sequelae (8).

References

1. Weir, RF. On restoring sunken noses without scarring the face. *N.Y. Med. J.* 1892; 56:449–454.
2. Tardy ME, Brown R. *Surgical anatomy of the nose.* Philadelphia: Raven Press: 1995.
3. Tardy ME. *Rhinoplasty: The art and the science.* Philadelphia: WB Saunders: 1997.
4. Meyer R. Secondary rhinoplasty. In Papel ID, Nachlas NE, *Facial plastic and reconstructive surgery.* St. Louis: Mosby Year Book: 1992.
5. Tardy ME, Walter MA, Patt BS. The overprojecting nose: anatomic component analysis and repair. *Fac Plast Surg.* 1993: 9(4):306–316.
6. Tardy ME, Patt BS, Walter MA. Alar reduction and sculpture: anatomic concepts. *Fac Plast Surg.* 1993; 9 (4):295–305.
7. Crumley R. Aesthetic surgery of the alar base. *Fac Plast Surg,* 1985; 5:135–142.
8. Tardy ME, Genach, SH, Murrell, GC. Aesthetic correction of alar-columellar disproportions. *Fac Plast Surg. Clin N.Amer.* 1995; 3 (4):359–406.
9. Sheen TH, Sheen AP. Aesthetic Rhinoplasty, ed. 2. St. Louis, C. V. Mosby, 1987.

Suggested Reading

Gunter JP, Rohrich RJ, Friedman RM. Classification and correction of alar-columellar discrepancies in rhinoplsty. *Plast Reconstruc Surg.* 1996; 97(3):643–648.

10 The Deviated Nose

S. S. Park

Contents

Introduction

There is no universally ideal nose, especially as one crosses ethnic and gender boundaries, although one consistent esthetic trait found across all cultures is a straight dorsum. Correcting the deviated nose is a formidable rhinoplastic challenge for many reasons. The frontal view is often seen in photographs but is not otherwise a common perspective during normal interpersonal encounters. For this reason, many individuals will notice small dorsal irregularities in photographs, which then prompt the surgical consultation. This true frontal view is the most challenging to perfect because even a subtle, focal area of fullness or depression can be conspicuous and readily detected as a dorsal asymmetry. Furthermore, correcting the twisted nose can be unpredictable because it relies on both sides of the nose healing in an identical way, with the same degree of swelling, scarring, and contracture.

In some ways, a rhinoplasty can be viewed as two operations: One on the left side and the other on the right. Although the same technical maneuvers may be performed on each side, the rate of healing and degree of scar contracture can vary and leads to unpredictability. Rhinoplasty is a *four-dimensional* operation. Manipulating the bony and cartilaginous framework in a three-dimensional space is the first challenge. The fourth dimension is time. This powerful force is an essential consideration in surgical planning and its recognition and appreciation has had a tremendous impact on contemporary rhinoplasty techniques.

There is a marriage between the cutaneous nasal deformity and the underlying anatomical cause, one that must be studied as a routine part of all preoperative analyses. After successfully identifying the external nasal problems, it is imperative to go the next step and investigate what bony or cartilaginous deformity is causing those findings. Such an exercise allows one to approach the surgical plan in a precise and targeted manner. This chapter will highlight the preoperative analysis and surgical repair of the deviated nose. The correction can be approached through a graduated algorithm that begins with a simple, minimally invasive maneuver and progresses toward destabilization and reconstruction. Representative cases will be used to demonstrate the analysis and rhinoplasty techniques.

Indications

The indications for repairing a twisted nose can fall under two general categories, i.e., cosmetic and functional. Naturally, the cosmetic group is integrally involved with the patient's perspective and complaints. Functionally, the twisted dorsum can be an active contributor to the cause of nasal obstruction and correcting this deformity is often an important part of restoring nasal patency. Most twisted noses are the result of blunt trauma, where the nasal skeleton is displaced and immediately apparent. While we often think of bony injuries with blunt trauma, significant distortion to the cartilaginous framework can also occur and may be amenable to immediate repair. Most long-standing nasal deformities can be related to a history of nasal trauma, albeit remote or minor, and occasionally forgotten by the patient. Relatively small injuries to the lower two thirds of the nose can disrupt the balance of intrinsic cartilaginous forces, which, over time, may result in progressive distortion and nasal twisting. Moreover, injuries at a younger age may influence the nasal growth centers and lead to asymmetrical development.

Iatrogenic dorsal deformities can occur during a dorsal hump reduction which inadvertently unmasks a midseptal deviation. Other rhinoplasty procedures can also heal and contract in an asymmetrical way and give rise to the twisted nose. The indications for a specific rhinoplasty maneuver to correct a dorsal deviation are dependent on the causes, they may be traumatic, iatrogenic, or idiopathic. A careful preoperative analysis of the structural aberrancy often dictates the approach and optimal surgical plan. At times, one must apply a stepwise approach such that a series of maneuvers are applied in a sequential fashion. For this reason, it is important to be facile with a host of surgical maneuvers before embarking on the repair of a twisted nose.

Contraindications

There are relatively few contraindications to performing this type of rhinoplasty. One may encounter philosophical contraindications to repairing the crooked nose, such as an individual who will be exposed to repeated trauma (e.g., the boxer or rugby player). Under these circumstances, the timing of surgery is more at issue than the surgery itself. There are circumstances where straightening the deviated nose may compromise the nasal lumen and be relatively contraindicated. This could occur with a patient who desires a straighter nose with the collapsed side being considered more esthetically pleasing. To create a symmetrical dorsum, the patient may request to have the normal side pinched medially, thus giving rise to an iatrogenic internal nasal valve obstruction.

Preoperative Considerations

Identifying the good rhinoplasty candidate is as important as the surgery itself. A thorough history should include a commitment to get to know the patient as a person, seeking to understand a few specific personality traits.

The *motivation* of individuals seeking a rhinoplasty can be diverse and some are considered healthy while others are felt to be unstable. Ideally, a patient should pursue a rhinoplasty only after adequate contemplation and understanding of the procedure. The motivating force should be personal wish to correct some specific deformity that is bothersome. After proper patient selection, a successful outcome can have far-reaching effects on self-image and self-esteem. Poor motivational factors include seeking cosmetic surgery to please others, correcting problems in their personal or professional lives, or in response to exogenous stresses in their lives.

The physical *expectations* must also be carefully evaluated to ensure that they are realistic and within the realm of surgical possibility. The single most essential step toward realistic expectations is clear communication between the surgeon and patient. There are physical limitations to some rhinoplasties, such as those relating to skin thickness or dramatic deviations to the dorsum, and these must be clearly defined preoperatively. It is also important to explain the balance between the nose and the face, such as the twisted nose on a person with preexisting facial asymmetry.

Psychological factors and personality traits can influence the outcomes and final patient satisfaction. A history of psychiatric illness, impulsive behavior, and use of mood-influencing drugs should prompt further investigation to determine psychological candidacy. Some traits interfere with the ability to accept one's body image while others cannot tolerate the change. The following are some common personality types that should alert the surgeon preoperatively:

1. The *dependant personality*: Overly compliant and leads the patient to interact in a subservient fashion to the surgeon.
2. The *passive–aggressive personality*: Nonconfrontational but may display self-deprecating behaviors.
3. *Obsessive-compulsive personalities*: Questions every detail yet remains indecisive, making effective communication difficult.
4. *Histrionic personality*: Charming and dramatic, but insists on special attention and responds in an exaggerated and inappropriate way.
5. *Paranoid personality*: Secretive, distrusting, and less tolerant of discomfort.

Age

Minors represent a special subset of patients as they may be brought to the surgeon by their parents. It is essential to determine who is seeking the cosmetic change and to ensure that the communication and instruction are mutual. The general teaching is that nasal cosmetic surgery should be delayed until age 15 for females and 17 for males. The two variables to consider before a pediatric rhinoplasty are *emotional maturity* and *completed pubertal growth* of the nasal skeleton. Both probably occur sooner in females than males.

Rhinoplasty in the older age group also involves unique emotional and anatomical factors. Older patients have lived with certain facial features for their entire lives and dramatic changes can be difficult to adjust to, occasionally having a negative impact on their self-image. As such, a conservative approach is further emphasized with this patient demographic. The older patient often has more brittle nasal bones, making osteotomies more challenging.

Body habitus is worth noting, particularly any preexisting facial asymmetries that can occur. A perfectly straight nose on a crooked face may not appear balanced.

Ethnicity and *gender* are important preoperative considerations for rhinoplasty but are less relevant in the management of the twisted nose because a straight dorsum is desirable in all cultures.

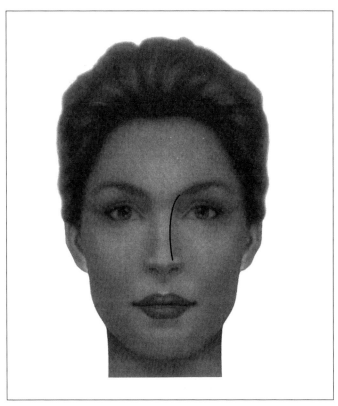

Fig. 10.**1**   The brow–tip esthetic line extending from the brow to the nasal tip seen in the esthetic dorsum.

Preoperative Analysis and Diagnosis

Normal Anatomy and Diagnosis

An accurate preoperative analysis of the deviated nose goes beyond recognizing the external deformity; it requires a deliberate investigation into the underlying cartilaginous and bony anatomy, and the complexity with which it shapes the nasal dorsum. Each area of the nasal skeleton is responsible for a discrete cutaneous subunit of the nose, such as the nasal bones defining the upper third, the dorsal septum and upper lateral cartilages shaping the middle third, and tip being supported by the lower lateral cartilages and anterior septal angle. Cutaneous deviations, on the other hand, can be the result of more than one anatomical structure. The ideal nose blends into the face without calling attention to asymmetry, imbalance, or disproportion, allowing the casual observer to be drawn to other areas that typically define facial beauty, such as the eyes. The esthetic dorsum is straight, remains in the midline of the face, and may have a subtle concavity that reflects a narrower middle vault. The "brow–tip line" is a useful landmark that helps define an esthetic dorsal contour. It begins from the medial brow, curving inferiorly along the dorsal border, gently blending with the tip-defining point. These lines should remain parallel and uninterrupted (Fig. 10.**1**).

It is often useful to evaluate the nasal dorsum in segments rather than just a gestalt from the frontal view. Dividing the nose into an upper, middle, and lower third can help with delineating discrete aberrancies. The *upper third* of the nose is

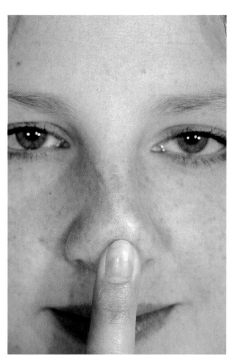

Fig. 10.**2**   Depressing the nasal tip helps identify the position of the anterior septal angle.

formed by the paired nasal bones and the frontal processes of the maxilla. The skin along the caudal border of the nasal bone is characteristically thin and allows small irregularities of bone, cartilage, or scar to be readily evident. Conversely, the skin and soft tissue at the nasion is much thicker and includes subcutaneous fat and the procerus muscle. Changes in the bony skeleton along this area tend to be camouflaged by the thicker overlying soft tissue which drapes between the higher riding glabella and rhinion. The nasal bones also define the appropriate width and dorsal projection to the upper nose. The bony septum is a minor contributor to the dorsum in normal circumstances but deviations to the upper third can involve the septum and must be considered. More will be discussed on this later in the chapter.

The *middle nasal vault* is normally slightly narrower than the upper or lower thirds and creates a gentle concavity to the brow–tip line. The middle third of the nose is shaped primarily by the dorsal septum and upper lateral cartilages. These structures are firmly adherent to one another and any intrinsic deviation to one will directly impact the other. The dorsal border of the normal septum should be straight and has a widened area that functions as physiological spreader grafts, contributing positively to the width of the middle vault as well as opening the internal nasal valves. Surgical reduction of the dorsal septum can create an iatrogenic narrowing of the middle vault with the "hour-glass" deformity occasionally seen in revision rhinoplasty. The upper lateral cartilages are also significant contributors to the dorsal width and provide support, symmetry, and fullness to the nasal sidewalls. Displacement of the upper lateral cartilage can create an imbalance to the natural concavity and the illusion of a twisted nose. The intimate relation between the upper lateral cartilage and dorsal septum is an essential consideration of the middle vault anatomy and

must be a part of the preoperative analysis for every twisted nose.

The *nasal tip* should appear elegant, indiscrete, and in the midline. While the tip is not often discussed with the twisted nose, it too can be deviated and contribute to dorsal irregularities. The midline position of the tip is dependent on both the lower lateral cartilages and caudal septum, especially the anterior septal angle. Like the middle vault, the culprit for a deviated tip may lie with either anatomical structure (or both) and a preoperative distinction is needed in order to develop a focused surgical repair. The anterior septal angle is often camouflaged by the thick tip skin and lower lateral cartilages, and palpation may be necessary to identify its position. When this caudal septum is deviated, it can bring the lower lateral cartilages with it and cause a passive tip deformity.

Analysis of Aberrant Anatomy

Evaluation of the twisted nose is a challenging aspect of rhinoplasty and is best done in a methodical and systematic manner. An accurate diagnosis is a prerequisite for developing a preoperative surgical plan that is direct and target oriented. For these reasons it is useful to evaluate the rhinoplasty patient with an algorithm that highlights some nuances that might otherwise go unnoticed. Preoperative nasal analysis should be organized and repeated several times.

First, multiple views of the nose are useful. Clearly, the frontal perspective is most revealing of dorsal deviations (and the most difficult to perfect surgically) but different abnormalities can be appreciated from the submental, oblique, and lateral views. Photography serves two important functions in terms of analysis. It allows for repetitive, preoperative analysis, including within the operating room. Second, the physical act of taking photographs allows a unique perspective of the patient not typically achieved during normal consultations. The camera's view finder, cropping, standardizing views, and the Frankfort horizontal all contribute to a form of tunnel vision that leads to an objective analysis of the nose, apart from room décor, attire, and emotional expression. For example, one often asks the patient to lower his/her chin and refrain from smiling, two interpersonal habits of human nature that are prevalent during the consultations but influence the analysis. A hypoplastic chin or preexisting alarcolumellar disproportion can be easily overlooked during an informal encounter but become readily apparent through a camera lens.

During the physical examination of a rhinoplasty patient, there are two useful tools that are occasionally omitted. *Palpation* of the nose is an invaluable asset that can reveal much in terms of bony and cartilaginous framework, stability, resilience, and soft-tissue problems. There are aspects of the nose that are best evaluated through careful palpation, such as the location of the anterior septal angle, the contour of the dorsal septum, tip support, and skin thickness (Fig. 10.**2**). During the examination, one must make it a point to investigate these areas and become familiar with the unique anatomy of each patient. A second useful tool when analyzing a twisted nose is to use a straight reference, such as a stick or cotton-tip applicator, in the precise midline of the face. With the midline clearly defined, one can inspect each third of the nose independently and better determine which component of the bony/cartilaginous framework is creating the cutaneous deformity (Fig. 10.**3**).

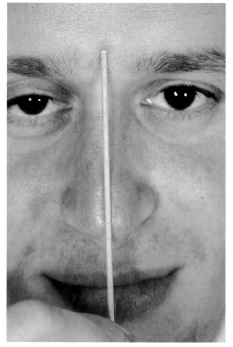

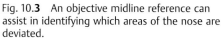

Fig. 10.**3**   An objective midline reference can assist in identifying which areas of the nose are deviated.

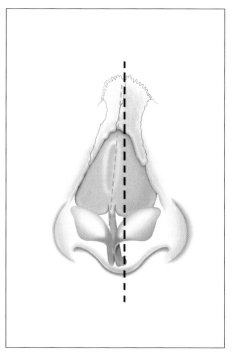

Fig. 10.**4**   A linear deviation to the nasal dorsum.

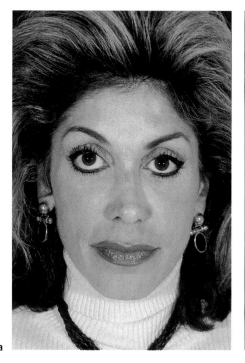

a

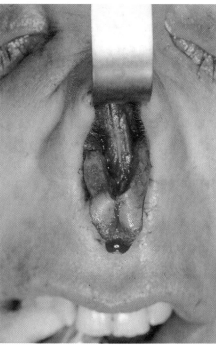

b

Fig. 10.**5**   (**a**) Nasal dorsum deviated the patient's left. (**b**) Linear deviation of the nasal bones and dorsal septum. Lower lateral cartilages remain in the midline.

The deviated dorsum comes in many forms and in no way can a single operation be universally applied to all patients. It is a critical to separate the cutaneous deformity of the nose from the underlying *structural cause* and anatomical pathogenesis. One must take a step backward from the cutaneous deformity to understand its cause, then proceed forward with a surgical repair targeting this framework problem. The nose with a bony deviation is entirely different from the collapsed upper lateral cartilage or the dislocated caudal septum, although both may re-

semble a "twisted nose." The nasal dorsum can be linear but deviated to one side, where all components of the nose are involved and need correction (Figs. 10.**4**, 10.**5**). The bony dorsum can have a solitary irregularity, usually in the paramedian position, that creates an asymmetry and the appearance of a twisted nose. The causes of such isolated lesions can be related to old bony fractures, including where small osteophytes have grown from the disrupted periosteum (Fig. 10.**6**). The remedy for such problems may be as simple as sharp excision or rasping of the lesion.

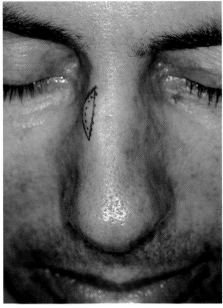

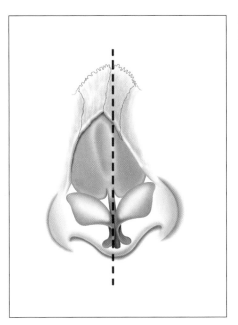

Fig. 10.**7**   Dorsal deviation secondary to displaced nasal bones.

Fig. 10.**6**   Bony overgrowth in the right paramedian location.

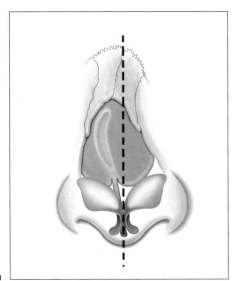

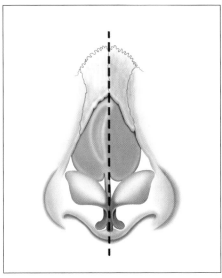

Fig. 10.**8**   (**a**) Twisted dorsum involving the upper and middle thirds, with a deviation of the nasal bones and dorsal septum. (**b**) Twisted dorsum limited to the middle third and the dorsal septum.

a

b

Some deviated noses are limited to the *upper third* and are the result of displaced nasal bones while the dorsal septum and lower two thirds are normal, as seen with nasal fractures (Fig. 10.**7**). Deflections of the bony pyramid, however, are not all identical and it is important to delineate 1) which side is aberrant, 2) the contour of the bone itself, and 3) potential involvement of the posterior bony septum. Bony deviations may involve only one side where an isolated segment is medially displaced. One must be alerted to the depressed nasal bone segment, as its repair may be unstable and require unilateral intranasal packing. Alternatively, these circumstances may be more efficiently managed with camouflage, onlay grafts.

Careful palpation of the bony pyramid is done to identify any intrinsic concavity or marked asymmetry in width to the nasal bones. This analysis will influence the location of osteotomies as well as the need for *intermediate* osteotomies. It is difficult to predict which bony *septal* deflections will hinder

realignment of the nasal pyramid and it is not uncommon to see significant endonasal deviations that do not interfere with dorsal repair. When the septal deviation is significant, it can be addressed either with endonasal closed reductions or percutaneous osteotomies.

The *twisted middle vault* is possibly the most complex in terms of preoperative assessment. The majority of cases involve a primary deviation to the dorsal septum and passive distortion to the upper lateral cartilages (Fig. 10.**8**). This anatomy is best appreciated with direct palpation of the dorsum as well as by tightening the nasal skin across the lateral nasal walls, which can outline the dorsal septum. Because the upper lateral cartilages are firmly adherent to the dorsal septum (in the primary nose), they are equally distorted and contributing to the external concavity. Releasing the fibrous attachments between these two structures will typically reveal a persistent defection to the septal cartilage and a correction of the upper lateral de-

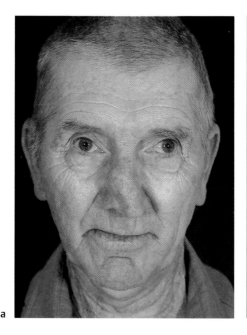
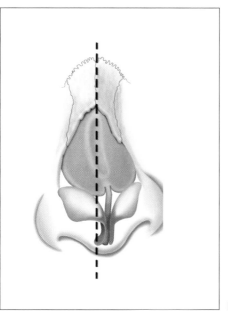

Fig. 10.**9** (**a**) Dorsal deformity involving the nasal tip. (**b**) Deviation of the caudal septum.

formity. This identifies the anatomical cause of the middle vault deviation and permits a targeted surgical correction. One should bear in mind that a twisted nose can be unmasked during a dorsal hump reduction when a preexisting midseptal deviation becomes the new dorsal strut. This iatrogenic twisted dorsum can be anticipated with careful intranasal inspection and corrected with traditional methods outlined below. A cartilaginous hump reduction also redefines the middle vault dorsum with an area of septal cartilage that is usually thinner, thus requiring prophylactic spreader grafts.

There are two instances of middle vault deviations where the upper lateral cartilages are the primary culprit rather than the dorsal septum. The upper lateral cartilage may be disarticulated off its supporting structures (usually the dorsal septum but occasionally the nasal bone) and the result is a gradual medial displacement and depression that creates a unilateral concavity. There will be a disruption of the esthetic brow–tip line on one side and the illusion of a twisted nose. When this occurs bilaterally and symmetrically, such as following a reduction rhinoplasty, it creates the typical "inverted V" deformity encountered during many secondary rhinoplasties. The second scenario is when the primary causes are with the size, shape, or form of the upper lateral cartilages themselves; although less frequent, there are times where an intrinsic upper lateral deformity exists with a concavity or buckling of cartilage. This sidewall asymmetry will be interpreted as a twisted nose and can be addressed directly, either through repair or camouflage.

The *lower third* may also be twisted to one side and create the appearance of a twisted dorsum. Tip position is dependent on numerous forces that must work in concert in order to hold the tip in the midline; a disruption of this balance of forces can lead to marked asymmetry. Lateral displacement may be due to a malposition of the caudal septum (particularly the anterior septal angle) (Fig. 10.**9**). Tip structure and stability is best assessed with careful palpation because simple inspection can be misleading in terms of the causative agent. It is not uncommon for the anterior septal angle to be significantly deflected

to one side and the cutaneous tip only slightly twisted. The caudal septum may be bowed or dislocated off the anterior nasal spine, causing deformities to both the columella and nasal tip. Similarly, marked asymmetry of the paired lower lateral cartilages can be associated with enough twisting of the tip such that the entire dorsum appears irregular.

The deviated nose can be associated with *functional problems* that are complex and related to pathology of the internal nasal valve, i.e., the area between the upper lateral cartilage and dorsal septum. Although this cross-sectional area represents a proportionally small amount of the intranasal lumen, it is responsible for a disproportionate amount of laminar airflow and small degrees of obstruction can quickly be symptomatic. Evaluating nasal obstruction related to the internal valve must be done carefully and systematically. The goal is to identify exactly where the level of obstruction is and to distinguish a static narrowing from a dynamic collapse, as their respective treatments are inherently different. Examination of the nasal airway must be done with minimal distortion or artificial support to the nasal sidewalls, especially that found with the nasal speculum. Dynamic collapse of the nasal sidewall is generally repaired with cartilaginous batten grafts placed precisely along the epicenter of collapse with the intent to reinforce that area and resist the collapsing force during nasal inhalation. The static narrowing at the internal valve is usually thought of as a problem involving malpositioned upper lateral cartilages, typically remedied with spreader grafts, flaring sutures, or butterfly type grafts (1, 2). The dorsal septum is an important player in the anatomy of the internal nasal valve and can contribute significantly to the cause of valve obstruction. Clinical obstruction can occur on either the concave or convex side of the septum and it is difficult to predict without careful intranasal inspection. On the convex side of the nose, the dorsal septum directly impinges on the internal valve from the medial side. When obstruction occurs on the concave side of the dorsum, the upper lateral cartilage is usually the culprit, being medially displaced, either through disarticulation off the septum or a buckling deformity. The dorsal septal deviation translates to a malformed upper lateral cartilage by virtue of its firm fibrous attachments. Similarly, a depressed nasal bone can cause both a cosmetic deformity to the dorsum as well as nasal obstruction at the level of the internal nasal valve. The displaced nasal bone brings with it the upper lateral cartilage and creates a secondary obstruction at the internal valve.

Surgical Correction

Once the precise anatomical cause of the external nasal deformity is understood, one can design an efficient surgical plan that is directed toward that specific aberrancy.

The surgical approach, i.e., *endonasal or external*, is primarily personal preference with some general considerations. The exposure must provide the surgeon with a level of comfort for consistent results. The columellar scar is not a significant deterrent, although more operative time and postoperative swelling are anticipated. One does not need to visualize the entire nasoskeleton for all techniques and, in fact, doing so may be detrimental to the outcome. While the cutaneous columellar scar may not be a concern, total nasal scarring, including that which occurs beneath the normal nasal skin from undermining and exposure, can be significant. Some of the dissection from an external approach occurs in normal areas of the nose. The act of "opening" the nose introduces a variable that may be avoided with the endonasal approach; scarring and contracture that occurs beneath the soft-tissue envelope will impact contour and may not occur symmetrically between the two sides. On some occasions, the healing process from the nasal exposure alone may be the cause of external deformity. For this reason, subtle deformities of the middle nasal vault that are corrected with small camouflage grafts may be better accomplished through the endonasal route, thereby avoiding the unpredictable contracture associated with degloving the nose. On the other hand, extensive and complex deformities may require more significant mobilization or reshaping of the cartilaginous framework. Releasing these structures from the overlying soft tissues may be advantages; partial adherence to the soft tissues may hinder reshaping of the cartilages. As a general guideline, when the cartilage needs to be aggressively reshaped rather than just augmented or trimmed, the external approach may have its advantages.

Upper Third Deviations

Osteotomies

Deviations of the upper third are usually repaired via osteotomies in order to realign the nasal bony vault to the midline. Not all twisted dorsa are managed with the same type of osteotomies (3). The preoperative analysis must identify which side is deviated and the individual contour of each bone. When both bones are relatively straight but deviated to the same side, bilateral lateral osteotomies may suffice, allowing the bony pyramid to realign as a single unit. Lateral osteotomies begin within the frontal process of the maxilla, usually around the head of the inferior turbinate, thus preserving a small ridge of bone in a lateralized position and

avoiding collapse of the lateral nasal wall (and valve obstruction). The path extends superiorly as the bone becomes thinner and easily fractured. The cut stops at the medial canthal area and is followed by a back fracture to the midline. One must avoid the tendency to carry the lateral cut too far superiorly, which could otherwise proceed into the frontal bone and create a "rocker deformity."

More significant deviations may require medial osteotomies through either an intercartilaginous incision (over the upper lateral cartilage) or transnasally by engaging the caudal border of the nasal bone, at its junction with the dorsal septum and upper lateral cartilage. This latter route requires a puncture of the intranasal mucosa but is associated with less soft-tissue dissection. The path of this bone cut flares laterally at its cephalic border and stops in the vicinity of the medial canthus. When only a single bone is displaced (usually medially), medial and lateral osteotomies performed unilaterally may be adequate to reduce the isolated segment. These situations are challenging because there is a tendency for the bone to collapse, especially if the periosteal attachments are disrupted. In these cases, intranasal packing may be needed, using either a resorbable material or a small finger cot. Systemic antibiotics are given in all cases of intranasal packing as prophylaxis against toxic shock syndrome. Ecchymosis following lateral osteotomies can be significantly reduced by digital pressure to the site for 3 minutes immediately after performing the cut. Most bleeding is from shredded periosteum and can be controlled with digital pressure. This single intraoperative maneuver *immediately* following the osteotomy can have a dramatic postoperative benefit in terms of bruising, swelling, and patient comfort.

Bony dorsal hump reduction in the context of a deviated pyramid must often be performed in an oblique orientation in order to permit adequate reduction of both sides. The longer nasal bone should have more resected from it with less bone resected from the deviated side, thus creating nasal bones of symmetrical width prior to realignment.

Intermediate Osteotomy

The intermediate osteotomy is a third bone cut placed vertically between the medial and lateral ones. Examination of the nasal bones can reveal two circumstances where such an osteotomy is indicated. When the contour of the nasal bone is irregular, either concave or convex, simple realignment to the midline can leave a persistent deformity to the dorsal or sidewall. Second, when there is marked discrepancy to the width of the two nasal bones, the wider bone will hinder the equal reduction of both sides and an intermediate osteotomy to that side is indicated. The intermediate osteotomy is performed following the medial and prior to the lateral bone cuts. It is a vertical cut that runs through the apex of the concavity (or convexity), creating two segments of bone that reduce independently (Fig. 10.**10**).

Bony Septal Deviations

Most deviations of the upper third can be adequately reduced through osteotomies but there are occasions where the posterior bony septum is sufficiently displaced as to hinder this realignment. The perpendicular plate of the ethmoid inserts to the undersurface of the nasal bones and may require direct at-

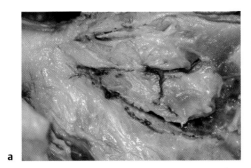

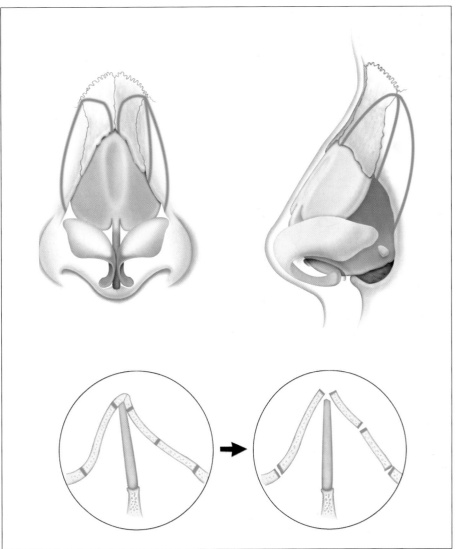

Fig. 10.**10**   (**a**) Cadaveric example of an intermediate osteotomy, positioned between the medial and lateral osteotomies. (**b**) Intermediate osteotomy used in a concave nasal bone.

tention. Most deviation of this portion of the septum can be gently fractured endonasally, allowing its reduction to the midline. It is imperative to recognize that its posterior/superior attachment is to the cribriform plate and aggressive manipulation in this area can risk a leakage of cerebral spinal fluid (CSF). For more significant deflections in this area, one can use a 2 mm percutaneous osteotome, inserted in the midline at the nasion, to create a controlled fracture of the bony septum.

It is not uncommon for the repair of a significantly twisted bony dorsum to fail over the ensuing months as the bones slowly drift back to their original position. While these late deviations are not as dramatic as the original deformity, they are problematic and may be the result of one of several factors. A septal deflection may have been overlooked and may be the source of asymmetrical tension on the nasal bones; severe deviations of the bony septum can influence the shape of the upper third of the nose. Second, overlying soft tissues, including the periosteum, can have some degree of *memory* that tends to pull the nasal bones back to the original position. Finally, deformities of the cartilaginous lower two thirds can certainly influence the upper third and must be addressed independently.

Camouflage Grafts

Sometimes the simplest and most direct means of improving the twisted dorsum is to place a graft that fills the depression, including to the middle third. They are used more often in the setting of a unilateral depression where the contralateral side is normal in width. Great care must be taken with these grafts because of the thin skin in this area and the risk of visible edges or contour irregularities. Placing the graft under the periosteum has the advantage of better camouflage of the edges and improved security. Supraperiosteal grafts have a tendency to be mobile but, in theory, viability may be enhanced due to vascularity from both sides of the graft.

A number of implant materials can be used for nasal camouflage but autogenous grafts remain the gold standard. Lightly crushed septal cartilage can be inserted through an intercartilaginous incision, placed in a subperiosteal pocket, and can have dramatic effects on the dorsal asymmetry. Other autogenous materials can be used in a similar way, including conchal cartilage and soft tissue/scar. Homograft costal cartilage is controversial and rarely needed in this area. Homograft acellular dermis is widely used as a nasal implant material and can serve this purpose nicely (4). There is some concern with long-

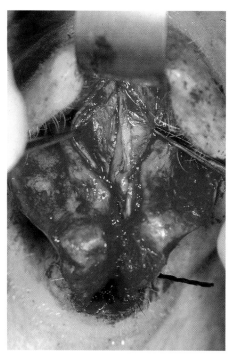

Fig. 10.**11** Spreader graft pocket between septal cartilage and upper lateral cartilage.

term partial resorption of this material, although it may be replaced with sufficient scar so as to maintain its esthetic effect. Alloplastic materials can also be used as camouflage grafts but one should recognize that the overlying skin is characteristically thin and graft extrusion is at risk.

Middle Third Deviations

Correcting the twisted middle vault can be one of the most unpredictable rhinoplasty challenges, often requiring a combination of techniques applied through an organized algorithm. Some surgical plans can be formulated preoperatively, but one must be prepared to progress to more aggressive techniques if others should fail.

Camouflage Grafts

Like the upper third, a middle vault concavity can often be improved with a small camouflage graft placed in a discrete pocket over the upper lateral cartilage, inserted endonasally through an intercartilaginous incision. A small disc of septal cartilage, lightly crushed to remove any intrinsic form, is an ideal graft for such purposes. The edges should be gently beveled in order to minimize the visibility of the graft borders. Creating the pocket is a critical step and should be done immediately superficial to the perichondrium and to precise dimensions in order to accommodate the graft without excessive mobility. Marking the skin should be done prior to infiltrating the local anesthetic. Suturing the graft in position is difficult endonasally but can be done with a small resorbable stitch through the center of the graft, and out percutaneously at the middle of the concavity. The suture can be taped to the adjacent skin and holds the graft in position for the first several days. Autogenous cartilage remains the standard implant for

such purposes, but other alternatives such as acellular dermis and some alloplastic materials are being used with some success (5). Resorption, infection, and extrusion must all be considered prior to implanting a graft, particularly under relatively thin nasal skin.

A *unilateral spreader graft* is a form of camouflage but more directly influences the causative anatomical structures. Despite an intrinsic deviation of the dorsal septum, the spreader graft, positioned between the concave septum and upper lateral cartilage, will laterally displace the upper lateral cartilage and correct the cutaneous deformity, i.e., the twisted middle vault. It can be considered as a camouflage technique because the septal deviation persists. Prior to utilizing this technique, one must diagnose the causative aberrancy and distinguish between a middle-third concavity versus a contralateral fullness and convexity. Failure to recognize this and inserting a unilateral spreader graft may generate an unnatural width to the middle vault that is equally conspicuous. The unilateral spreader graft is placed in a small pocket between the upper lateral cartilage and dorsal septum, taking care not to violate the mucosa and enter the nasal cavity (Fig. 10.**11**). If this does occur, the perforation should be directly repaired prior to placing the grafts. Septal cartilage is ideally suited for such grafting, although conchal cartilage is an acceptable alternative. When using ear cartilage, one often needs two separate pieces, sutured to one another with their concavities facing each other. In this way, each cartilage serves as a splint to the other and a straight graft is created. Costal cartilage may be a second alternative but is rarely needed. Alloplastic materials are at risk of extrusion due to the thin mucosal barrier intranasally. Grafts are carefully carved to an adequate width, which is usually thicker than first impression. The length of the spreader graft should span the entire vertical length of the upper lateral cartilage, occasionally extending between the caudal borders of the nasal bones. The grafts are usually secured by suture in a mattress fashion. Care must be taken when placing these sutures because if they are too far posterior they may pinch the upper lateral cartilages together, effectively narrowing the internal nasal valve (Fig. 10.**12**).

Straightening the Dorsal Septum

The most anatomical method of correcting the twisted dorsum is to directly alter the dorsal septum. This is often done through a sequence of steps:
- Beginning with a complete release from the *extrinsic binding structures* (bony septum, overlying soft tissues, septal perichondrium, upper lateral cartilage),
- Followed by a controlled release of *intrinsic tension forces*, and finally
- External splinting, or
- Resection and reimplantation.

Realigning the dorsal septum is readily accomplished through the external approach, giving direct access to the area of need and allowing accurate trimming and suturing.

The deviated dorsum may be a linear deformity to one side. When the dorsal strut is straight but misaligned, it may need to be detached from the posterior bony septum and maxillary crest in order to allow it to swing back to the center (Fig. 10.**13**). The critical bony/cartilaginous junction ("keystone area") should be resecured with a permanent suture in order to

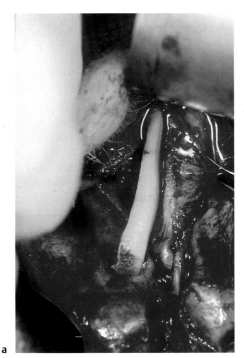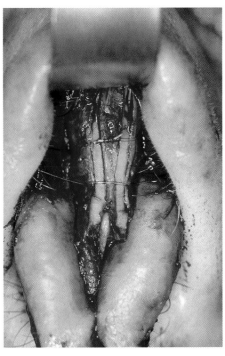

a   b

Fig. 10.**12** (**a**) Insertion of a right spreader graft. (**b**) Suture fixation.

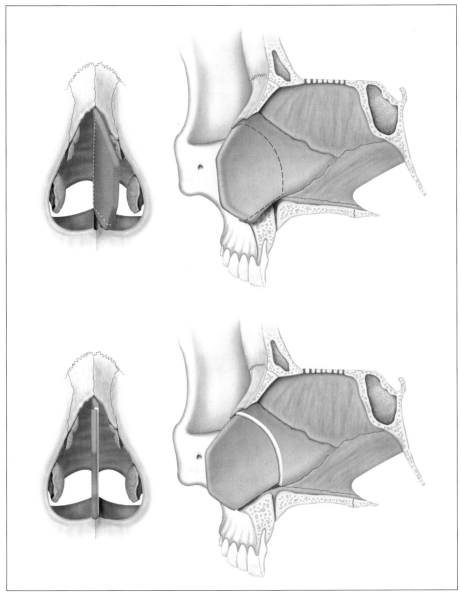

Fig. 10.**13** Disarticulation of the bony–cartilaginous junction for realignment of quadrilateral cartilage.

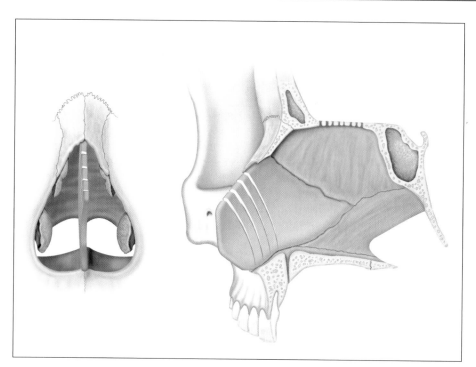

Fig. 10.**14**   Full-thickness incisions to correct significant intrinsic deformity of the cartilaginous septum.

avoid future loss of support and saddle deformity. To do this, one should leave a small knuckle of posterior cartilage through which one can pass a suture. Even when other complex deviations exist in the remaining dorsal septum, if the proximal area along the bony junction is off center it should be addressed first as one proceeds from a superior to inferior direction.

The first step in correcting the twisted dorsal septum is to detach it from the upper lateral cartilages bilaterally. The firm fibrous attachments may themselves be contributing to the warped configuration and a complete release is an essential prerequisite for straightening the alignment.

Secondly, the perichondrium on the *concave* side of the septum is then elevated, thus releasing a binding force to the septal deviation. These two maneuvers may be sufficient to correct a dorsal deformity of the cartilaginous septum, particularly one that involves the anterior septal angle (6). This dissection also allows an accurate intraoperative analysis of the remaining intrinsic deviations to the dorsal septum.

Following release of the extrinsic attachments, persistent deviations are then addressed with partial thickness incisions on the concave side which will further release the constricting forces and help to straighten the cartilage. Relying on the partial thickness incisions alone for significant reshaping may not provide the longevity one desires, and the cartilaginous deviation may recur. One possible mechanism for the relapsing deformity may have to do with the many small, wedge-shaped spaces created as the cartilage bends open. Cartilage has a characteristically low metabolic rate and the healing of these tissue voids occurs with scar formation and wound contracture (7). The contracture represents numerous small forces that may deform the cartilage once again. Mattress sutures placed across the deviated dorsum can stabilize the correction. Permanent suture material is used and the longitudinal part of the suture should be on the convex surface. When placed this way, tightening the suture will bend the cartilage in a favorable way and serve to reinforce the dorsal strut. Persistent deviations may require multiple, full thickness, vertical, car-

tilaginous incisions which allow the twisted septum to realign in a straight configuration (Fig. 10.**14**). There is a moderate degree of structural destabilization from this maneuver and splinting is often indicated.

The autogenous dorsal septal splint serves two functions: It can further straighten the bowed cartilage, and also restore support to a weakened structure. The ideal material is thin but rigid enough to maintain cartilaginous alignment; posterior bony septum is readily accessible and functions well in this regard. It should be directly sutured in a mattress fashion to the dorsal septum after small burr holes have been created in the bone. Wider splints, for example, double cartilaginous spreader grafts, can be used to splint and camouflage simultaneously. These grafts are secured in position with mattress sutures that resuspend the upper lateral cartilages as well.

There are occasions when extensive and complex deformities of the cartilaginous septum exist and the above measures prove inadequate. On these occasions it may be necessary to excise the entire septum, reorient it such that the new dorsum is a straight strut, and suture it back into place. This is an aggressive maneuver as it is difficult to control the dorsal projection in a precise manner. It is helpful to leave a small strip of cartilage along the posterior bony junction for suturing. The upper lateral cartilages must be carefully resuspended to the neodorsum, often with bilateral spreader grafts to ensure appropriate width to the middle third. If the caudal strut is equally distorted, it may also require resection and reimplantation.

The twisted dorsum can be due to a unilateral fullness of the middle vault, rather than a concavity on the other. These deformities are more amenable to a volume reduction of the involved side via shave excision of the convex dorsal septum. This maneuver is always followed by a resuspension of the upper lateral cartilage (Fig. 10.**15**). The resected cartilage can be transplanted to the contralateral side if indicated. Many dorsal deformities require combined techniques for accurate realignment of the cartilaginous framework and correction of the external deformity.

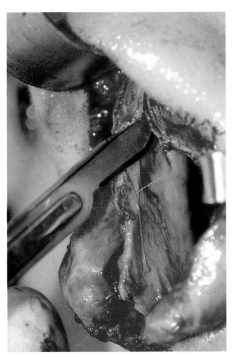

Fig. 10.**15**   Shave resection of the lateral border of the dorsal septum.

Tip Deviations

Tip displacement can be the sole deformity of a twisted dorsum. Surgical maneuvers of the lower lateral cartilages are covered elsewhere in this text and apply to correction of the deviated dorsum as well. While most tip deformities are the result of aberrancies of the lower lateral cartilages, the septum, particularly the anterior septal angle, can have a significant role in dorsal twisting. The anterior septal angle can be straightened by a number of methods. On occasion, simply elevating the perichondrium from the concave side will release the binding force and allow the cartilage to spring back to the midline. Partial thickness incisions on that side will further break up the intrinsic tension forces and permit the cartilage to realign.

Alternatively, the deviation of the caudal septum may be due to an isolated fracture rather than a broad area of concavity. In these circumstances, it is best to excise the fracture line, mobilize and reduce the displaced segment, and fixate with sutures (Fig. 10.**16**). Splinting with a small bone graft extended from the middle third down to the anterior septal angle, similar to methods described above, will usually be effective in reinforcing this area.

Functional Repair

Correcting the twisted dorsum for functional purposes follows many of the same principles as cosmetic rhinoplasty, but the focus is on the intranasal anatomy rather than the cutaneous form. A twisted upper third with collapse of a nasal bone may be the cause of nasal obstruction and correctable with osteotomies that lateralize the bone, and indirectly the upper lateral cartilage. The acute nasal fracture may create nasal obstruction from the displacement of the caudal portion of the nasal bone

along with the upper lateral cartilage. Conversely, nasal obstruction from acute nasal trauma may occur on the contralateral side, i.e., the convex side, due to displacement of the septum. Standard septoplasty techniques are employed with attention to the dorsal septum.

Long-standing deviations to the middle third of the nose can be associated with nasal obstruction on either the concave or convex side. When the clinical obstruction occurs on the convex side of the nose, it is usually due to the deformity of the dorsal septum and its direct impingement on the internal nasal valve. The surgical correction of the dorsal septum is often best achieved through the external route, giving direct access to this area of the septum. The intrinsic cartilaginous bow must be realigned and is done in a step-wise fashion, beginning with release of the binding forces (intrinsic and extrinsic), followed by splinting. When the obstruction is on the concave side, one must focus on lateralizing the nasal sidewall away from the septum. This is accomplished with batten grafts, spreader grafts, and flaring sutures.

The spreader graft is very effective in correcting a cutaneous concavity, but its contribution toward expanding the internal valve cross-sectional airway is less convincing (8). The technique for inserting a *functional* spreader graft is identical to a cosmetic one with greater emphasis on adequate graft width in order to shift the upper lateral sufficiently. The flaring stitch is placed across both upper lateral cartilages in a horizontal mattress fashion, using the dorsal septum as a fulcrum, and directly widening the internal valve (9).

Placing a batten graft is one of the more common surgical maneuvers used to support the nasal sidewall and improve function at the middle vault area. Autogenous grafts are used nearly exclusively and both septal and conchal cartilage work well. The natural curvature of the conchal graft lends itself particularly well to supporting the lower third of the nose. These grafts do not need to be particularly thick or wide, but it is critical that they have adequate length to rest on the bony pyriform aperture, thus pulling the sidewall tissues out laterally (Fig. 10.**17**). It is common for a combination of techniques addressing the twisted dorsal septum, collapsed upper lateral cartilage, and flaccid lateral wall soft tissues to be employed.

Principles of Postoperative Care

General principles of postrhinoplasty care are applicable to many types of facial plastic procedures. The initial few days can be associated with significant periorbital swelling, ecchymosis, epistaxis, and congestion. At times the swelling can be the primary source of discomfort during the convalescent period. Tremendous benefit comes from diligent and prompt use of ice packs to the eyes and consistent head elevation during the first two to three days. Bags of ice cubes tend not to be as effective as either crushed ice or bags of frozen peas. Strenuous activities are generally avoided for two weeks and contact sports for six weeks. Following these principles, along with digital pressure after osteotomies, can significantly minimize the postoperative ecchymosis, and on occasion eliminate it altogether.

Dense intranasal packing following rhinoplasty was once the standard of care in an effort to maintain compression on septal flaps as well as minimizing epistaxis. Precise suture

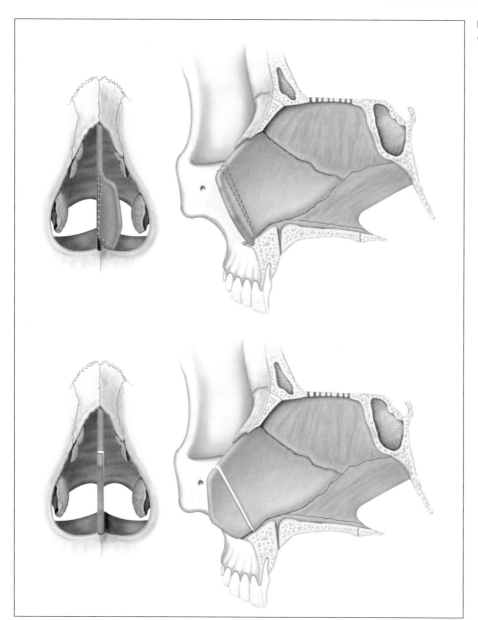

Fig. 10.**16**   Resection of septal fracture with reduction of the caudal septum.

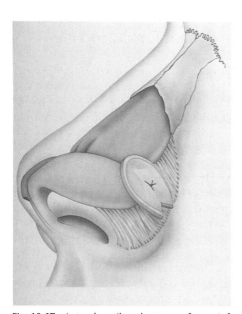

Fig. 10.**17**   Lateral cartilage batten graft to reinforce nasal sidewall. Note the nonanatomical placement.

techniques for reapproximating septal flaps have obviated the need for this type of postoperative packing. Intranasal crusting can be minimized by maintaining a moist environment through humidifiers, saline nasal sprays, and ointments in both nasal vestibules. Topical nasal decongestants and steroid sprays may also be of some short-term benefit. The external rhinoplasty dressing serves to minimize postoperative swelling, obliterate the dead space beneath the soft-tissue envelope, and remind the patient to avoid trauma. This type of bandage is usually kept in place for five to seven days. There is a role for long-term nasal taping with patients in whom a moderate amount of soft-tissue dissection was performed, especially when debulking of soft tissues occurred. In these circumstances, it is practical to have the patient reapply his/her rhinoplasty dressing themselves in the evening. Some degree of recurrent deviation of the bony and cartilaginous skeleton can occur postoperatively. This can present in the form of recurrent twisting as well as widening of the nasal bones. Instructing the patient to perform daily nasal exercises can help mold the nasal bones during the healing period, particularly by applying more pressure to a given side.

Complications

Acute complications are not common, but include such things as excessive epistaxis, infection, nasal obstruction and congestion, unexpected pain, or massive swelling and ecchymosis. In general, these types of complications are found in all nasal procedures and are best managed on an individual basis. Later complications can arise as healing progresses and include such items as intranasal synechia or progressive airway obstruction from either lateral nasal wall collapse or septal deformities.

The most troublesome and common long-term complication specific to the twisted nose is recurrent deformity. When significant dorsal twisting exists, it may be worthwhile to forewarn patients that recurrent deformity is a distinct possibility and that revision procedures may become necessary. In some patients with tremendous dorsal deformities and asymmetrical intrinsic forces, the postoperative period is associated with a degree of memory to the tissues and subsequent recurrent deformity. This can occur at both the bony and cartilaginous portions of the nasal skeleton. Another reason for recurrent deviations relates to the external surgical approach and normal wound contracture. The "shrink wrap" effect that occurs beneath the nasal skin is powerful, ongoing, and not necessarily symmetrical. Subtle variations in this process will lead to recurrent twisting. Third, when the dorsal strut is realigned via partial thickness incisions, recurrent warping occurs unless properly buttressed with a graft. Although these partial thickness incisions create a dramatic effect on the operating table, they leave triangular spaces that heal with second intention and wound contracture. These small contractile forces may be the source for recurrent deviations to this cartilaginous structure.

Small dorsal irregularities are another complication prevalent in twisted nose rhinoplasty. Cartilaginous grafts are used liberally as either splints or camouflage grafts during the correction of the twisted nose. The skin along the middle vault is characteristically thin and the continued contracture of the nasal envelope will allow these cartilaginous edges to become visible. In anticipation of this potential complication it may be worthwhile inserting a soft-tissue filler to serve as a barrier between the skin and cartilage, thus buffering the edges of these grafts. Autogenous fascia, acellular dermis, and rarely alloplastic materials can be used for this purpose. Once the irregularities become evident, they can be selectively trimmed through an endonasal approach, but this remains technically challenging under the thin overlying skin.

Conclusion

Rhinoplasty for a twisted nose is a particularly challenging and diverse operation. Great emphasis should be placed on the preoperative analysis, recognition of the cutaneous deformity, diagnosis of the exact anatomical cause, and a step-wise approach toward surgical repair. Long-term results are essential in recognizing the success and shortcomings of various rhinoplasty maneuvers, particularly since recurrent twisting is not uncommon after many years. Finally, it is imperative for the rhinoplasty surgeon to have a large array of surgical maneuvers in his armamentarium because unsuspected cartilaginous abnormalities can be uncovered intraoperatively. Under these circumstances, one must be able to proceed with more aggressive techniques, including a complete resection, destabilization, and rebuilding of the nasal framework.

Representative Cases

Case 1: Mild Dorsal Deviation

A 33-year-old woman complains of bilateral nasal obstruction and the twisted appearance of her nose. On frontal view, her dorsum is slightly twisted with a concavity on her right. The nasal bones have a palpable ridge in the left paramedian area. The nasal tip is somewhat wide and bulbous. On lateral view, her dorsum is overprojected and represents both bony and cartilaginous structures. Her tip is slightly ptotic and has good projection. Intranasal examination shows narrowing to both nasal valves as well as a dynamic collapse to the nasal sidewall (Fig. 10.**18**).

Intraoperatively, there is a twisted contour to her dorsal septum and narrowing along the internal nasal valve (Fig. 10.**19**).
Surgical repair was done with selective mucosal elevation of the right mucoperichondrium, release of both upper lateral cartilages, and a right unilateral spreader graft. Additional maneuvers included rasping of her bony ridges and lateral osteotomies to maintain balance to the upper third of her nose. She had bilateral cartilaginous batten grafts to the sidewall to reinforce that region. A flaring suture was placed across the upper lateral cartilages to further support the internal nasal valve. She has a bilateral cephalic trim and placement of an interdomal suture to refine her nasal tip (Fig. 10.**20**).

Postoperatively, she was satisfied with the improved esthetics and nasal function (Fig. 10.**21**).

Case 2: Severe Dorsal Deviation

A 38-year-old woman complains of the twisted nose and asymmetrical nasal tip. She had a reduction rhinoplasty roughly eight years ago. On frontal view, the nasal bones are seen to be slightly deviated to her left with a significant twisted deformity to the middle third, with the concavity on her right. Her tip also has a twisted and asymmetrical appearance. Sharp bossae are palpable with tip-defining points at uneven levels. On lateral view, the dorsum is underprojected with a low radix. Tip projection is adequate although slightly rotated cephalically (Fig. 10.**22**).

Palpation of her dorsum reveals c-shaped configuration involving the upper and middle thirds (Fig. 10.**23**).

Intraoperatively, the upper lateral cartilages were disarticulated off the dorsal septum, which in turn showed a twisted configuration. There were tip bossae at uneven levels and a fracture through the left intermediate crus (Fig. 10.**24**).

Surgical repair to her dorsum was accomplished by dissection of the mucoperichondrium off both sides of the dorsal

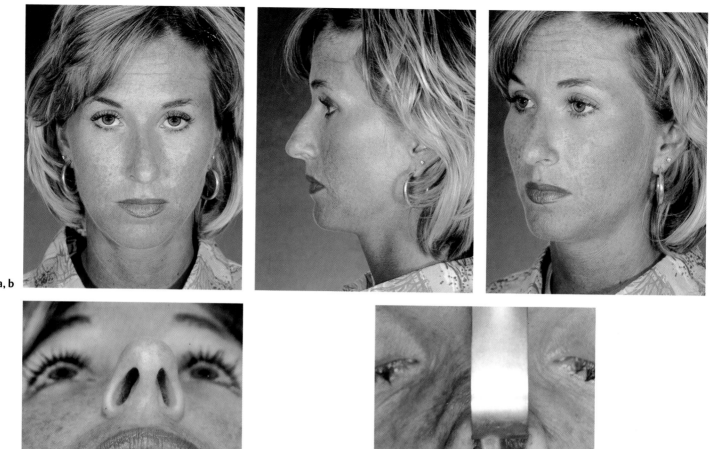

a, b

c

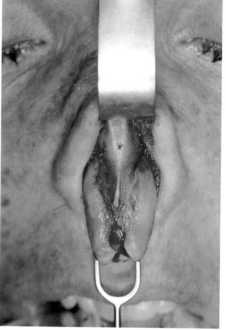

d

Fig. 10.**18** (**a**) Preoperative frontal view. (**b**) Lateral view. (**c**) Oblique view. (**d**) Submental view.

Fig. 10.**19** Intraoperative view showing intrinsic deviation to the dorsal ▷ septum.

septum followed by full-thickness incisions in order to release the intrinsic deviation to this area of her septum. The superior bony–cartilaginous junction was separated to allow the quadrilateral cartilage to reduce to the midline. Bilateral spreader grafts were used as splints. A dorsal onlay graft with septal cartilage was also utilized. Additionally, lateral osteotomies were performed to realign the upper third of her nose. The tip was addressed with a vertical dome division and excision of the bossae. These areas were closed primarily. An interdomal suture was also placed to maintain support and symmetry (Fig. 10.**25**).

One year postoperatively, she is satisfied with nasal contour and tip. She denies problems with nasal obstruction (Fig. 10.**26**).

Case 3: Fractured Dorsum and Twisted Tip

A 45-year-old woman comes in with complaints of her nasal deformity, in particular the twisted appearance of her dorsum, as well as bilateral nasal obstruction. She had a reduction rhinoplasty roughly 15 years previously. On frontal view, one can see and palpate her dorsal septum projecting through the upper lateral cartilages as well as between the nasal bones. The nasal tip is deviated to her left and her dorsum appears to deviate to her right. On lateral view, her tip is somewhat ptotic, with loss of support. The upper two thirds of her nose have adequate projection. The lower lateral cartilages show obvious

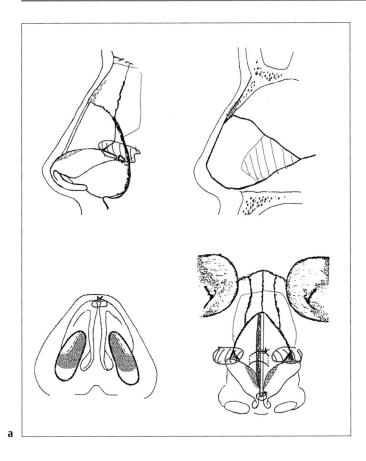

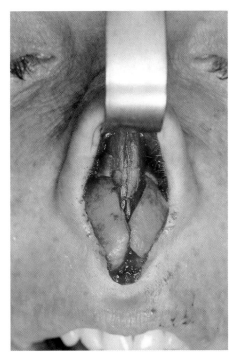

Fig. 10.**20** (**a**) Schema of the operative procedure. (**b**) Intraoperative view showing elevation of right mucoperichondrium, spreader graft, flaring stitch, and batten grafts.

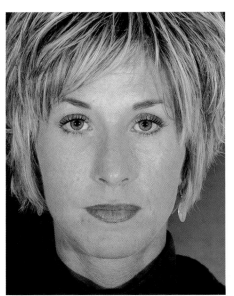

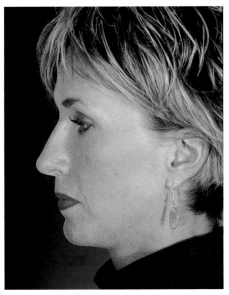

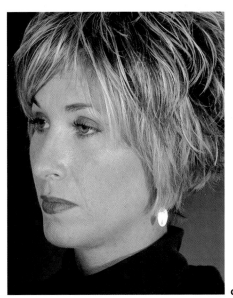

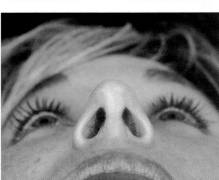

Fig. 10.**21** Eighteen months postoperatively. (**a**) Frontal view. (**b**) Lateral view. (**c**) Oblique view. (**d**) Submental view.

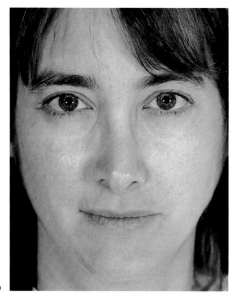
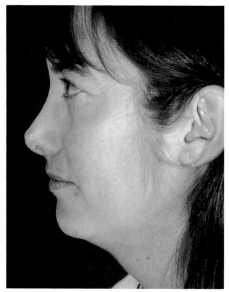
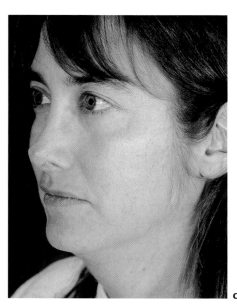

a, b

c

Fig. 10.**22**   (**a**) Preoperative frontal view. (**b**) Lateral view. (**c**) Oblique view. (**d**) Submental view.

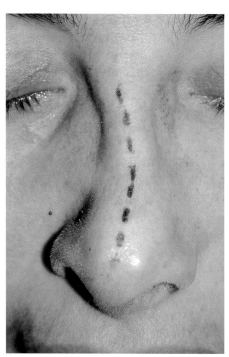

d

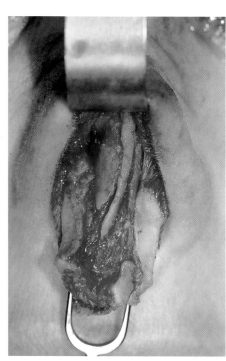

Fig. 10.**24**   Intraoperative finding of deviated dorsum and disarticulated upper lateral cartilages. Note bossae to lower lateral cartilages.

Fig. 10.**23**   Deviated dorsum with concavity on right.

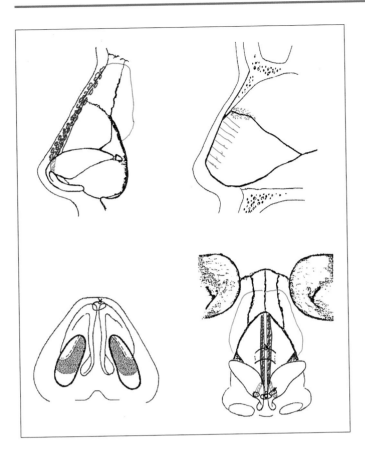

Fig. 10.**25**   Schema of operative procedure.

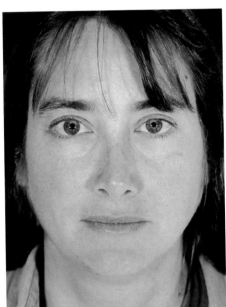
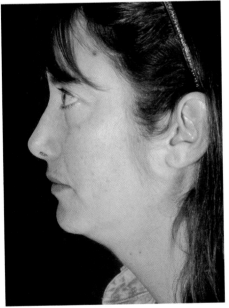
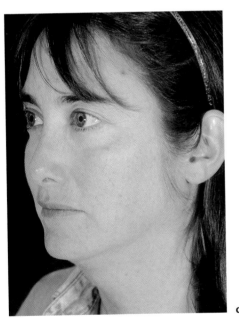

a, b

d

Fig. 10.**26**   One year postoperatively. (**a**) Frontal view. (**b**) Lateral view. (**c**) Oblique view. (**d**) Submental view.

c

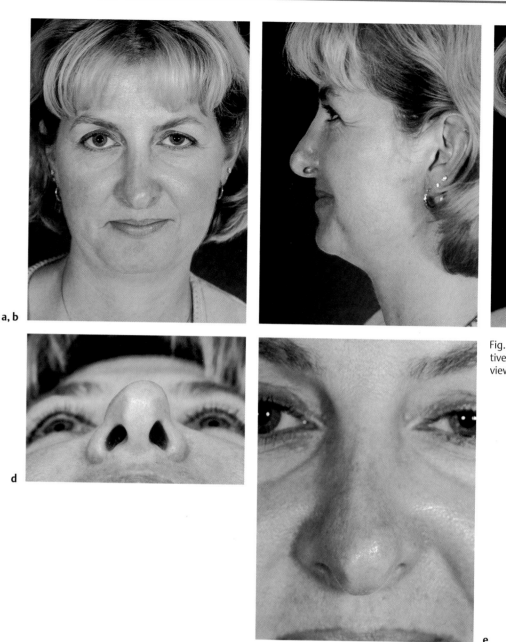

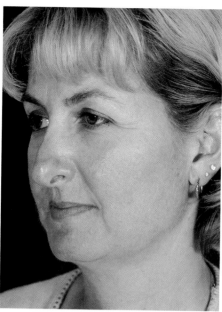

Fig. 10.**27** (**a**) Preoperative view. (**b**) Preoperative lateral. (**c**) Oblique view. (**d**) Submental view. (**e**) Close-up frontal view.

asymmetry with tip-defining points at uneven levels. There is fullness to her left supra tip area that can be palpated. On base view, the nasal tip appears to deviate to her left (Fig. 10.**27**).

Intraoperatively, one can see a disarticulation to her caudal septum with a significant deviation of the superior portion to her right. The dorsal septum was projecting through the upper lateral cartilages and the nasal bones. The lower lateral cartilages show an asymmetrical, overresection of both lateral crura that failed to adequately address the intermediate crura. The two intermediate crura were overlapping one another, creating the asymmetrical tip (Fig. 10.**28**).

Her rhinoplasty plan included a resection of the redundant dorsal septum with open reduction of this fracture line. This was reapproximated primarily and fixated with suture. The tip was made more symmetrical by equalizing the remaining lower lateral cartilages and creating a left vertical dome division with overlapping lateral crural segments. Interdomal sutures and a columella strut helped to stabilize the tip-defining points in the midline and at even levels. Lateral sidewall batten grafts were placed bilaterally to support that area. The septal cartilage was used as a dorsal onlay graft and sutured into position (Fig. 10.**29 a–c**).

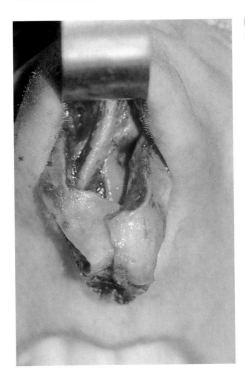

Fig. 10.**28** Intraoperative view showing the fracture of the dorsal septum with deviation of the septum to the right and nasal tip to the left.

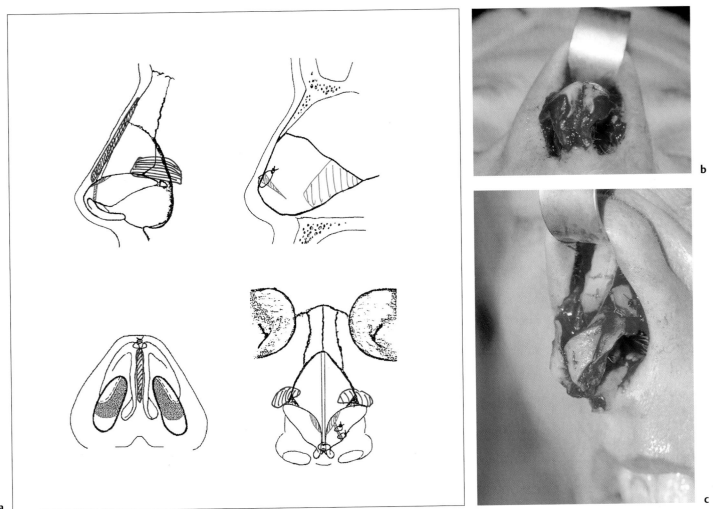

Fig. 10.**29** (**a**) Intraoperative maneuvers. (**b**) Symmetry to the lower lateral cartilages. (**c**) Dorsal onlay graft.

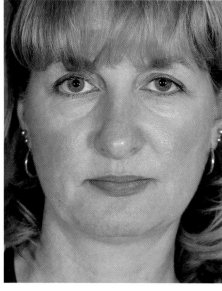
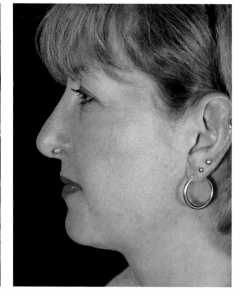
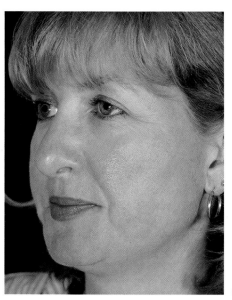

a, b

c

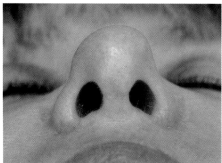

d

Fig. 10.**30**   One year postoperatively. (**a**) Frontal view. (**b**) Lateral view. (**c**) Oblique view. (**d**) Submental view.

One year postoperatively, she continues to show increased fullness on her right but there is improvement in the dorsum as well as nasal function (Fig. 10.**30**).

Case 4: Functional Obstruction from Deviated Dorsum

A 30-year-old woman comes in complaining of a twisted nose and left-sided nasal obstruction. On frontal view, the left middle third of her nose is unusually wide and full. Her nasal tip is slightly bulbous and ptotic. On lateral view, her dorsum is somewhat overprojected. The posterior septal angle was dislocated off the anterior nasal spine and rested in her left vestibule (Fig. 10.**31**).

Endonasally, the right airway was widely patent. The left lumen was obstructed at the level of the internal nasal valve. Palpation of her dorsum shows her nasal bones to be straight; however, there was a twisted deformity to her dorsal septum with the concavity on her right (Fig. 10.**32**).

Intraoperatively, one finds a complex deformity of the cartilaginous septum. The dorsal strut is twisted with a concavity on the right. The caudal strut is twisted with the posterior septal angle displaced to her left. The concavity to her dorsal septum was creating the obstruction to her left internal valve (Fig. 10.**33**).

The surgical plan included a complete release of the extrinsic binding forces to the cartilaginous septum. The left lateral aspect of her dorsal strut was thinned via sharp exci-

sion. A right unilateral spreader graft was then placed to serve as a dorsal splint. A flaring suture was subsequently used to further open the internal valve. The tip was refined with an interdomal suture and tip graft. A columella strut was also placed for additional support (Fig. 10.**34**).

Eighteen months postoperatively, she reports a significant improvement in her nasal function and is satisfied with the improved dorsal alignment (Fig. 10.**35**).

References

1. Sheen JH. Spreader graft: A method of reconstructing the roof of the middle nasal vault following rhinoplasty. *Plast Reconstr Surg.* 1984; 73:230.
2. Park SS. Treatment of the internal nasal valve. *Facial Plast Surg Clin N Am.* 1999; 7(3):333–345.
3. Most SP, Murakami CS. Nasal osteotomies: anatomy, planning, and technique. *Facial Plast Surg Clin N Am.* 2002; 10(3):279–285.
4. Lovice DB, Mingrone MD, Toriumi DM. Grafts and implants in rhinoplasty and nasal reconstruction. *Otolaryngolog Clin N Am.* 1999; 32(1):113–141.
5. Romo T, McLaughlin LA, Levine JM, Sclafani AP. Nasal implants: autogenous, semisynthetic, and synthetic. *Facial Plast Surg Clin N Am.* 2002; 10:155–166.
6. Gibson T, Davis B. The distortion of autogenous cartilage grafts: its cause and prevention. *Br J Plast Surg.* 1958; 10:257.
7. Krizek TJ, Cram AE. Transplantation in plastic surgery. In Smith JW, Aston SJ, eds. *Grabb & Smith's Plastic Surgery.* Boston: Little, Brown: 1991:91–106.
8. Schlosser RJ, Park SS. Surgery for the dysfunctional nasal valve. *Arch Facial Plast Surg.* 1999; 1:105–110.
9. Park SS. The flaring suture to augment the repair of the dysfunctional nasal valve. *Cosmetic Ideas and Innovations.* 1997; 1120–1122.

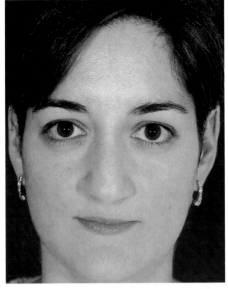

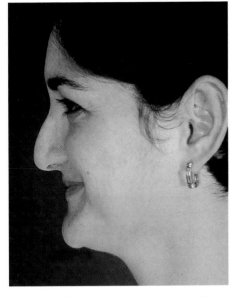

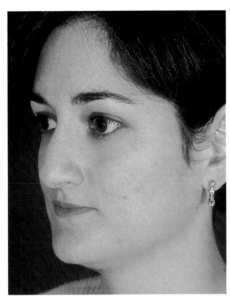

b

c

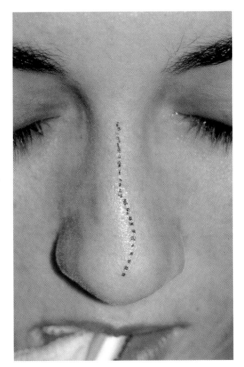

d

Fig. 10.**31**   (**a**) Preoperative frontal view. (**b**) Lateral view. (**c**) Oblique view. (**d**) Submental view.

Fig. 10.**32**   Palpation of the dorsum reveals a twisted deformity to her dorsal strut.

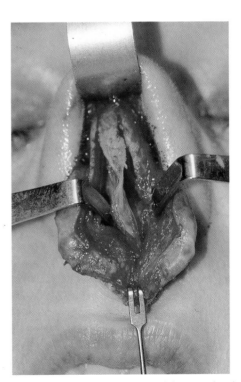

Fig. 10.**33**   Intraoperative view of the complex deformity of the quadrilateral cartilage.

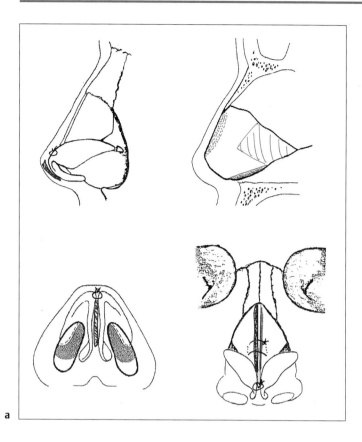

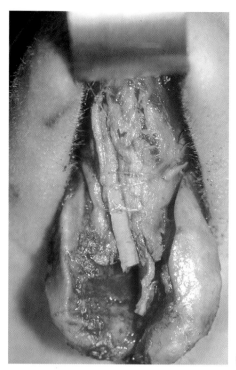

Fig. 10.**34** (**a**) Surgical plan. (**b**) Intraoperative view of right unilateral spreader graft and flaring stitch. A shave excision of the left dorsal septum was also performed.

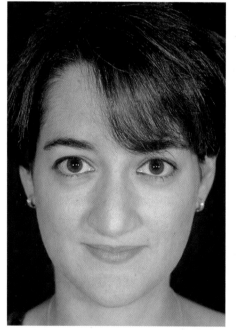

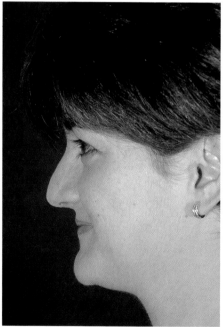

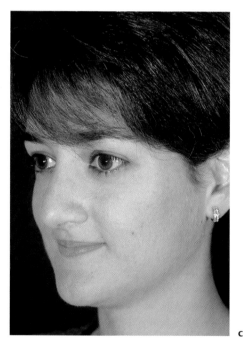

Fig. 10.**35** Eighteen months postoperatively (**a**) Frontal view. (**b**) Lateral view. (**c**) Oblique view. (**d**) Submental view.

11

The Functional Tension Nose, The Overprojected Nose

H. Behrbohm

Contents

Introduction

Definition of Terms

The functional tension nose is characterized by an excess of material in the cartilaginous nose. The basic problem is excessive length of the septal cartilage in the basodorsal direction combined with hyperplasia of the upper lateral cartilages. Both the septal and lateral cartilages develop embryologically from a common rudiment (16). It is common, therefore, to find combined hyperplasia which frequently affects the alar cartilages as well. This overgrowth leads to a general elevation of the nasal dorsum. The nasal pyramid is narrow and resembles a high, narrow, pointed gothic arch. Due to the firm attachments between the septum and upper lateral cartilages and the membranous attachment of the alar cartilages, the changes in the nasal dorsum are always accompanied by typical deformities of the nasal tip. This marks the difference between the functional tension nose and the *humped nose*, in which the dorsal hump is bony or cartilaginous in varying proportions. The shape of the nasal tip is usually unchanged. The hump in itself does not cause nasal airway problems, unless it is posttraumatic and associated with septal deviation.

A *pseudohump* exists when the distance from the nasal tip to the facial plane is too small, causing the dorsum to move above the level of the nasal tip.

The term *tension nose* always refers to a combined morphological and functional problem.

Due to the excess cartilage, the *functional tension nose* is often disharmonious in relation to the face. It is too large and too high, i.e., *overprojected*. The nasal tip alone may be overprojected, independently of the overall size of the nose (Figs. 11.**1a, b**, 11.**2a–d**).

Building on the tripod model of Andersen and its modification by McCullough and Mangat, Parell and Becker identified four key factors in the pathogenesis of the functional tension nose: Excessive height of the septum, anteroinferior rotation of the tip, narrowing of the tip, and excessive length of the lateral crura of the alar cartilages (1, 12, 13).

The functional tension nose also tethers the upper lip, causing abnormal exposure of the maxillary gingiva (18).

Various surgical techniques have been described for relieving tension on the alar cartilages. These techniques focused mainly on the resection of the dome area (15), portions of the lateral crura (10), or the upper and lower alar cartilages (13). Bull stressed the importance of a hyperplastic *anterior nasal spine* in the overprojected nasal tip and recommended resecting the spine to retroposition the tip (5).

Measurement of Overprojection

Joseph used the *profile angle* as a measure of nasal projection. He defined it as the angle formed by the intersection of two straight lines: One line tangent to the glabella and chin, and a second line tangent to the nasal dorsum. He stated a normal range of 23–37°. By measuring the angles in portraits painted by various famous artists (e.g., Holbein, da Vinci, Reynolds, Gainsborough), Joseph determined an average profile angle of 30° (11) (Fig. 11.**3**).

Goode recommended the ratio of nasal length, measured as the distance between the nasion and pronasale, and projection measured between the alar groove and the pronasale for evaluating underproject or overprojection of the nose and nasal tip. He defined the normal range as a ratio of 0.55–0.60 (7).

Baud described a method of profile analysis in which he drew a circle around the face with a radius from the external auditory canal to the pronasale (tip-defining point). He then checked the relationship between three key profile points (the *pronasale*, *pogonium*, and *frontal hairline*). Ideally, the three key points are located on the path of the circle (see Chapter 5, Preoperative Management). He used three sectors and sector angles to analyze the profile (3). Our own modification of this method is described in Chapter 5. In our experience, the facial circle should be centered on the lateral roof of the external auditory canal (the *porion*).

We have had good experiences with a simplified and modified form of this method in routine situations, as it permits a rapid assessment of nasal projection in relation to the chin and forehead. The following questions can be answered:

- Is the nose or tip overprojected?
- Does the patient have maxillary or mandibular prognathism?

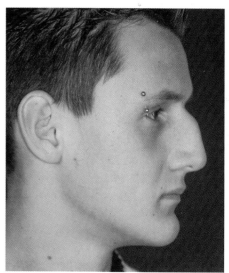 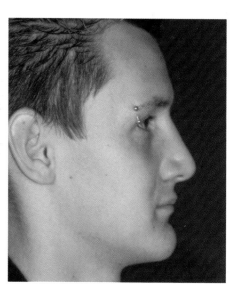

a   b

Fig. 11.**1**   Dorsal hump. (**a**) Before, and (**b**) three years after septorhinoplasty.

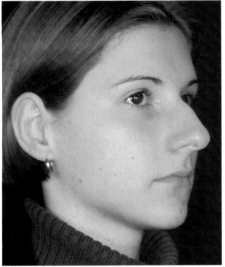
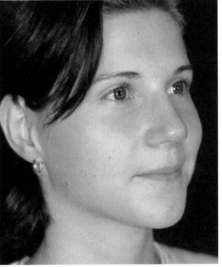

a

b

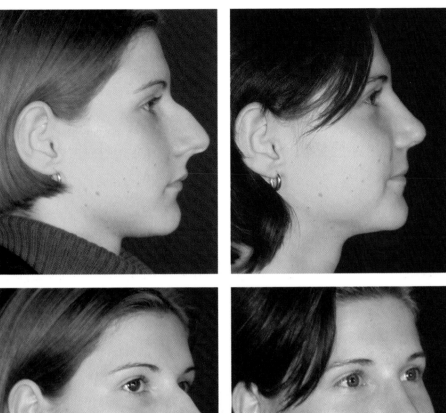

Fig. 11.2 (**a, c**) Woman with typical functional tension nose and overprojected nose due to hyperplasia of multiple structural elements. The anterior septal angle projects past the tip-defining point. The tip shows poor definition, with absence of a double break, the nasal dorsum features an osseocartilaginous hump. The nasolabial angle is obtuse and poorly defined. The upper lip appears shortened. (**b, c**) Appearance three years after septorhinoplasty.

c

d

- How does the forehead affect the profile (high or sloping forehead)?

Digital image processing can be used, for example, to predict whether reducing the tip projection, causing a relative anterior displacement of the pogonion toward the circle, will provide sufficient improvement to the profile, or whether chin augmentation should be recommended (4, 8) (Fig. 11.**4**).

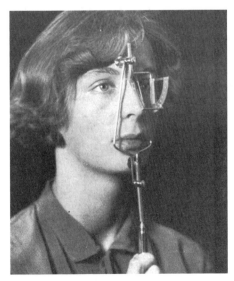

Fig. 11.**3** Joseph developed a "profilometer" for directly measuring the profile angle, without the need for a lateral photograph.

Indications

The surgical treatment of the overprojected nose or functional tension nose has both functional and esthetic indications. Both indications are based on the same morphological causes, and they are separated here purely for didactic reasons.

Functional Indications

The nares display typical changes: They are narrow, have a slit-like rather than oval shape, and terminate in a high "gothic" vestibule. The alar lateral crura and upper lateral cartilages are

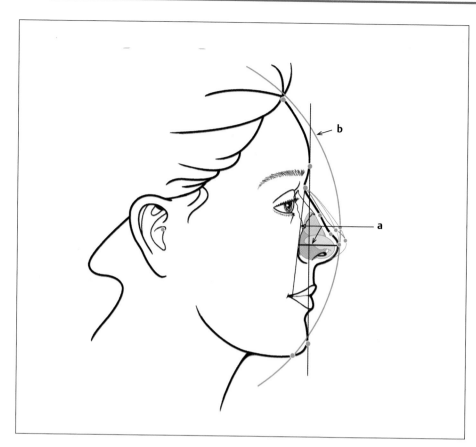

Fig. 11.**4** Methods of determining projection.
(**a**) Method of R. Goode. (**b**) Modified method
of C. Baud. Within the facial circle = normal
nose. Outside the facial circle = overprojected
nose.
- (black) – normal nose
- (red) – functional tension nose without
  overprojection
- (blue) overprojection tip
- (green) overprojected functional tension
  nose

Compare with figure 5.**3**

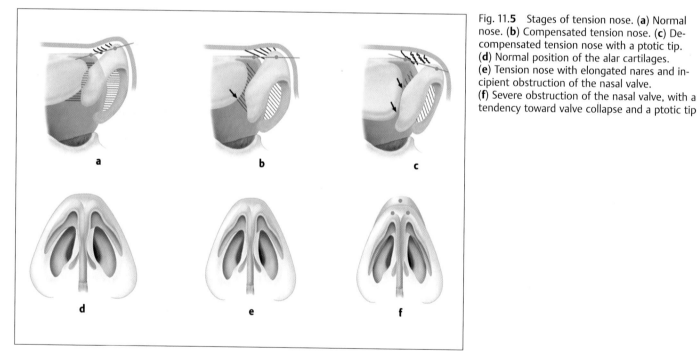

Fig. 11.**5** Stages of tension nose. (**a**) Normal
nose. (**b**) Compensated tension nose. (**c**) De-
compensated tension nose with a ptotic tip.
(**d**) Normal position of the alar cartilages.
(**e**) Tension nose with elongated nares and in-
cipient obstruction of the nasal valve.
(**f**) Severe obstruction of the nasal valve, with a
tendency toward valve collapse and a ptotic tip

medialized, causing stenosis of the nasal valve. The nasal valve
is formed by the junction of the free caudal margin of the
upper lateral cartilage with the septal cartilage. The normal
nasal valve opens at an angle of approximately 15°. This angle
is decreased in the functional tension nose, which in itself
leads to obstructed nasal breathing. Forced inspiration causes
the nasal valve to narrow and collapse, causing further airway

obstruction (Fig. 11.**6**). Even a mild degree of high septal deviation in this situation will produce marked aerodynamic effects
and exacerbate the nasal obstruction. Today the term *nasal
valve* (see Chapter 5) is distinguished from *nasal valve area*,
which includes the membranous attachment to the free cranial
margin of the alar cartilage and the functionally important
head of the *inferior turbinate*.

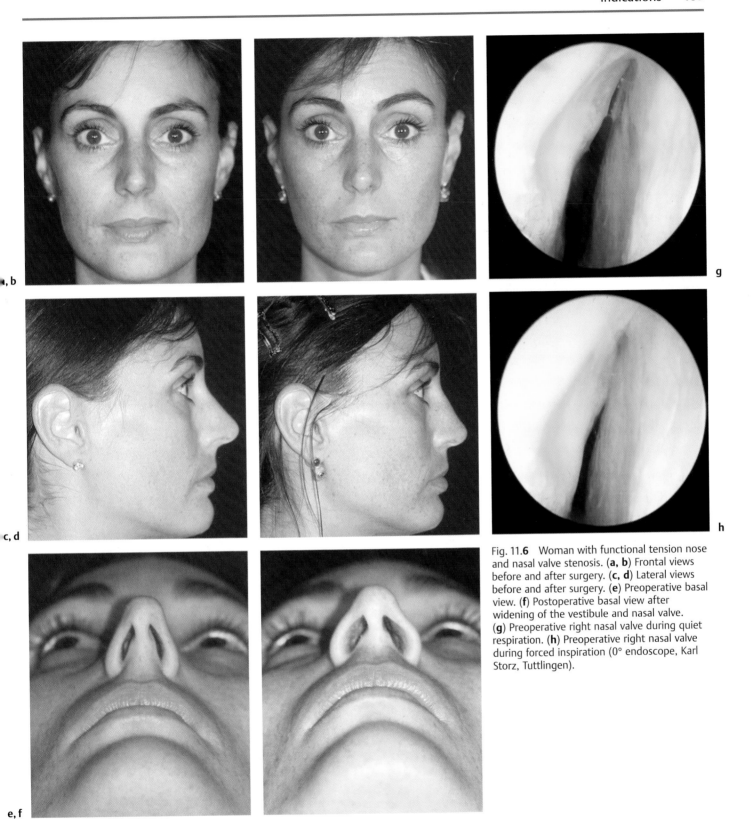

a, b

c, d

e, f

g

h

Fig. 11.**6** Woman with functional tension nose and nasal valve stenosis. (**a, b**) Frontal views before and after surgery. (**c, d**) Lateral views before and after surgery. (**e**) Preoperative basal view. (**f**) Postoperative basal view after widening of the vestibule and nasal valve. (**g**) Preoperative right nasal valve during quiet respiration. (**h**) Preoperative right nasal valve during forced inspiration (0° endoscope, Karl Storz, Tuttlingen).

Esthetic Indications

The functional tension nose is characterized by hyperplasia of the septal cartilage. Typically the septal cartilage is too long in its dorsobasal dimension, elevating the upper lateral cartilages and cartilaginous nasal dorsum. The cartilaginous dorsum is typically convex or may form a hump, which blends proximally with a bony hump at the rhinion. The nasofrontal angle is reduced, depending on the size of the hump. Not infrequently, hyperplasia of the individual cartilages is also combined with increased longitudinal growth, creating the impression of a long nose.

Functional tension nose is associated with typical changes in the supratip area, depending on the anatomical situation.

The *supratip point* moves to the level of the *tip-defining points*, and tip definition is lost.

Elastic fibers in the nasal tip area pass from the *corium layer* of the skin to the corium of the nasal vestibule (9). The skin in this area is relatively immobile. If the hyperplasia of the caudal septum can no longer be compensated by the elastic and collagen fibers of the skin over the nasal tip and the connective tissue fibers between the septum, alar cartilages, lateral cartilages, and membranous septum, then the tip-defining points will droop below the level of the supratip point (at the level of the anterior septal angle). This drooping of the tip is called *ptosis*.

If we draw a straight line from the tip-defining point to the supratip point, we find that the angles of the *nasal tip tangents* are reversed when compared with the "ideal" nose. Although this discrepancy in the levels of the tip and supratip areas may be no more than 1–2 mm, it has a significant impact on nasal tip esthetics (Figs. 11.**5**, 11.**6 a–h**).

Contraindications

Contraindications for septorhinoplasty for a functional tension nose or an overprojected nose or tip are based on functional and esthetic considerations. Other contraindications may be due to underlying conditions (e.g., coagulation disorders, hypertension) or systemic diseases (diabetes mellitus). The patient's skin and connective-tissue type may prohibit the use of certain operative techniques. For example, very thin skin through which the contours of the alar cartilages can be seen preoperatively would contraindicate grafting procedures on the tip.

An overprojected nose with a convex dorsum may be an ethnic feature. It may be very desirable to preserve this convexity at operation. We have also seen cases in which the patient desired straightening of the nasal dorsum but her family did not. The operation should not be scheduled until an agreement has been reached.

Functional Contraindications

- Good to very good nasal breathing by rhinomanometry.
- No stenosis or collapse of the nasal valve, no inspiratory alar collapse.
- Function should not be sacrificed for morphological change. If significant reduction of the dorsum is needed, the surgeon should use spreader grafts, for example, or alternative techniques to establish a functioning nasal airway.

Esthetic Contraindications

- Adverse effects on the overall profile. For example, a high nasal dorsum "lightens" a heavy, massive chin, even in prognathism. Lowering the dorsum in this case would further accentuate the lower half of the face.
- The correction of an overprojected nose, possibly combined with a mentoplasty, can radically alter the facial appearance. If the patient does not want this, the surgery may be contraindicated.

Preoperative Preparations and Prerequisites

Inspection

As with every nose, facial proportions should be considered in the assessment of the functional tension nose, especially the position of the chin, forehead, maxilla, and mandible in the three standard views: *frontal, lateral,* and *basal.*

When the tension nose is viewed from the front, the bony and cartilaginous framework appears thin and the nasal base is narrow. The skin of the supratip and tip area is tight, pale (hypoemic), and relatively immobile. The nasal dorsum and tip are usually narrow. The infratip triangle is usually too long.

In the basal view, the nares appear narrow and slitlike rather than elliptical, and they terminate in a high "gothic" vestibule. The alar lateral crura and upper lateral cartilages are medialized (see Fig. 11.**6**).

Typical associated profile changes are described in the section on Esthetic Indications above.

Palpation

Especially in patients with a functional tension nose, palpation of the external and internal nose yields information that is important for surgical planning. It is easier to palpate tension than to see it.

- External nose: Size, shape, and resilience of the alar cartilages; palpation of the anterior septal angle; tip recoil and tip support.
- Internal nose: Anterior septum, anterior nasal spine, membranous septum, medial crura, and footplates.

Function Studies

Active anterior rhinomanometry should be performed to objectify the subjective sensation of obstructed nasal breathing. This study is based on the synchronous recording of the narinochoanal pressure difference ΔP (in Pa) and of the nasal airflow $\dot{V}$ (in cm³/sec) (4, 6).

If there are signs of nasal valve stenosis, Bachmann recommends the dilatation test. Spreading open the upper part of the valve with a small cotton ball can demonstrate the pathological significance of the morphological or functional valve stenosis. The dilatation curve in this case is better than the resting curve (2).

Informed Consent

The preoperative consultation with the patient is held at least 24 hours before the operation and is preferably conducted by the surgeon or a physician representing him/her, following the recommendations given in Chapter 5. The doctor and patient review the agreed surgical goals, preferably aided by clinical photographs or drawings, and the patient is informed about all possible complications. The points that have been reviewed are documented.

The patient signs a consent form stating that all necessary information has been presented (verbally and in writing), that the patient understands all of this information, and that he/she consents to the operation.

Photographic Documentation and Computer Simulation

Patients with an overprojected nose or nasal tip often want to have the desired surgical result simulated preoperatively on a computer screen so that they can see their "new" nose and appreciate the overall effect of the operation on the face. This wish is justified, given the radical effect that this type of surgery can have on the patient's appearance. Opinions differ as to the value of graphics programs in preoperative planning. We offer our patients this option and have had positive experience with it.

One advantage is that the doctor and patient have 20–30 minutes in which they can thoroughly discuss and review the surgical goals. During this time the doctor can learn a great deal about the patient's wishes. Only those changes that can actually be effected in the nose should be simulated on the computer. The simulated image is not the blueprint for judging the success of the operation, but only a tool for comprehension and planning. Consequently, we do not save the simulated image but document the desired result in a diagram.

Laboratory Tests

The routine workup includes a simple blood count (Hb, platelets, leukocytes). Coagulation parameters (Quick prothrombin time [PT], partial thromboplastin time [PTT], and thrombin time) are also determined.

Patients are asked about the use of cardiovascular medications or "blood thinners." If patients report the use of non-steroidal anti-inflammatory agents (e.g., aspirin, acetylsalicylic acid), a platelet function test is indicated. If this test is delayed, the operation should be postponed. The workup should include an allergy test if there is evidence of perennial or seasonal allergy.

At least a plain radiograph of the paranasal sinuses should be obtained prior to any septorhinoplasty. If sinus disease is present, the sinuses should be evaluated by coronal computed tomography (CT).

Function studies consist of active anterior computerized rhinometry with a decongestion test and olfactometry with a threshold and identification test. Patients with middle ear ventilation problems or otitis media should be assessed with tonal audiometry and tympanometry.

Postoperative Measures

Doyle splints are used to stabilize the nasal septum. They are removed on the third to fifth postoperative day. Merocel packs can be left in the ethmoid for two to three days, but intranasal packs should be dispensed with whenever possible. Steristrips are affixed to the external nose, placing light traction or pressure on the nasal tip according to requirements. The nasal dorsum can be padded with gelatin sponge (Gelform).

The internal nose is treated with nasal oil (e.g., GeloSitin, Coldastop) and an isotonic saline spray (e.g., Emser Sole Spray, Rhinomer). Intranasal crusts are removed under endoscopic control. Further details on postoperative care are presented in Chapter 15.

Preoperative Analysis

Although the nose consists of only a few structural elements, the variations in their size, arrangement, and interrelationships lead to countless shapes and nuances. Ultimately, no two noses are alike. The preoperative morphological analysis of an overprojected nose or a functional tension nose is essential for a successful operation. Through inspection and palpation, the surgeon can determine which structural elements are the major causes of the overprojection or tension deformity of the nasal inlet. Hyperplasia is rarely confined to a *single* structure, but often only a few features are chiefly responsible for the overprojection.

Although the operation focuses on the main anatomical problem based on this morphological analysis, the surgical correction of an overprojected nose always requires more or less extensive changes in multiple structural components of the nose in order to achieve the most natural and harmonious result.

Because an overprojected nose is always a result of hyperplasia, surgical treatment consists mainly of a series of resections.

Principles of Surgery for the Overprojected Nose and Tension Nose

1. Reduction or resection of hyperplastic structural elements
2. Selective weakening of tip support mechanisms as described by Tardy (19) (Figs. 11.**7**, 11.**8 a–f**)

Principal Causes of Overprojection

Hyperplasia of the Anterior Nasal Spine

An overprojected tip may be caused by an overdeveloped anterior nasal spine, either alone or combined with other hyperplasias. The hyperplastic nasal spine pushes the anterior septum upward.

The nasolabial angle is obtuse and obscured. The upper lip is tethered and appears shortened. There is concomitant downward rotation of the tip. Hyperplasias of the caudal septum and nasal spine can be differentiated by careful external and internal palpation (Figs. 11.**9**, 11.**10 a, b**).

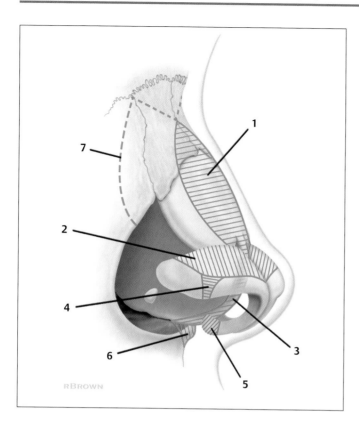

Fig. 11.**7** Typical steps involved in surgical correction of the overprojected nose.
1. Lowering the nasal dorsum.
2. Cranial volume reduction.
3. Shortening the caudal septal margin.
4. Wedge excision from the lateral alar cartilages.
5. Resection of the footplates.
6. Removal of the nasal spine.
7. Curved lateral osteotomies.

Figs. 11.**7**–11.**20**
Red shading—different steps of operative correction

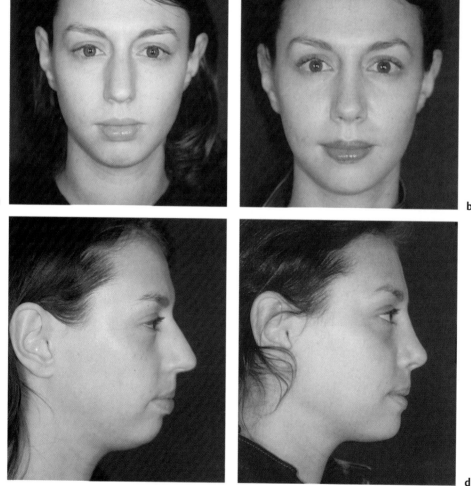

Fig. 11.**8** Woman with an overprojected nose and functional tension nose, before and three years after surgery. (**a**) Frontal view: Washed-out contour between the nasal pyramid and facial plane. (**b**) Postoperative appearance. (**c**) Preoperative lateral view: Overprojection, retrognathism. (**d**) Postoperative appearance after steps 1, 2, 3, 4, 6, and 7 in Fig. 11.**7**. (**e, f**) Preoperative and postoperative half profile.

Fig. 11.**8 e, f** ▷

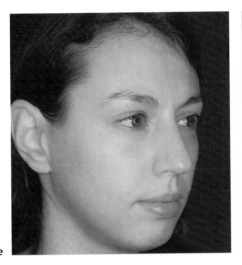

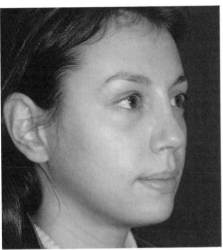

Fig. 11.**8 e, f**

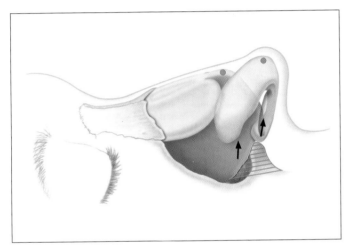

Fig. 11.**9**   Overprojected nasal tip due to hyperplasia of the anterior nasal spine.

Fig. 11.**10**   Lateral views (**a**) before and (**b**) two years after surgery.

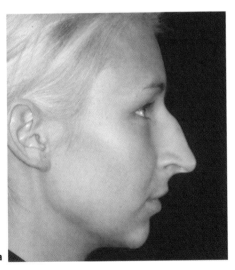

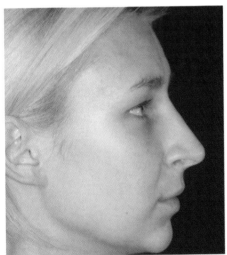

Hyperplasia of the Alar Cartilages

Hyperplastic alar cartilages may be the sole cause of an over-projected and usually bulbous nasal tip. Usually the cartilage is very elastic and there is firm connective tissue. The nasolabial angle is not affected (Figs. 11.**11**, 11.**12 a, b**, 11.**13 a, b**).

Excessive Length of Medial Crura (Columellar Hyperplasia)

Elongated medial crura that are wedged between the nasal tip and spine lead to typical changes in the alar–columellar region. Usually there is concomitant hyperplasia of the anterior septal cartilage. It is typical to find increased lateral exposure of the nares with vestibular skin show. A harmonious double break is absent. The intermediate crus of the alar cartilages is lengthened, causing excessive length of the infratip triangle (Figs. 11.**14**, 11.**15 a, b**).

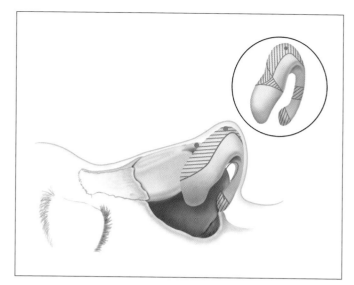

Fig. 11.**11**   Overprojected nasal tip due to hyperplasia of the alar cartilages.
Red shading: possible operative steps for retroposition of the nasal tip.

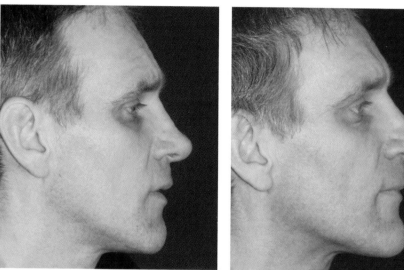

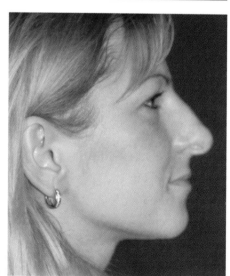

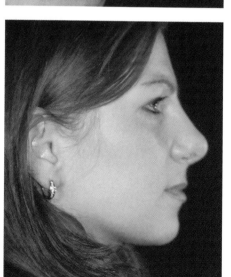

Fig. 11.**12**   Patient with an overprojected nose due to alar cartilage hyperplasia. (**a**) Before and (**b**) three years after surgery.

Fig. 11.**13**   Patient with an overprojected tip due to alar cartilage hyperplasia. (**a**) Before and (**b**) four years after surgery.

a

b

a

b

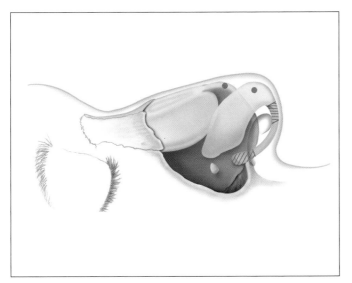

Fig. 11.**14**   Overprojection of the nose due to columellar hyperplasia with elongated medial crura.

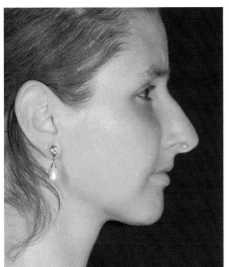
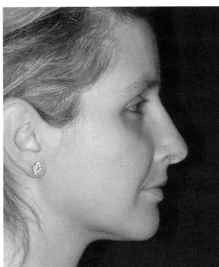

a   b

Fig. 11.**15**   Lateral views (**a**) before and (**b**) two years after surgery.

Hyperplasia of Septal Cartilage in the Dorsobasal Direction, Hyperplastic Vomer, Pollybeak Deformity

Hyperplasia of the septal cartilage in the dorsobasal direction leads to elevation of the cartilaginous nasal dorsum. A similar effect can result from an overdeveloped vomer. Due to the elevation of the supratip area, the tip loses definition and has an amorphous appearance. The anterior septal angle is above the tip-defining point.

A postoperative *pollybeak* can result from insufficient shortening of the dorsal septal cartilage. Postoperative scarring, especially in thick skin, can also lead to pollybeak deformity (Figs. 11.**16**, 11.**17 a, b**, 11.**18 a, b**).

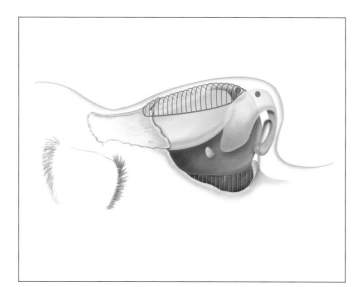

Fig. 11.**16**   Overprojection of the nose due to hyperplasia of the septal cartilage in the dorsobasal direction.

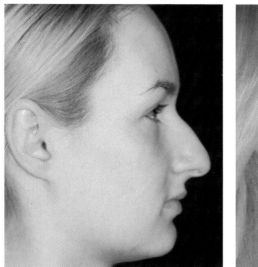
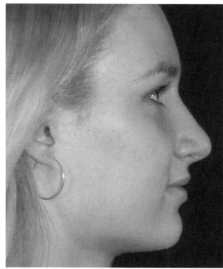

a

b

Fig. 11.**17**   Lateral views (**a**) before and (**b**) two years after surgery.

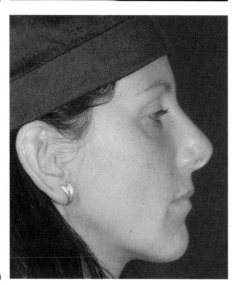
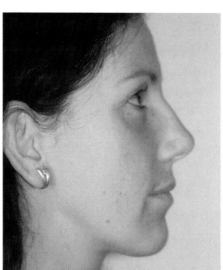

a

b

Fig. 11.**18**   (**a**) Pollybeak deformity seven years after a previous operation. (**b**) Appearance three years after revision surgery.

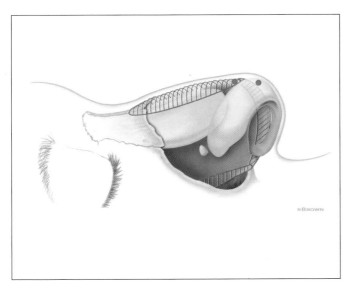

Fig. 11.**19** Overprojection of the nose due to hyperplasia of the septum in the craniocaudal direction.

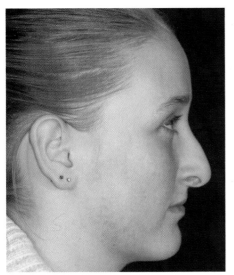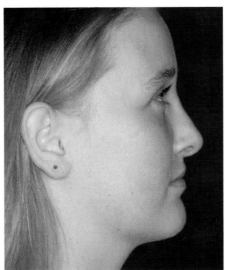

Fig. 11.**20**   Lateral views (**a**) before and (**b**) four years after surgery.

a   b

Hyperplasia of Septal Cartilage in the Craniocaudal Direction

Hyperplastic septal cartilage that shows marked caudal extension leads to a typical clinical picture. Usually the cartilage is also hyperplastic in the dorsobasal direction. The nasal tip is poorly defined. The anterior septal angle (supratip point) is above the level of the tip-defining points. The tip is caudally rotated and ptotic. The appearance is similar to that of columellar hyperplasia due to excessively long medial crura. The difference can be appreciated by palpating the firm caudal septal cartilage and distinguishing it from the membranous septum. As with columellar hyperplasia, there is marked vestibular skin show and a deficient double break (Figs. 11.**19**, 11.**20a, b**).

Operative Strategy

Preoperative analysis of the morphological problems of the nose is the basis for an efficient operation. This analysis is essential for identifying the structural elements of the nose that require critical modification and reorientation and for planning the approach, which should be as invasive as necessary and as noninvasive as possible.

The preferred approach for correcting the functional tension nose or overprojected nose is the *delivery approach*. This is a closed approach that provides excellent exposure for direct, symmetrical modification of the alar cartilages. Several techniques can be used in this approach for retroposition of the nasal tip:

- Cranial volume reduction with or without resection of the tip-defining points (complete strip);
- Wedge excision from the lateral alar cartilages, reapproximating the stumps with sutures;
- Releasing, modifying, or reorienting cartilage tension by cross-hatching, morselizing, or incising.

In approximately 15% of our patients with an overprojected or tension nose, we use an open approach. The indications for this approach are as follows:
- Significant overprojection requiring a dome resection,
- Severe asymmetry of the nasal tip,
- Revision surgery.

Central Role of the Septum

The nasal septum is of key importance in the surgical correction of the functional tension nose. By reducing the septal height, changing the position of the anterior septal angle, shortening the caudal septal margin, or beveling the anterosuperior margin, the surgeon can selectively modify the shape, position, and esthetics of the nasal tip (4, 8).

The operation begins with exposure of the septal cartilage. The transfixion incision is better for this purpose than the traditional hemitransfixion. Tip support can be weakened and reduced in two ways through this approach:
- Dividing the membranous septum,
- Releasing the footplate attachments to the caudal septal margin.

The preferred three-tunnel technique of Cottle has the advantage of preserving the nutrient connections between the cartilage and mucoperichondrium. The risk of postoperative septal hematomas is reduced, and there is less scarring and less tendency toward redeviation.

If it is necessary to correct septal deviation in addition to shortening the septal cartilage in the dorsobasal or craniocaudal direction, it can be helpful to create two superior tunnels. In this way the surgeon can fully expose the septal cartilage and assess its deformities and tensions. It is common to find dual sites of anterior and posterior stenosis. With two superior tunnels, these sites can be corrected under vision by scoring or cross-hatching both sides. It is our impression that this facilitates rotation of the septal cartilage between the alar cartilages and the actual "trimming" of the mobilized and basally shortened cartilage. The risk of perforation is thereby in principle increased, but this can be prevented by avoiding mucosal lesions at corresponding sites.

Intranasal Septal Resection

Basal Strip

A septum that is too long in the basodorsal direction can be relaxed by resecting a basal strip only 2 mm wide. The effect of this on the nasal tip and supratip area should be checked at each step in the operation. The effects vary considerably in different patients, ranging from no visible change to a marked decrease in projection or a saddle depression in the supratip area.

Anterior Septal Margin

Shortening the anterior septal margin by 2–4 mm may be necessary if the septum is too long (see Fig. 11.**20**). This can affect the tip rotation. Cranial rotation is produced by shortening the cranial or caudal septal margin between the medial and ante-rior septal angle. Another option is to shorten the entire anterior margin or, if the nasolabial angle is obscured, shorten the basal portion.

Swinging Door

The septal cartilage can be detached 2 mm in front of the perpendicular plate to expose and access the bony septum. Experience has shown that approximately 30% of the causes of nasal obstruction are located in that region. Bony spurs and ridges also have indirect effects on the anterior septal cartilage. If they are left alone, nasal breathing will continue to be obstructed and there will be a danger of incomplete relaxation of the septal cartilage.

Treating the Septal Cartilage

The intrinsic tension of the basally and cranially mobilized septal cartilage can be altered by scoring, careful morselizing, cross-hatching, or incising. The cartilage should be scored on the concave side to lengthen and "open up" the shorter curvature on that side. This is supported by small wedge excisions on the opposite side (19).

Reimplantation

All cartilage that is removed from the nose should be treated externally and reimplanted to help stabilize the nasal dorsum and tip. The position of both structures should be permanently and predictably maintained after the operation. This can also prevent septal flutter during phonation and forced respiration. The removed fragments are compressed by applying careful, controlled pressure with a cartilage crusher. This alters the bending properties of the cartilage without seriously damaging it or compromising its mechanical strength. Fibrin glue can be used to reattach the cartilage fragments and seal the mucosal pouch (see Chapter 12, The Saddle Nose).

Principles of Profile Correction and Hump Removal

We use a closed approach in approximately 85% of our patients with an overprojected nose or tip or functional tension nose. The delivery approach, unlike the cartilage-splitting approach, permits specific measures for retroposition of the nasal tip. These include resections to reduce the alar cartilages themselves as well as incisions to weaken the tip support mechanisms. By delivery of the alar cartilages, the surgeon can modify the *three* most important factors that determine tip support and projection:
- The size, shape, and resilience of the medial and lateral crura of the alar cartilages,
- The attachment of the crural footplates to the caudal septum,
- The connective-tissue attachment between the upper lateral and alar cartilages.

The nasal tip is corrected first, followed by the dorsum. The advantage of the delivery approach is that it allows the surgeon to evaluate the effects of each step in the operation on the

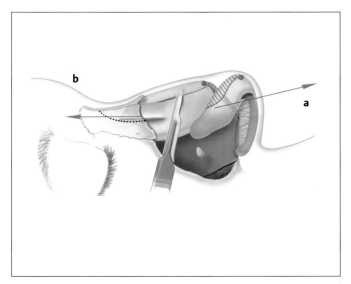

Fig. 11.**21** Surgical techniques used in fractionated lowering of the nasal dorsum. (**a**) Lowering the cartilaginous dorsum. The cut is aimed at the top of the naris. (**b**) The osteotome is applied at a low angle for resecting the bony dorsum.

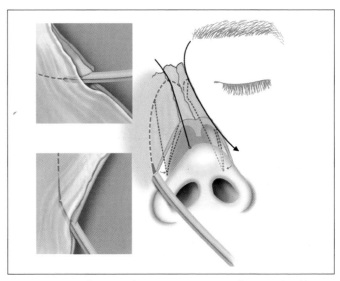

Fig. 11.**22** Laterally curved osteotomies using the minichisel/osteotome.

tense contours of the external nose. Also, it preserves the system of elastic and collagen fibers in the skin of the nasal tip for enhanced tip support.

It is logical to correct the nasal tip first, as this sequence allows the surgeon to evaluate fine changes in the nasal tip at each step of the operation. When the desired tip projection and rotation have been achieved, the height of the nasal dorsum can be adjusted. A large hump is the only situation in which it may be better to deviate from this sequence.

Resection of the cartilaginous and bony nasal dorsum should be done in the extramucous plane to avoid intraoperative and postoperative bleeding. Injuries to the nasal mucosa during lowering of the nasal dorsum or hump removal are a particularly common source of bleeding. The mucosa can be separated from the dorsum using an elevator.

An osseocartilaginous hump should be removed piecemeal. The bony component is usually smaller. With a piecemeal technique, the osteotome can be positioned at a more precise angle for shaping the nasal dorsum than with an en bloc resection (Fig. 11.**21**).

The larger, cartilaginous portion of the nasal dorsum has a more important effect on the supratip area, tip area, and dorsal region. After the cartilaginous dorsum has been lowered with a No. 15 blade, the Rubens osteotome can be used. Generally less bony hump is removed due to the differences in skin thickness at the nasal root, rhinion, and tip. Fractionated, piecemeal hump removal is the best technique for achieving a straight dorsum or obtaining a slightly convex contour in the rhinion area.

Based on our own recommendations, a minichisel was developed for medially and laterally curved osteotomies that combines the features of a chisel and an osteotome. It has two different bevels and a very slight bend in the shaft. Due to this design, the surgeon can predefine the cutting curve of the instrument, similar to the curve traced by a skate blade in speed skating (Fig. 11.**22**).

The removal of large humps or marked lowering of the nasal dorsum always carries a risk of postoperative valve ste-

nosis. This can be avoided by the liberal use of spreader grafts placed in the extramucous plane.

Complications

Possible complications relate to the hazards of the selected approach and the various steps in the operation. A closed endonasal approach causes less tissue trauma than an open approach and is associated with less edema, swelling, and ecchymosis. The less trauma is inflicted, the more quickly postoperative swelling will subside. The most aggressive instruments are rasps. They should be used only sparingly to smooth irregularities.

Potential complications include infection, hemorrhage, and the displacement of mobilized cartilage and bone. Injury to the orbit from a minichisel is possible in theory, but the author is unaware of any cases reported to date.

Infection

The larger the wound area and the longer the operation, the higher the risk of infection. Atraumatic technique reduces this risk, as small hematomas are associated with less danger of infection.

Bleeding

Dissections should proceed strictly in the surgical plane (see Chapter 1, The Dual Character of Nasal Surgery). This can prevent bleeding and minimize swelling.

The nasal mucosa should be preserved as scrupulously as possible. Mucosal injuries are the most frequent cause of significant postoperative hemorrhage.

Dislocations

The surgically modified cartilage and bone should be securely fixed in their new position and stabilized. Significant long-term scar traction (e.g., on onlay grafts) is a concern. Cartilage should be fixed with sutures, and bone should be stabilized with splints or a nasal cast.

The complications of endonasal endoscopic microsurgery are reviewed in Chapter 1.

References

1. Anderson JR. The dynamics of rhinoplasty. In *Proceedings of the Ninth International Congress in Otorhinolaryngology, Excerpta Medica*. International Congress Series 206. Amsterdam, Excerpta medica: 1969.
2. Bachmann W. Klinische Funktionsdiagnose zur behinderten Nasenatmung. *HNO*. 1983; 31:320–326.
3. Baud C. *Harmonie der Gesichtszüge*. La Chaux-de-Fonds: Clinique de la Tour: 1967.
4. Behrbohm H, Hildebrandt Th, Kaschke O. *Funktionell-ästhetische Chirurgie der Nase*. Tuttlingen: Endo-Press: 2001.
5. Bull TR. The over-projected nasal tip. In Nolst Trenité, Kugler, *Rhinoplasty*. The Hague: XX. 1998:167–169.
6. Enzmann H. Vergleich rhinomanometrischer Verfahren. *HNO*. 1983; 31:327–331.
7. Goode R. cited by Tardy (1996)
8. Hildebrandt Th, Behrbohm H. Functional aesthetic surgery of the nose. The influence of the septum on the aestetics of the nasal tip. Media-Service, CD ROM: 2001.
9. Lang J. *Klinische Anatomie der Nase, Nasenhöhle und Nebenhöhlen*. Stuttgart: Thieme: 1988.
10. Lipsett E. A new approach to surgery of the lower cartilaginous vault. *Arch Otorhinolaryngol*. 1959; 70:42.
11. Joseph J. *Nasenplastik und sonstige Gesichtsplastik nebst einem Anhang über Mammaplastik und einige Operationen aus dem Gebiete der äußeren Körperplastik*. Leipzig: Curt Kabitzsch: 1934.
12. McCullough EG, Mangat D. Systematic approach to correction of the nasal tip in rhinoplasty. *Arch Otolaryngol*. 1981; 197:12–16.
13. Parell JG, Becker GD. The "tension nose". *Facial plastic surgery*. 1984; 1:81–86.
14. Powell N, Humphreys B. *Proportions of the aesthetic face*. Stuttgart: Thieme: 1984.
15. Safian J. *Corrective rhinoplastic surgery*. New York: Paul B. Hoeber: 1934.
16. Rettinger G. Formfehler der Nase. In Naumann, Helms, Herberhold, Kastenbauer, eds.*Oto-Rhino-Laryngologie in Klinik und Praxis*. Stuttgart: Thieme; 1992:141–149.
17. Simons RL. Nasal tip projection, ptosis and supratip thickening. *Ear Nose Throat J*. 1982; 61:452–455.
18. Tardy ME, Walter M, Patt BS. The overprojecting nose: Anatomic component analysis and repair. *Facial Plastic Surgery*. 1993; 9:306–316.
19. Tardy ME. *Rhinoplasty: The art and the science. Vol I und II*. Philadelphia: W.B. Saunders: 1996.
20. Webster RC. Advances in surgery of the tip: Intact rim cartilage techniques and The tip-columella-lip esthetic complex. *Otolaryngol Clin North Am*. 1975; 8:615–644.

12

The Saddle Nose—Causes and Pathogenesis, Approaches and Operative Techniques, Principles of Tissue Replacement in the Nose

H. Behrbohm

Contents

Introduction

The term *saddle nose* denotes a polycausative condition that is associated with destabilization or destruction of the bony or cartilaginous structures of the nose. In old textbooks on otorhinolaryngology, saddle nose was most often described as a feature of congenital syphilis (28).

Today, osseous forms of saddle nose are rare and usually result from dysplasia of the nasal bones or from nasal or midfacial trauma. The cartilaginous saddle nose is a more frequent concern for rhinologists. The central problem in this condition is serious structural compromise caused by a loss of anterior septal cartilage between the rhinion (keystone area) and the "septal pedestal" at the level of the premaxilla and anterior nasal spine (4).

Frontal trauma to the nose can lead to septal cartilage necrosis as a result of septal hematoma or septal abscess. Meanwhile, cartilage fragments may be displaced and weaken the mechanical properties of the septal cartilage or may produce a sharp, angular septal deviation or transverse deviation. Combined injuries to the bony and cartilaginous nose lead to lateralization of the *nasal bones* or portions of the *maxillary frontal process*. This creates an *open roof*, often with disruption of the osseocartilaginous junction at the *rhinion* (keystone) and the formation of a visible stepoff (*inverted V*) between the cartilaginous and bony nasal segments. Cartilaginous saddle nose can also result from the overresection of septal cartilage in a septoplasty—a common legacy from the age when the Killian resection was widely practiced.

Depending on their size and location, septal perforations cause a loss of cartilage substance, leading to concavity of the cartilaginous nasal dorsum and retraction of the lower columella ("hidden columella"). Other causes may be Wegener granulomatosis, cocaine abuse, trauma from nose picking, atrophic rhinitis sicca (often combined with an anterior septal deviation), or polychondritis (6).

A change in the septal cartilage is almost never the sole cause of saddle nose, however. Saddling is a multifactorial process in which the destabilization of the septum incites changes such as separation or settling of the upper lateral cartilages, and cranial tip rotation or loss of tip projection and support. For this reason, stable reconstruction of the cartilaginous septum is the critical challenge in the operative treatment of saddle nose deformity. Saddle nose is a typical example of the inseparable link between morphological and functional abnormalities in the nose and the task that is faced by corrective nasal surgery.

The depression of the supratip area leads to widening of the nasal valve with a caudal drift of the upper lateral cartilages. The increased nasal valve angle is accompanied by hyperplasia of the inferior turbinates (ballooning phenomenon). The result of these changes is always an impairment of nasal breathing.

The surgical treatment of saddle nose has a reconstructive character. Many patients will bring in old photographs of themselves to demonstrate the original shape of their nose. In contrast to most other operations in esthetic nasal surgery, where the object is to modify an existing form, the usual goal in saddle nose surgery is the restoration of a former state (Fig. 12.**1**).

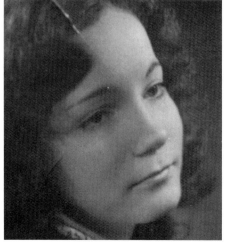
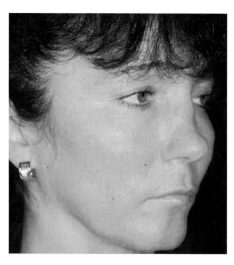
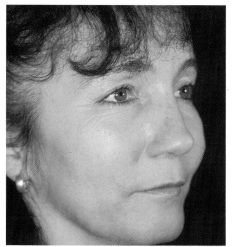

a, b
c

Fig. 12.**1** Woman with posttraumatic saddle nose. (**a**) Teenage photograph of the patient. (**b**) Preoperative appearance. (**c**) Appearance four years after operative treatment.

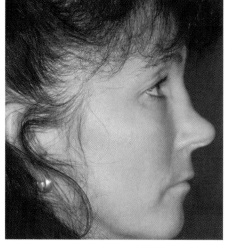
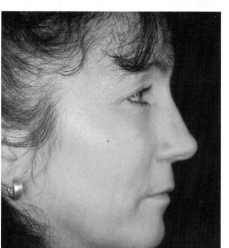

d
e

The surgery of saddle nose requires expertise in the selection, procurement, and placement of suitable grafts or implants for tissue replacement in the nose (see the section on Guidelines for Tissue Replacement in the Nose below).

Many different techniques have been described for the surgical correction of saddle nose. The state of the art is particularly well represented by the works of Tardy, Meyer, Rettinger, Nolst Trenité, Aiach, and others (2, 21, 22, 25, 29).

Indications

The goal of a saddle nose correction is not just to reconstruct the nasal dorsum. A more important goal is to restore the supportive framework of the nose in order to improve nasal breathing and achieve stable long-term results.

Form and function are almost always equally compromised in saddle nose deformity, and both must be included in the plan of operation in order to achieve acceptable results.

Our discussion of functional and esthetic indications in separate sections is done purely for didactic reasons.

Functional Indications

The indication for septorhinoplasty on functional grounds is based largely on the degree of nasal breathing impairment. Severe impairment often leads to pathological sequelae such as pharyngitis, laryngitis, and bronchitis. Septal deformities, usually following septal fractures, lead to paranasal sinus ventilation problems with recurrent or chronic sinusitis, which in turn may cause headaches and facial pain. Septal perforations can cause drying of the mucosa and olfactory compromise, depending on their size.

Esthetic Indications

Saddling leads to typical external changes in the nose relating to depression of the cartilaginous dorsum, especially in the supratip area. Depending on the cause, there are typical pathogenic mechanisms that affect the face as a whole and especially the proportions of the profile.

Figure 12.**2** illustrates these typical changes in a woman with posttraumatic saddle nose. The frontal view demonstrates a broadened nasal dorsum. The rhomboid of the nasal tip is broadened. We look in vain for the *supratip point* formed by the anterior septal angle. The result is a broad, poorly defined tip. A *hidden columella* is apparent in the frontal view. The infratip triangle is shortened. The result is a general coarsening of the facial features.

The lateral view shows saddling of the nasal dorsum in the supratip area. The tip is rotated upward and has lost projection. As a result, the chin appears to jut forward.

A *pseudo-saddle nose* is caused by an overprojected tip combined with a concave nasal dorsum. The facial circle is useful for determining the position of the tip and helps in differentiating between a true and pseudo-saddle nose (see Chapter 5, Preoperative Management).

A *pseudohump* occurs when the cartilaginous nasal dorsum is depressed below the rhinion. In contrast to a true hump, the nasofrontal angle is not increased.

The hidden columella is most apparent in the three-quarter profile view (Fig. 12.**2 a–f**).

Contraindications

Contraindications for septorhinoplasty exist in patients with florid granulomatous inflammations that have caused cartilaginous destruction, as in Wegener granulomatosis or polychondritis. The top priority in these cases is to diagnose the underlying disease. It is often difficult to make a histological diagnosis in Wegener disease. The excisional biopsy should always be taken from the margin of the septal perforation and should include normal-appearing mucosa along with the granulations. If possible, reconstruction should be deferred until remission has been achieved with pharmacological therapy.

Pirsig reported on the successful reconstruction of saddle nose in cases of Wegener granulomatosis and ectodermal dysplasia using extranasal incisions and auricular cartilage (24).

Saddle nose reconstruction following a prior septal operation is most successful when it is delayed for approximately nine months after the initial surgery so that the new operation can be planned on the basis of definitive, scarred defects. Operating too early before wound healing is complete and stabilizing or destabilizing the result of the previous operation will also jeopardize the revision outcome. Traumatic saddle nose in boxers should not be corrected until the patient has retired from the ring. Often, however, professional boxers will already have problems with obstructed nasal breathing at the start of their career. In these cases a compromise may be struck between functional improvement and reasonable esthetic improvement without extensive mobilization of the nasal skeleton.

Preoperative Preparations and Prerequisites

History

History-taking in saddle nose patients should include any prior history of trauma. Besides the mechanism of a nasal injury, the timing of the injury provides important causative clues. If the trauma affects the cartilaginous growth zones of the pediatric nose, saddling may result from the inhibited growth of specific nasal cartilages. The traumatized adult nose is characterized by the displacement of initially normally developed cartilages.

The rhinological history should also probe for signs of cartilaginous diseases, previous nasal operations, and underlying diseases.

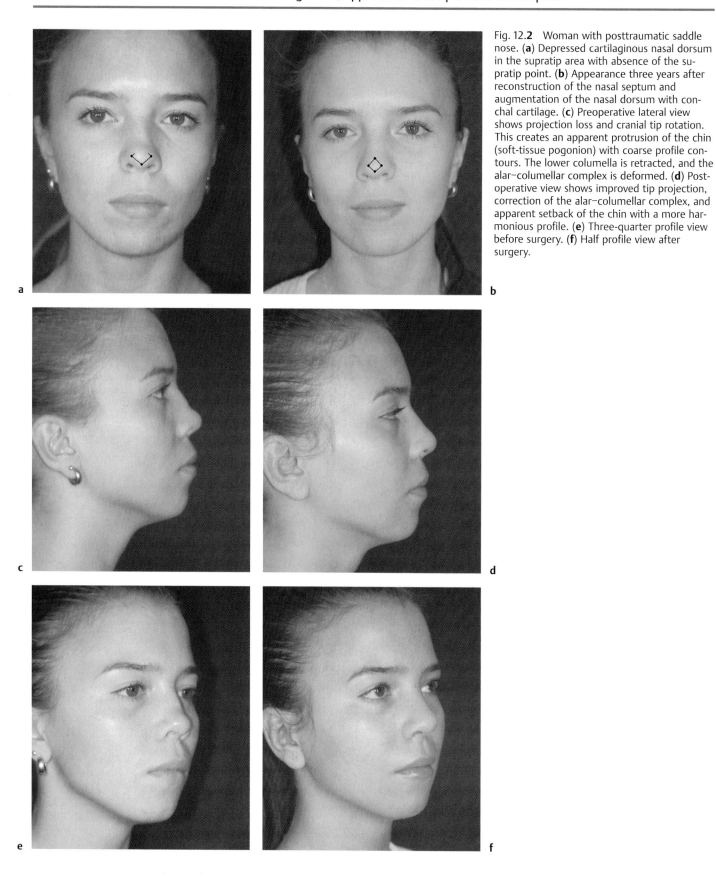

Fig. 12.2 Woman with posttraumatic saddle nose. (**a**) Depressed cartilaginous nasal dorsum in the supratip area with absence of the su-pratip point. (**b**) Appearance three years after reconstruction of the nasal septum and augmentation of the nasal dorsum with con-chal cartilage. (**c**) Preoperative lateral view shows projection loss and cranial tip rotation. This creates an apparent protrusion of the chin (soft-tissue pogonion) with coarse profile con-tours. The lower columella is retracted, and the alar–columellar complex is deformed. (**d**) Post-operative view shows improved tip projection, correction of the alar–columellar complex, and apparent setback of the chin with a more har-monious profile. (**e**) Three-quarter profile view before surgery. (**f**) Half profile view after surgery.

Inspection

Saddle noses present characteristic external features that vary with the underlying pathogenic mechanisms.

Frontal View

The following changes may be seen as isolated findings or in various combinations: The nose appears generally broadened. This may be most conspicuous in the supratip area or may affect the entire nasal dorsum. If the nasal bones are displaced or lateralized, hypertelorism is noted. Often this impression is strengthened by ruptured medial palpebral ligaments. Epicanthal folds result from a disproportion between the skin and the reduced nasal height. An open roof contributes to widening of the nasal dorsum. The "inverted V" is a sign that the connection between the cartilaginous and bony nose has been disrupted.

Lateral View

The nasal dorsum is depressed. The tip is usually rotated upward or occasionally downward, causing a loss of projection. If the cartilaginous anterior septal margin is absent, the columella is retracted cephalad (*hidden columella*) with deformation of the alar–columellar complex. The columella is shortened. The upper lip appears too long.

Basal View

The nasal base and nares are broadened. The nares assume a more horizontal alignment and have a round or transverse oval shape. The columella is shortened. The angle between the septum and lateral alar cartilages is obtuse.

Nasal Endoscopy

The nasal valve is broadened. The inferior turbinates are hyperplastic, and the upper lateral cartilages show caudal displacement (*ballooning phenomenon*).

The septum can be inspected for cartilaginous defects (*soft septum*) with the endoscope and a cotton applicator. Granulations and perforations can be evaluated and biopsy specimens taken. Precise information on how much cartilage is still present is just as important as the size of a septal perforation.

Palpation

Important information can be gained in saddle nose patients by external and internal palpation of the nose.

External Palpation

The nasal dorsum is palpated for irregularities, bony and cartilaginous defects, and an open roof. Trauma will often leave sharp-edged irregularities resulting from displaced fragments of nasal bones. Selection of the operative technique is guided by the palpation of tip support in connection with the anterior septal angle.

Internal Palpation

Internal palpation of the nose can furnish information on the anterior septum, its anterior margin, and the presence of cartilaginous fractures or defects in the anterior septum.

Laboratory Tests

Saddle nose patients should be assessed with a simple blood count and basic coagulation studies (Quick prothrombin time [PT], partial thromboplastin time [PTT], platelets). The blood group is not routinely determined because hemorrhage requiring a transfusion is extremely rare. If the patient should require a transfusion because of heavy bleeding, the blood group can be quickly determined in a hospital setting.

In patients with septal perforations and granulomatous inflammations, *interleukin 6* is a more sensitive marker than *c-reactive protein* in assessing the acuteness of the inflammation.

If an autoimmune disease such as Wegener granulomatosis is suspected, the lungs should be investigated by plain radiography and computed tomography (CT). Laboratory tests are done to check for signs of progressive renal failure (*cystatin C, creatinine*). When Wegener granulomatosis is present, tests will reveal anticytoplasmic antibodies directed against plasma granules of neutrophilic polymorphonuclear leukocytes and monocytes (*ACPA/ANCA*) (9, 11).

Patients with elevated transaminases should undergo more precise coagulation testing (*platelet function test*) prior to surgery. Members of high-risk groups such as homosexuals, drug users, and prostitutes should be tested for HIV.

Preoperative Analysis

Saddle nose can result from a variety of causes. Three pathogenic mechanisms have been identified for the most common types of saddle nose:

Type I Pathogenic Mechanism of Saddle Nose

Loss of nasal dorsum support from the anterior septum leads to a loss of cartilaginous dorsal height. There may be lateralization, spreading, or separation of the upper lateral cartilages, depending on the depth of the saddling. With depression of the dorsal septal margin, an important tip support mechanism is compromised. This leads to depression of the supratip area and anterior septal angle. As this occurs, the rhomboid of the nasal tip loses its *supratip point*, and the tip becomes amorphous. Because tip support is deficient, the tip rotates upward. If residual cartilage is preserved in the caudal septum near the caudal margin, this remnant can still provide adequate tip support. The loss of projection in the nasal tip results from cranial rotation due to deficient support of the supratip area.

This cranial rotation leads to a loss of tip projection. The nasolabial angle is broadened (> 110°). The loss of structural support from the septal cartilage causes the caudal portions of the lateral cartilages to sag, with broadening and deformation

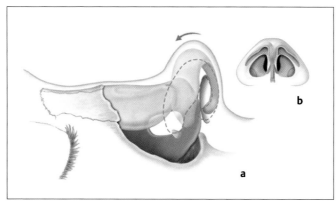

Fig. 12.**3**   (**a**) Cartilaginous saddle nose has resulted from cartilage loss in the area indicated, with preservation of the caudal septal margin. Note the depression of the cartilaginous nasal dorsum and the cranial tip rotation with loss of projection. (**b**) Typical changes in the nasal base with broadening of the nasal valve and compensatory hyperplasia of the inferior turbinates.

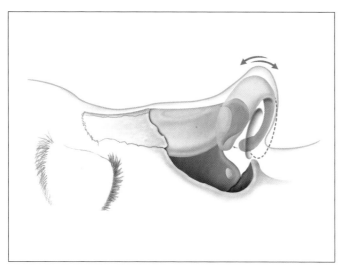

Fig. 12.**4**   Cartilaginous saddle nose with destruction of the caudal septal margin. The lower columella is retracted upward ("hidden columella"), and the alar–columellar complex is deformed.

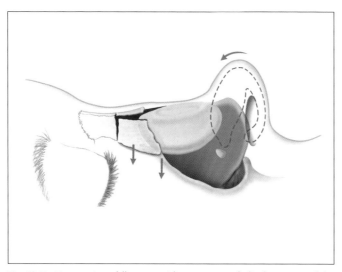

Fig. 12.**5**   Traumatic saddle nose with an open roof, displacement of the nasal bone fragments, and disruption of the osseocartilaginous junction ("inverted V") at the rhinion or keystone area.

of the nasal valve angle (ballooning phenomenon). There is compensatory hyperplasia of the inferior turbinates.

Viewed from the front, the central nasal dorsum appears broad and blends smoothly with a poorly defined tip (Fig. 12.**3**).

Type II Pathogenic Mechanism of Saddle Nose

This type is based on extensive cartilage defects in the septum or an absence of cartilage at the caudal septal margin. Absence of the anterior cartilaginous septum leads to a lack of support of the dorsal septal margin. There is no membranous septum to stabilize the medial crura of the alar cartilages, and the caudal septal margin is unable to secure the footplates of the medial crura. The columella is retracted upward (*hidden columella*). The tip loses projection due to the complete loss of tip support. The tip may rotate upward or downward, depending on whether the forces exerted by scar formation and tissue contraction act chiefly on the nasal dorsum and supratip area or the caudal septal margin. Because the depression of the cartilaginous dorsum and dorsal septal margin and the basal movement of the upper lateral cartilages create a greater loss of static support, the tip usually rotates upward, compounding the loss of projection.

The broadened central portion of the nose in this situation is accompanied by a broadened tip. Because of the lax membranous attachment between the upper lateral and alar cartilages, the anterior margins of the upper lateral cartilages slip downward while the alar cartilages are displaced laterally. The columella is shortened (Fig. 12.**4**).

Type III Pathogenic Mechanism of Saddle Nose

Displaced fractures of the nasal bones or maxillary frontal process combined with trauma to the cartilaginous nose can disrupt the attachments of the upper lateral cartilages to the nasal bones in the *keystone area*.

"Keystone" is an architectural term for the central stone that is wedged in place at the apex of an archway. If the keystone were removed, the archway would collapse.

Describing the osseocartilaginous attachment at the level of the rhinion as the keystone area underscores the essential load-bearing importance of this area. A traumatic avulsion of the cartilaginous nose from the nasal bones leads to an inverted V-shaped depression that is difficult to correct. In contrast to the type I and II mechanisms, the cranial portion of the upper lateral cartilage or the entire lateral cartilage is shifted downward.

Associated changes in the cartilaginous dorsum and nasal tip result from the mechanisms described above.

The bony nasal pyramid is depressed, and the dorsum already appears broadened at the bony level (Fig. 12.**5**).

Surgical Strategy

The surgical treatment of saddle nose is reconstructive in nature. While the patient with an overprojected nose, for example, wants to have something altered, most patients with saddle nose are interested in having their former appearance restored. Often the patient will bring in old photographs to give the surgeon an idea of the desired result.

The most important surgical goal in saddle nose is to reconstruct a stable septum. All other reconstructive measures are adjuncts. The main consideration, then, is how to carry out the reconstruction. The surgeon can determine the approximate extent of the cartilage defect by carefully probing the septum with a soft cotton applicator, guided by a 0° wide-angle endoscope. Besides identifying the missing cartilage areas, the surgeon can also gain information on the size and resilience of the remaining cartilage. Important points to note are the size of the cartilage defects and the cartilage remnants that are still present.

Only small defects can be reconstructed by the local transfer of residual cartilage.

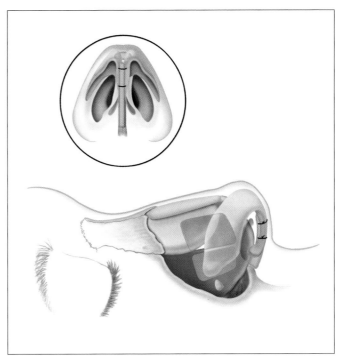

Fig. 12.**6**   Reconstruction of saddle nose.

Reconstruction for Minor Saddling of the Cartilaginous Dorsum with a Circumscribed Defect in the Cartilaginous Septum and Normal Tip Support

The options in this situation are reconstruction with posterior septal cartilage or with cartilage harvested from the conchal cavity.

Reconstruction of the anterior septum with material from the posterior septum is possible if there is residual cartilage of sufficient quantity and quality. The septal cartilage is fully exposed by making a hemitransfixion incision and developing two superior and inferior tunnels.

Using this technique, the "fontanelles" formed by duplications of the mucosa at cartilage defects can be visualized without tension and sharply divided with a No. 15 blade. The remaining posterior cartilage is divided basally and dorsally with a pair of Heymann nasal scissors and elevated with a Freer elevator at its junction with the perpendicular plate. It can be mobilized then and removed en bloc. Once removed, the piece of cartilage can be placed on a small carving bench for measuring and modification.

Mild deviations can be corrected by carefully morselizing the cartilage or scoring it on the concave side. While the anterior cartilage piece should not be morselized, the posterior cartilage can be enlarged by careful compression with a Rubin morselizer.

After external preparation of the cartilage pieces is completed, a mucoperiosteal flap is medialized by the insertion of a Doyle splint. Using fibrin glue, the surgeon replaces the cartilage pieces like mosaic tiles and glues them to the medialized mucosa. A defect located at a very caudal level can be repaired with a large piece of cartilage fitted into a columellar pocket. The columellar pocket is developed by passing a pair of curved Cottle scissors from above in a downward direction between the medial crura of the alar cartilages and carefully spreading open the connective tissue in the vertical plane (Figs. 12.**6**, 12.**7a–f**).

The cartilage piece is secured inferiorly with a 4–0 polydioxanone suture (PDS) on a straight needle. Since the tissue will undergo scarring and shrinkage, the cartilaginous dorsum should be augmented with a dorsal onlay graft, even with mild degrees of saddling. A hemitransfixion incision extending to the anterior septal angle can provide atraumatic access for graft placement. A supraperichondrial recipient bed can be created on the depressed nasal dorsum with a pair of fine Joseph scissors, keeping strictly below the vascular plane of the superficial musculoaponeurotic system (SMAS).

The connective tissue should be carefully dissected using either a blunt spreading technique or sharp division when scars are present. The recipient bed should be scarcely larger than the actual graft size. While a tight pocket cannot prevent scar contractures, it will allow the dorsal graft to heal in an optimum position. Fibrin glue (Beriplast) can be used for graft fixation. Larger onlay grafts should be introduced through a bilateral intercartilaginous incision with a superior hemitransfixion.

Reconstruction for Deep Saddling of the Cartilaginous Dorsum with Extensive Cartilage Losses or Septal Perforations and Adequate Tip Support

Conchal cartilage makes a suitable graft material for reconstructing the cartilaginous nasal septum. This material is less stable than septal cartilage, however, and should be morselized very carefully.

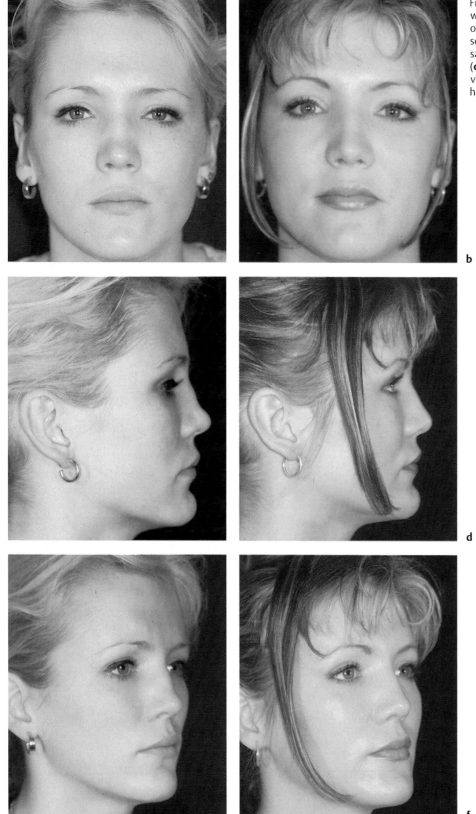

Fig. 12.**7** Saddle nose in a woman who underwent septoplasty several years earlier. (**a**) Preoperative appearance. (**b**) Three years after septal reconstruction with placement of a dorsal onlay graft of autologous conchal cartilage. (**c, d**) Preoperative and postoperative lateral views. (**e, f**) Preoperative and postoperative half profile.

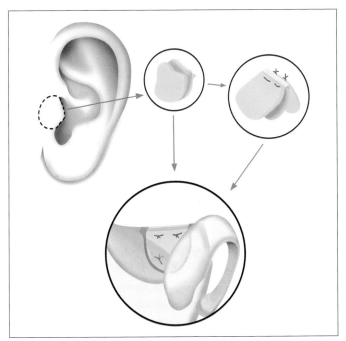

Fig. 12.**8** Reconstruction of a circumscribed depression in the supratip area with a butterfly graft from the tragus.

Harvesting the Donor Cartilage

Three ultrathin needles are placed below the margin of the conchal cavity, and the posterior sites of emergence are marked with methylene blue. A retroauricular skin incision is made, and a skin flap is raised. The cartilage is divided, and the conchal cartilage is carefully dissected from the anterior conchal skin. The skin on the anterior side of the conchal cavity is more adherent to the cartilage than on the posterior surface of the auricle. The conchal cartilage graft is circumscribed and removed.

The open approach can be used to reconstruct the nasal dorsum in patients with deep saddling. If the nasal dorsum appears broad or if an open roof is present, two paramedian and laterally curved osteotomies are performed with miniosteo-

tomes. The upper lateral cartilages are detached from the superior margin of the septum. The apposed mucosal layers are sharply separated, dissecting onto the nasal floor at the level of the anterior nasal spine, premaxilla, and vomer. Cartilage islands that are encountered are removed and set aside. Then the harvested, straightened conchal cartilage is placed on the nasal floor and attached to the connective tissue of the nasal spine anteriorly with a PDS suture.

The two upper lateral cartilages are pulled upward with two-prong hooks and fixed with two fine needles. After checking the position of the upper lateral cartilages on the supporting neoseptum, the surgeon secures them with two prolene sutures. The conchal cartilage above the upper lateral cartilages is cut off with a pair of Fomon nasal scissors (Figs. 12.**8**, 12.**9 a, b**).

Circumscribed saddling of the supratip area can be corrected with a *butterfly graft*. The graft is composed of conchal cartilage with both perichondrial layers dissected off the graft but attached at one edge. The cartilage is placed in the supratip area with the perichondrial "wings" spread symmetrically over the upper lateral cartilages and secured with PDS sutures or fibrin glue. The graft is supported by the lateral cartilages, which anchor it to stabilize the supratip area (Figs. 12.**10**, 12.**11 a–g**).

Reconstruction of the Nasal Dorsum with Severe Loss of Tip Support

Cartilage harvested from the sixth or seventh rib is suitable for the reconstruction of saddle nose with severe loss of tip support. Good results have been achieved with autografts and allografts. Only central cartilage should be used ("balanced grafts") to prevent subsequent warping and displacement of the implants (12).

Two pieces are cut from the central portion of the cartilage, and the dorsal onlay graft and columellar strut are carved from these pieces. The dorsal graft is fashioned so that it extends from the tip area to the cranial part of the bony nasal pyramid. The sides are beveled to eliminate visible or palpable ridges. The columellar graft is placed against the nasal spine or,

Fig. 12.**9** Frontal views (**a**) before and (**b**) four years after circumscribed saddle correction with a butterfly graft.

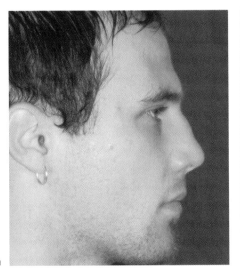
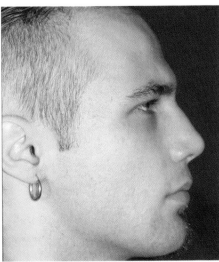

a   b

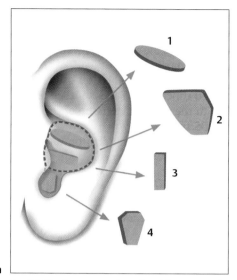

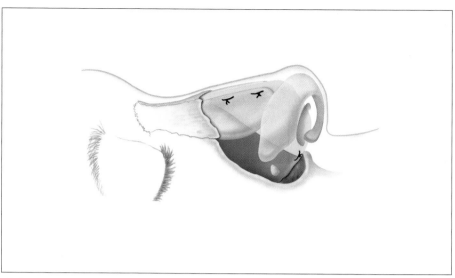

Fig. 12.**10**   Reconstruction of saddle nose with conchal cartilage.
1 – onlay graft, **2** septal graft, **3** columellar strut, **4** shield or tip grafts

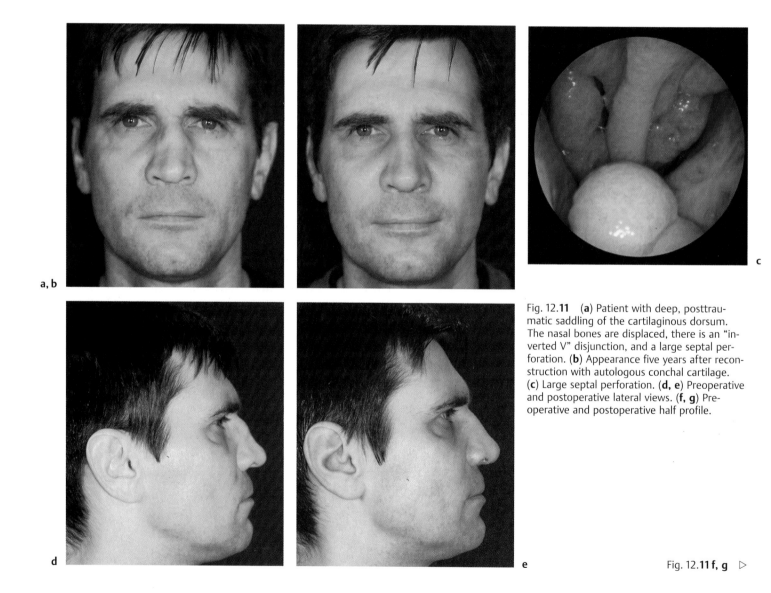

Fig. 12.**11**   (**a**) Patient with deep, posttraumatic saddling of the cartilaginous dorsum. The nasal bones are displaced, there is an "inverted V" disjunction, and a large septal perforation. (**b**) Appearance five years after reconstruction with autologous conchal cartilage. (**c**) Large septal perforation. (**d, e**) Preoperative and postoperative lateral views. (**f, g**) Preoperative and postoperative half profile.

Fig. 12.**11 f, g**   ▷

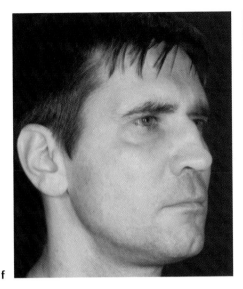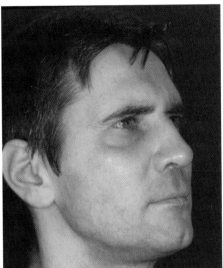

Fig. 12.**11 f, g**

f   g

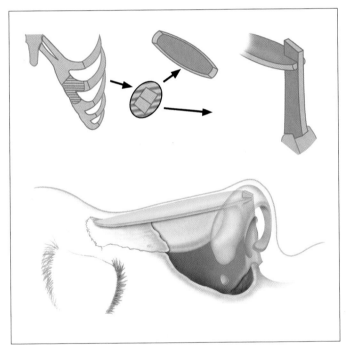

Fig. 12.**12**   Reconstruction of saddle nose with costal cartilage.

if nasal lengthening is desired, farther anteriorly on the upper alveolar crest.

The grafts are connected with tongue-and-groove joints. This provides a firm connection that is also flexible enough to yield to scar traction and provide some residual mobility of the tip (Figs. 12.**12**, 12.**13 a–d**).

Guidelines for Tissue Replacement in the Nose

The basic types of material available for cartilage replacement in saddle nose reconstruction are autografts, allografts, and synthetic implants.

Graft Requirements

Graft and implant materials must satisfy various requirements. They should have good biocompatibility or be biologically inert. They must cause no local or systemic toxicity. The graft should undergo minimal absorption in the body and should not alter its shape or position in the recipient bed. The material should be quickly and safely accessible, available in the necessary quantities, and economical. It is advantageous if the material is easy to shape and use, with mechanical properties (resilience, load-bearing ability) that closely approximate those of the original tissue (5).

With cartilage implants, "balanced cross–section" costal grafts should be used to allow for the special deformation properties of the cartilage (12). The tension in septal, conchal, or tragal cartilage grafts can be altered by cross-hatching, morselizing, or scoring on the concave side.

Allografts and synthetic implants must be autoclavable. The current consensus is that allografts should no longer be used in the facial region.

Synthetic Implants

New implant materials have constantly been developed and utilized for tissue replacement in reconstructive surgery. The history of nasal implants began in 1828 with gold and silver (Rousset). Paraffin was used in 1904 (Eckstein), ivory in 1925 (Maliniac), cork in 1931, marble in 1939 (Zeno), and acrylate in 1948 (Wolf) (20).

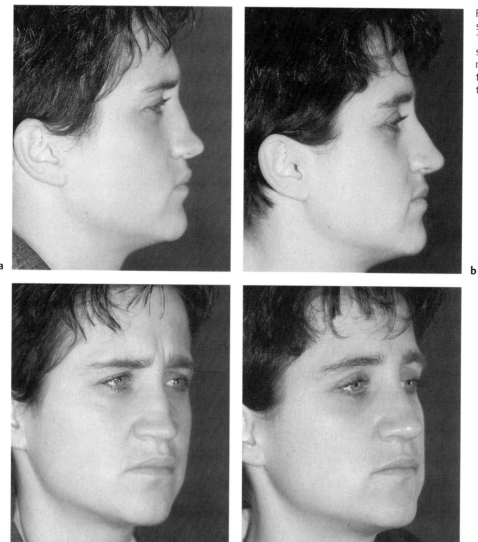

Fig. 12.**13**   (**a**) Woman with cartilaginous saddle nose following severe nasal trauma. There is a complete loss of tip projection and support. (**b**) Appearance three years after nasal reconstruction with autologous costal cartilage. (**c, d**) Preoperative and postoperative three-quarter profile.

Synthetic implants must meet rigorous criteria (26). These include chemical and thermal stability that permit autoclaving, dimensional stability, minimal foreign body reactions, and the absence of cytotoxic, antigenic, and carcinogenic properties. Polyvinylchloride (PVC), polyamide (Nylon), polyvinyl alcohol (Ivalon), and polyurethane (Perlon) are among the materials that do not meet these criteria due to inadequate chemical stability. These materials should no longer be used as implants.

Cement materials (biocement, ionomer cements such as aluminum oxide ceramic, and hydroxyapatite cement) are too brittle for use in flexible areas that are exposed to functional stresses, such as the cartilaginous nose. Cements have proved effective for bone replacement. Use in soft tissues and cartilage is contraindicated, however, due to poor adhesion and undesired motility of the cement implant (5, 21) (Fig. 12.**14a–d**).

Materials that do meet these requirements include polytetrafluoroethylene (PTFE, Teflon), expanded polytetrafluoroethylene (ePTFE, Gore-Tex), polyethylene terephthalate (Dacron), polyethylene, and silicone (27)

The reactions of these synthetics in tissues show basic differences that make particular materials suitable or unsuitable for implantation in certain regions in the body. Some im-

plants, such as silicone, are biologically *inert*, meaning that their surface does not stimulate the ingrowth of connective tissue. Other materials, such as macroporous Gore-Tex, are *incorporable*, meaning that they are receptive to tissue ingrowth.

Silicone becomes encapsulated by a fibrin layer without bonding to the adjacent tissue. Microtrauma, especially in the mobile cartilaginous nose, causes motion to occur at the interface between the implant and its surroundings, leading to microhemorrhage, edema, and inflammatory reactions around the implant. As a result of this, silicone implants are susceptible to infection in the nose and should not be used in cartilaginous reconstructions (Fig. 12.**15a, b**).

Studies have shown that thin-walled implants composed of the biocompatible materials PTFE (Teflon) and ePTFE (Gore-Tex) become permeated by connective tissue (16, 17). This ingrowth is dependent on the porosity of the plastic material. Macroporous structures with a pore size of 100–150 μ are the most favorable.

The incorporation of biocompatible plastics occurs in three stages:

1. Exudation: The surface pores become filled with microclots after implantation. The prosthesis is covered by a fibrin film.

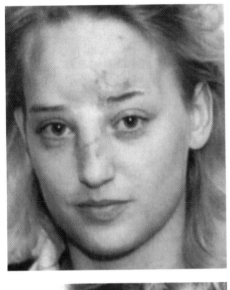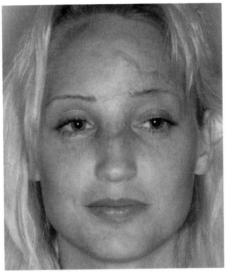

a   b

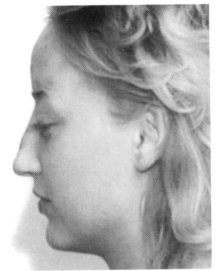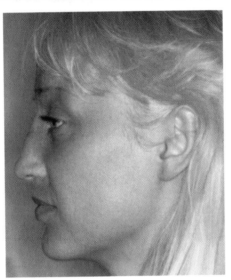

c   d

Fig. 12.**14** (**a**) Posttraumatic broad nose accompanied by absence of the outer table over both frontal sinuses. (**b**) Appearance 10 years after reconstruction of the frontal defect with bioceramic and septorhinoplasty with closure of the open roof deformity. (**c, d**) Preoperative and postoperative lateral views.

2. Absorption: Histiocytes, fibroblasts, and capillaries proliferate and form granulation tissue. This tissue covers the outer surface of the implant and grows from there into the pores.
3. Organization: The granulation tissue is replaced by connective tissue from the surface into the pores. The initially disorganized connective tissue is replaced by collagen fibers (Fig. 12.**16**).

New synthetic materials for tissue replacement in the nose are usually greeted with initial enthusiasm. Later there are reports of expulsions and complications, dampening the early expectations. In retrospect, no synthetic material has been able to fulfill all expectations, and so the rhinosurgeon should always regard new materials with a certain skepticism. This is the only way to safeguard patients from implants that will not yield positive intermediate- and long-term results.

It is certain that new synthetic implant materials will continue to be developed. Organ replacement with a biocompatible material that can be carved to any shape and is available in unlimited quantities is a fascinating concept.

It may be, however, that advances in tissue engineering for nasal cartilage replacement will slow this trend. There

have already been several case reports on the successful reconstruction of the nasal septum following a childhood abscess (8). Tissue engineering for cartilage generation is based on the use of biodegradable polymers as a temporary scaffold for differentiated chondrocytes or precursor cells (7). The cells are harvested, propagated in culture, seeded onto the scaffold in vitro, and then transplanted. While in the body, the differentiated cells should produce their tissue-specific matrix constituents, generating a tissue that has virtually the same morphological and functional properties as the original cartilage.

A compromise to avoid implantation hazards is to implant an incorporable material (e-tetrafluoroethylene) at an inflexible site, such as the retroauricular area, and then use the incorporated implant to augment the nasal dorsum approximately six weeks later (1).

In our experience there is always sufficient endogenous tissue available for reconstructing the nose, and consequently there is little reason to implant synthetic materials in the nose.

Autologous tissue should be used whenever possible. Autologous cartilage continues to be the gold standard for plastic reconstructive surgery of the nose (23). The most popular graft types are listed below.

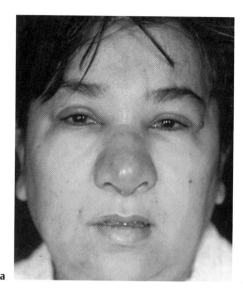

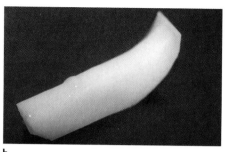

b

Fig. 12.**15**   (**a**) This patient presented with infection six years after the insertion of a silicone implant (in Thailand). (**b**) Silicone implant after removal.

Fig. 12.**16**   Section through the wall of an ▷ ePTFE prosthesis, completely permeated by connective tissue, showing distinct capillary structures (from 16).

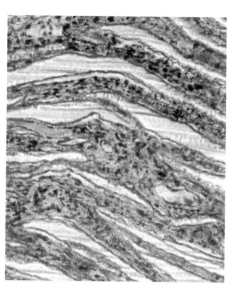

a

Autologous Grafts

Septal Cartilage (Autologous, Isotopic Graft of First Choice)

Cartilage from the posterior septum should always be used when it is available in sufficient quantity. It should be harvested behind a line between the rhinion and anterior nasal spine, leaving intact the cartilage that is essential for dorsal support.

Septal cartilage has good stability and resilience. Tension can be removed by cross-hatching, incising, or gentle morselizing with an atraumatic Adson forceps or Rubin morselizer. Septal cartilage is easier to morselize than conchal cartilage, for example. It is more stable to pressure and will alter its bending properties under gentle pressure without fraying. Generally, however, the properties of the cartilage should be altered as little as possible.

Other advantages of septal cartilage are that its properties are identical to those of the tissue being replaced, and it can be quickly and safely harvested through one approach.

Alar Cartilage

Pieces of alar cartilage, usually from the upper lateral crura, can be used for augmentation of the nasal dorsum or tip. Because of their thinness, they are principally used as onlay grafts for superficial contour modification rather than as supporting grafts for the nasal dorsum.

Conchal Cartilage (Autologous, Heterotopic Graft of Second Choice)

Considerable amounts of conchal cartilage can be harvested from the conchal cavity and tragus.

Conchal Cavity

Conchal cartilage is excellent for cartilage replacement in the nose and is the material the author uses most frequently for that purpose. This is because septal cartilage is rarely available

in sufficient amounts for the reconstruction of saddle nose deformity. Conchal cartilage is dimensionally stable, resilient, and provides good mechanical support for use in the nose. It can be harvested quickly and safely and is easy to carve (15, 29).

Another advantage is that conchal cartilage has a variety of intrinsic convexities and concavities that are useful for reconstructing specific areas in the nose (see Fig. 12.**10**).

Conchal cartilage is suitable for the replacement of septal cartilage, upper lateral cartilage, and alar cartilage. It can be used in the form of a shield graft, tip graft, or columellar strut.

The cartilage is exposed through a retroauricular approach. The skin on the posterior side of the auricle is loosely attached to the perichondrium by abundant connective tissue. The skin on the anterior side is tight and immobile. Often it is best to leave connective tissue on the cartilage when the graft is harvested, as this will help in the correction of larger defects.

As a general rule, conchal cartilage should be harvested and used without perichondrium. In children, however, a perichondrial layer can be left on the graft to exploit the chondroplastic potential of the cartilage (29).

Conchal cartilage is usually easy to carve with a scalpel. It is extremely difficult to morselize, however, as it will fray when the least pressure is applied. The cartilage heals without difficulty and undergoes very little resorption (15). During use, the surgeon should take advantage of the intrinsic shapes and curvatures of the cartilage.

Tragus

Tragal cartilage is harvested through an approximately 12-mm incision made with a No. 15 blade just behind the anterior border and directed toward the external meatus. The cartilage can be used along with two small perichondrial flaps, which are quickly dissected, and has the same uses as cartilage from the conchal bowl. The perichondrium is thin but very tough. It can be used to camouflage an inverted V in the nasal dorsum, as in cases where the keystone area has been injured during the reconstruction of a traumatic saddle nose. The perichondrium undergoes less postoperative swelling than fascia.

The perichondrial layers can be mobilized on both sides and left on one end of the cartilage, where it can be fixed with

PDS sutures. The tragus can be used in this way as a butterfly graft to reconstruct circumscribed cartilage defects in the supratip area.

Costal Cartilage

The use of costal cartilage is indicated in saddle nose reconstruction when there has been extensive loss of nasal supporting structures with a lack of tip support. Septal or conchal cartilage may lack sufficient strength in this type of situation.

The cartilage is harvested from the sixth or seventh rib through a 4- to 5-mm skin incision placed over the right rib or in the inframammary crease in women. The perichondrium is incised, and the costal cartilage is harvested within the perichondrium. The surgeon should be alert to possible pneumothorax by wetting the pleura with a few drops of sterile water and consulting with the anesthesiologist. The rib cartilage should be balanced, i.e., only the central portions of the cartilage should be used for grafting.

The disadvantage of the long, stiff rib graft is its unnatural consistency in the nasal dorsum. The nose becomes rigid, and even a perfectly healed graft may cause a foreign body sensation.

Fascia

In principle, adequate amounts of autologous temporal fascia or fascia lata can be quickly harvested through an incision placed in the scalp or the lateral thigh.

Temporal Fascia

Temporal fascia is available in sufficient quantities. An incision made in the scalp above the auricle provides the best access. The fascia should be sharply divided inferiorly, elevated and separated from its muscle fibers with a Joseph elevator, and then harvested with a pair of small, preferably ball-tipped scissors. The less damage caused to muscle fibers, the more bloodless and atraumatic the graft removal.

The consistency of the fascia varies greatly in different individuals, depending on the connective-tissue type.

Fascia lata

Fascia lata is the toughest fascia in the body. It consists of an approximately 5-cm-wide strip extending between the greater trochanter and lateral epicondyle of the femur. The course of the fascia lata must be considered in the harvesting of graft material. After the fascia is removed, the defect should always be repaired to prevent the herniation of muscle tissue.

Bone

Bone has probably been the most widely used material for augmentation of the nasal dorsum in saddle nose over the past 100 years (20). The harvesting of iliac bone is a painful procedure. Iliac bone transplanted to the bony nose requires a stable, well-vascularized bed; otherwise it will be resorbed (18).

The bone (especially its cancellous portion) does undergo resorption in the mobile cartilaginous nose.

Allografts
Cartilage

Cartilage tissue from the septum, concha, or rib can be stored by various methods (Merthiolate, Cialit, alcohol, freeze-drying, dehydration, gamma irradiation). In principle, allograft cartilage, or "banked cartilage," is comparable to autologous cartilage in its mechanical strength, its low degree of resorption, its susceptibility to infection, and its deformation properties (14).

Merthiolate-preserved cartilage behaves like devitalized tissue. It is partially resorbed at the edges and is also replaced and ensheathed by connective tissue (10).

Fascia and Dura

Fascia lata and dura mater are used in the form of lyophilized or dehydrated banked material. The tissue must be rehydrated before use. After implantation, the tissue is broken down by resorption and replaced by connective tissue. This transformation depends on the size of the graft and the properties of the recipient bed (scarring, mechanical stresses, blood supply).

AlloDerm

AlloDerm is banked human skin that has been freed of epidermis and cellular constituents. The remaining protein matrix is freeze-dried (12, 19, 30).

The applications of this material in septoplasty include augmentation of the nasal dorsum and the camouflage of an inverted V.

Fibrin Glue

Fibrin glue is a physiological two-component adhesive (Beriplast). In principle, it mimics the final stage of blood coagulation. Fibrinogen is polymerized by thrombin to produce fibrin. The latter is cross-linked by factor XIII to form a stable fibrin clot. The glue contains a small amount of aprotinin (fibrinogen solution) to protect the fibrin clot from premature degradation in vivo.

The glue is excellent for attaching onlay grafts, fascia, perichondrium, and similar materials used for camouflage.

Principles of Implantology in the Nose

The successful transplantation of autograft or allograft cartilage is influenced by the following factors: The type of cartilage, its storage and preservation, the volume and surface area of the graft, the methods used to harvest and prepare the graft, the biological characteristics of the recipient bed (rigid or flexible part of the nose, deep or superficial), the condition of the operative field, the connective-tissue type, the surgical technique, and the postoperative mechanical stresses to which the graft is exposed (14).

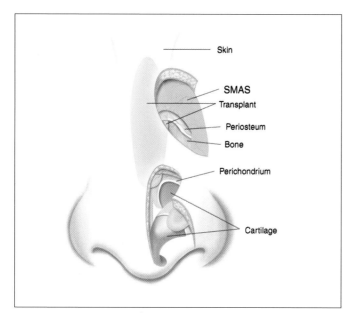

Fig. 12.**17**   Deep and superficial grafts in the nose.

The principal dangers of cartilage implantation in the nose are graft resorption, deformation (warping), and infection.

The graft material of first choice is always viable autologous cartilage. If it is not available, allograft tissue should be used. We have experienced no problems with infection, intolerance, or inflammation associated with the use of autologous cartilage grafts.

Harvesting Graft Material

Atraumatic harvesting of the graft material is essential for the successful transplantation of autologous cartilage. Septal cartilage should be dissected in the subperichondrial plane, conchal cartilage in the supraperichondrial plane. The tissue should not be injured or crushed during removal. Perichondrium does not protect the graft from resorption and should be dissected off the cartilage (14) unless it is intended to have a chondroplastic function in children, in which case it should remain on the graft (29).

Following hemostasis with fine bipolar forceps, the donor site must be absolutely dry. This is necessary to prevent hematoma formation, which can become a major problem in postoperative care.

The conchal cavity should be packed with pledgets after graft harvest to promote adhesion of the skin layers.

The harvested material is prepared for use on a small carving bench that has a millimeter scale. After the size of the recipient defect has been measured with a rhinoplasty template, the necessary size and shape of the graft are precisely marked using a color marker. Then the cartilage is carved with a No. 15 blade while it is held with a blunt Adson forceps. Either that instrument or a Rubin cartilage crusher can be used to morselize the cartilage. Tension can be removed from the graft by cross-hatching, scoring, or incisions on the concave side to avoid graft deformation in the recipient bed.

Preparing the Recipient Bed

The quality of the recipient bed is critical for the fate of the graft and thus for the long-term success of the operation.

The size of the recipient bed should closely match the graft size to prevent subsequent displacement. When cartilage is implanted to broaden and stabilize the nasal valve or to reinforce collapsing alar cartilage, it may even be wise to make the recipient pouch slightly too small to maintain a certain basic tension in the graft. We have found that a rhinoplasty template or other measuring device is an indispensable aid for matching the sizes of the graft and recipient bed.

Deep implants in the nasal dorsum have a supporting function and provide for the structural replacement of cartilage or bone substance. They should be placed between the perichondrium and the vascular SMAS layer, from which they will derive their vascular supply. Injuries to the SMAS lead to hemorrhage. Hematomas can result in graft infection as well as heavy scarring that can jeopardize graft healing. Superficial grafts are used for contouring the external nose, which requires a direct subcutaneous graft placement. The surgeon must decide case by case whether to attach the grafts with sutures or fibrin glue. We use absorbable suture material almost exclusively for graft fixation—usually polydioxanone and less commonly polypropylene (Prolene).

When revision surgery is performed, care should be taken to dissect the tissues in a way that will not subject the implant to scar traction. (Fig. 12.**17**).

Postoperative Care

In patients who have undergone reconstructive nasal surgery with grafts, it is essential to rest the operative area for several days after the surgery. This is aided by starting the patient on a liquid diet, progressing later to semisolid foods. Ice goggles can be worn in the postoperative period to reduce soft-tissue swelling.

The nasal septum is stabilized with a flexible silicone stent (Doyle) for five to seven days. The nasal dorsum is immobilized with a plaster cast, thermoplastic splint, or metal splint. The length and size of the nasal dressing are varied according to its desired effect.

Draining secretions and clots are aspirated from the nose with semiflexible plastic suction probes with fingertip control (Micro-Flex probes, Pennine, UK).

The nasal mucosa is kept moist by spraying it with an isotonic saline solution. Since the mucosa tends to dry out after intranasal surgery, this replacement is important for the postoperative functional regeneration of the mucociliary apparatus. Options include nasal oils (GeloSitin), isotonic saline sprays (Emser Sole Spray, Rhinomer), or the inhalation of isotonic saline solution. Ultrasonic waves can generate a fine, relatively homogeneous mist that can deliver droplets smaller than 5 µm to the nasal and paranasal sinus mucosae (3).

If splints or packs are left in the nose for more than three days, an antibiotic (cephalosporin) should be administered for six days. Treatment with an herbal mucolytic agent (e.g., Gelomyrtol forte) for two to three weeks has also proved beneficial.

This product has deodorizing, bacteriostatic, mucolytic, and secretomotor properties.

Complications

The main complications associated with the use of grafts for saddle nose reconstruction are infection, expulsion, displacement, and resorption.

The best way to prevent infection is to avoid using allografts in the nose. Other critical factors are the use of autologous tissue and an atraumatic technique for harvesting the graft and preparing the recipient bed. Infected synthetic implants will eventually have to be removed. In Asia, silicone implants are still widely used in reshaping the broad, flat Asian nose.

Minimally displaced autologous grafts in the nasal dorsum or the slight warping of a graft can be managed with minor corrections of the nasal dorsum. For greater degrees of graft displacement, a revision procedure should be scheduled at eight to nine months.

Bleeding may occur from the richly vascularized nasal mucosa during the immediate postoperative period. The source of the bleeding should be identified endoscopically so that it can be selectively coagulated. If intranasal packs are needed to control the bleeding, they should be placed by the surgeon under endoscopic guidance.

A postoperative septal hematoma should be drained by opening a suture (e.g., in the hemitransfixion incision) without delay. A loose pack will support the fixation of the mucosa to the septal cartilage.

Postoperative infections are rare. Initially they can be treated with empirical antibiotics, followed later by specific antibiotic therapy. To date, we have not had to remove a cartilage graft because of postoperative infection.

References

1. Adamson P. Controversies in septorhinoplasty—one problem—one goal—one solution. Course in functional aesthetic septorhinoplasty, Ulm, June 2002.
2. Aiach G. *Atlas of rhinoplasty. Open and endonasal approaches.* St. Louis: Quality Medical Publishing, Inc: 1996.
3. Behrbohm H, Kaschke O, Nawka T. *Endoskopische Diagnostik und Therapie in der HNO.* Stuttgart: G. Fischer: 1997.
4. Behrbohm H, Hildebrandt T, Kaschke O. *Funktionell-ästhetische Chirurgie der Nase.* Tuttlingen: Endo-press: 2000.
5. Brunner FX. Implantatmaterialien – was hat sich wo und wann bewährt? *Eur. Arch. Oto.Rhin.Laryng.* 1993; Suppl I:XX.
6. Buttgereit F, Kaschke O, Krause A, Burmeister G-R. Protrahiert ver-laufende Polychondritis als Ursache für progrediente Nasendeformität, subglottische Trachealstenose und Innenohrschwerhörigkeit. *Laryngo-Rhino-Otol.* 1997; 76:46–49.
7. Bücheler M. Tissue Engineering in der Hals-Nasen-Ohrenheilkunde, Kopf- und Halschirurgie. *Laryngo-Rhino-Otol.* 2002; 81 (suppl. 1):61–80.
8. Fussenegger M, Wieser S, Meinhart J, Muhr T, Eckmayr A. Nasenseptum-rekonstruktion nach Abszess im Kindesalter. *Otorhinolaryngol Nova 2001*; 11:257.
9. Ganzer U, Donath K, Schmelzle R. Geschwülste der inneren Nase, der Nasennebenhöhlen, des Ober- und Unterkiefers. In Naumann HH, ed. *Oto-Rhino-Laryngologie in Klinik und Praxis.Teil 2.* Stuttgart: Thieme: 1992.
10. Gammert C, Masing H. Langzeiterfahrungen mit konserviertem Knorpel in der Wiederherstellungschirurgie der Nase. *Laryng.Rhinol.* 1977; 56:650–656.
11. Gesierich P. Personal Communication
12. Gibson T, Dawis W. The distorsion of autogenous cartilage grafts; Its cause and prevention. *Brit. J. plast. Surg.* 1958; 10:257.
13. Gryskiewicz JM, Rohrich RJ, Reagan BJ. The use of alloderm for the correction of nasal contour deformities. *Plast. Reconstr. Surg.* 2000; 106:561–570.
14. Hellmich S. Fehler und Gefahren bei der freien Knorpeltransplantation im Gesichtsbereich. *HNO.* 1982; 30:140–144.
15. Jovanovic S, Berghaus A. Autogenous auricular concha cartilage transplants in corrective rhinoplasty. Practical hints and critical remarks. *Rhinology.* 1991; 29:273–280.
16. Kaschke O. Untersuchungen zur Entwicklung eines epithelisierten, alloplastischen Tracheaersatzes. Dissertation. Humboldt University. Berlin. 1993
17. Kaschke O, Gerhardt H-J, Böhm K, Wenzel M, Planck H. Die Epithelisierung poröser Biomaterialien mit isolierten respiratorischen Epithelzellen in vivo. *HNO.* 1995; 43:80–88.
18. Kastenbauer ER. Fehler und Gefahren bei der Knochentransplantation *HNO.* 1982; 30:145–147.
19. Livesey SA, Herndon DN, Hollyoak MA. Transplanted acellular allograft dermal matrix: Potential as a template for the reconstruction of viable dermis. *Transplantation.* 1995; 60:1.
20. Mackay IS. Augmentation rhinoplasty In Nolst Trenité G, Kugler, *Rhinoplasty.* The Hague: Kugler Publications: 1993.
21. Meyer R. *Secondary rhinoplasty. Including reconstruction of the nose.* 2nd edition. Berlin: Springer: 2001
22. Nolst Trenité GJ. *Rhinoplasty. A practical guide to functional and aesthetic surgery of the nose.* The Hague: Kugler Publications: 1993.
23. Park SS. Reconstruction of nasal defects larger than 1.5 centimeters in diameter. *Laryngoscope.* 2000; 110:1241–1250.
24. Pirsig W, Penz S, Lenders H. Repair of saddle nose deformity in Wegener's granulomatosis and ectodermal dysplasia. *Rhinology.* 1993; 31:69–72.
25. Rettinger G. Rekonstruktion ausgeprägter Sattelnasen. *Laryngo-Rhino-Otol.* 1997; 76:672–675.
26. Scales JT. Discussion on metals and synthetic materials in relation to soft tissue; tissue reaction to synthetic materials. *Proc R Soc Med.* 1953; 46:647.
27. Schultz-Coulon H-J. Fehler und Gefahren bei der Implantation von Kunststoffen im Gesichtsbereich. *HNO.* 1982; 30:148–155.
28. Steurer O. *Körner-Steurer: Lehrbuch der Ohren-, Nasen-, Rachen-und Kehlkopf-Krankheiten.* München: Verlag v. JF Bergmann: 1944.
29. Tardy ME. *Rhinoplasty: The art and the science. Vol. II.* Philadelphia: W.B. Saunders: 1997.
30. Vacanti CA, Langer R, Schloo B, Vacanti JP. Synthetic polymers seeded with chondrocytes provide a template for new cartilage formation. *Plast Reconstr Surg.* 1991; 88:753–759.

13 Nasal Trauma

O. Kaschke

Contents

Introduction

The nose is the most prominent facial element. The fracture of the nasal pyramid is one of the most frequent bone fractures of the human body. The energy required to cause a fracture is lower than for other facial bone fractures. More than 50% of all facial fractures are injuries to the nose. In the course of increasing incidents of injuries to the facial area, the resulting mostly complex consequences pose great challenges for the trauma specialist, who, with his assessment and treatment, is responsible for the reconstruction of form and function (24, 26).

For nasal injuries, one can differentiate based on the type, direction, and energy volume of the impinging trauma between superficial soft-tissue injuries with lacerations of the skin and soft tissue, burns and frostbite, and fractures of the cartilage and bony framework and structure. High levels of energy striking the face often result in extensive and combined injuries.

Not infrequently, injuries and especially fractures of the nose are considered minor injuries in an average clinical day and often treated with insufficient diagnostics as well as inadequate care. The incidence of posttraumatic deformities that have not only unaesthetic but also functionally unacceptable consequences is high. In many cases, the necessary revision septorhinoplasty has proved to be difficult. Therefore practicable guidelines for the optimal medical care of acute nasal trauma are necessary. Currently there are still discrepancies with regard to the timing and methodology involved in posttraumatic management. Posttraumatic repositioning of nasal bone fractures implemented early are generally carried out as simple, contained manipulations, resulting in cases requiring the corrective medical care of either rhinoplasty or septorhinoplasty. The data for frequency vary between 14% and 50% (6, 18, 24).

Trauma-Relevant Anatomy of the Nose

A detailed anamnesis, in particular of the trauma event, as well as an exact clinical examination, are especially important for the assessment of the injury. In doing so, precise knowledge of the fundamental anatomy is virtually essential for the surgeon. The osseous architecture of this compact region includes the twin nasal bones, front process of the maxilla, the maxillary process of the frontal bone, the lacrimal bone, the lamina papyracea of the ethmoid bone, the sphenoid bone, and the vomer. Fitted into this structure are the cartilage elements of the quadrangular cartilage of the septum and the upper and lower lateral cartilages of the external nose. The midfacial bony structures are reinforced by vertical and horizontal buttresses. The upper horizontal buttress is formed by the lower anterior rim of the sinus and the upper orbital rim, while the lower orbital rim functions together with the zygomatic bone as the lower horizontal buttress (Fig. 13.1). The twin nasoethmoidal complex functions as a "central element" and forms the vertical buttress together with the frontal process of the maxillary bones and the lateral interior angle of the frontal bone. Only the thickened posterior edges of the nasal bones are components of the buttresses, but they protect the further dorsally located thin bones of the medial orbital wall. The central element is also the fixation point for the medial canthal tendon, which guarantees support for the bulb and the eyelids (Fig. 13.2). Tears to this support signify a traumatic telecanthus and a rounding of the medial canthus. However, the function of the M. orbicularis oculi is not influenced by a mobile canthal tendon. In contrast, impairment of the lacrimal sac drainage

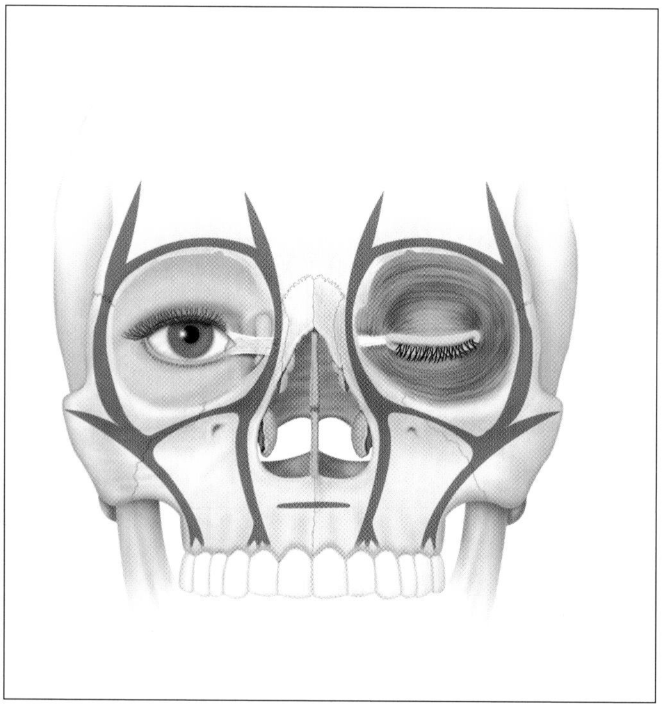

Fig. 13.1 Horizontal and vertical columns constitute a static, supportive function in the midface. The vertical supporting column forms the central element; the upper horizontal column is formed by the frontal bone and the upper margin of the orbita; the lower horizontal column is formed by the lower orbital margins. The medial canthal tendon enters the bone of the medial canthus region that is part of the central element. An external portion of the tendon extends to the surface of the nasal bone.

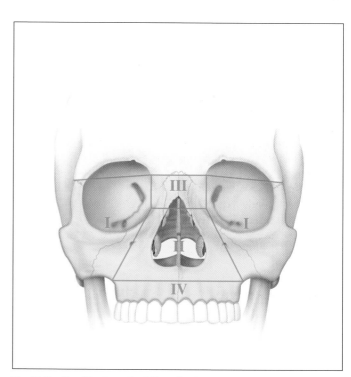

Fig. 13.2 Classification of midface fractures:
I = zygomatico–orbital complex
II = naso–maxillary complex
III = naso–ethmoidal complex
IV = dento–alveolar complex

can result, because this is surrounded by portions of the canthal tendon (33).

The nose as a central and prominent facial element can function as an energy absorber and thus as protective buffer of the viscerocranium. The cartilage portions have a high level of flexibility, and traumata with a low amount of energy can be partially absorbed without permanent damage. The variously thick bone structures determine the predilection sites of fractures, but the different bone thickness also has an influence on the extent of the fracture. Thus, older people with osteoporotic bones have comminuted fractures more frequently whereas in children dislocative fractures are rare, but here greenstick fractures predominantly occur (4).

The anatomical relations are significantly different in children in comparison to adults. The bones are shorter and the cartilage portion is larger. Additional protection is given because the bones are embedded in thicker soft tissue. Also, the nose is less prominent than in adults, which reduces the trauma consequences as the striking energy is distributed across a larger surface (27). On the other hand, various anatomical growth zones in the child's nasal skeleton are strongly influenced. Consequently, the potential for growth impairment and problems with the development of the nasal framework and septum exist following trauma (22).

Classification of Nasal Trauma

The embedding of the nose in the midface requires that nasal fractures must be considered in the classification of midfacial fractures. In the classification according to LeFort, bony injuries of the nose exist in types II and III (Fig. 13.**3**). The classification according to Becker and Austermann is divided into central, lateral, and centrolateral midfacial fractures (Table 13.**1**). Isolated nasal bone fractures are included in the midfacial fractures, whereas the fractures of the naso-orbito-ethimoid complex are synonymous with the centrolateral fractures. For isolated central nasal fractures, the categorization according to Simmen has been well-established, divided into types I–IV. This categorization takes the direction of the trauma into consideration and specifies the trauma consequences on the osseous and cartilaginous system. In the classification according to Becker and Austermann, these fracture types are included in the category of central midfacial fractures of nasomaxilliary and nasoethmoidal types. A classification of the viscerocranium fractures with regard to the supporting structure xmechanism seems sensible from a functional perspective but has generally not yet been accepted (4).

Isolated Central Nasal Fractures

Type I corresponds to the unilateral depression of the nasal bone (Fig. 13.**4**). Fractures of this type are caused by the effect of a lateral impact with only low or moderate energy. An untreated fracture is apparent by an asymmetrical nasal pyramid, a damaged esthetic eyebrow line, and the potential presence of a low level of protuberance formation on the rhinion (Fig. 13.**5**). The lamina perpendicularis and the septum cartilage remain intact in this type of fracture. The osseouscar-

tilage connections of the nasal bone and the upper lateral cartilages remain intact as well.

Type II is the multiple fracture of the nasal pyramid as a consequence of a frontolateral blunt trauma. The nasal bones and the lamina perpendicularis are fractured and the external fragments dislocate laterally. This fracture type results in a destruction of the central buttress with fracture and dislocation of the septum, whereby the osseouscartilage connections are predominantly separated. The dislocation of the septum structures can occur along the entire length of the nose (Fig. 13.**6**). The long-term consequences are osseouscartilaginous slanted noses with an occasional severely deviated and frequently also subluxated septum cartilage (Fig. 13.**7**). Intranasal avulsions of the mucosa and dislocation of cartilage fragments are very frequently observed. In the late phase, pronounced deformations and deviations are visible.

Type III is the consequence of direct frontal traumas, in which bilateral fractures and depressions or dislocations of the nasal bone occur. The lamina perpendicularis and the septum cartilage also frequently fracture as a result of the usually severe depressions. A separation of the connection between the nasal bones and the cephalic rim of the upper lateral cartilages often results as well. For this degree of injury a relatively high level of energy is necessary (Fig. 13.**8**). The long-term consequences of a nontreated fracture is expressed by a lowering and widening of the nasal pyramid, usually with a palpable protuberance formation on the bridge of the nose but also a saddle formation due to the lack of anchoring of the septum in the K-region (Fig. 13.**9**). Often a concha head avulsion at the height of the piriform aperture and mucous membrane avulsions with exposure of the cartilage is apparent endonasally. In addition, a deviation of the septum usually forms in the dorsal section. In the case of low trauma energy, only a

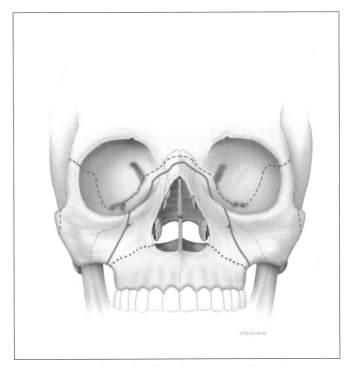

Fig. 13.**3** Fracture lines of midface fractures according to LeFort types I–III.

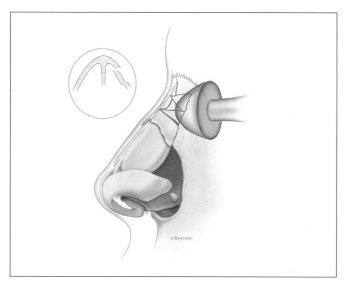

Fig. 13.**4**   Nasal fracture type I. Impression of the lateral bony nasal wall caused by a lateral impact.

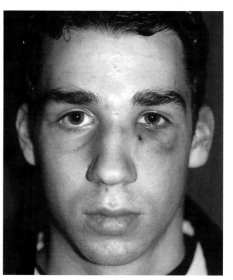

Fig 13.**5** Central type I left nasal bone fracture. The impression of the left nasal bone is masked by the accompanying soft-tissue edema and hematoma, but can be clearly felt by palpation.

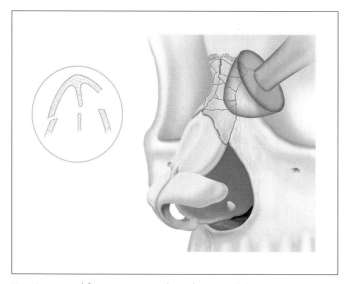

Fig. 13.**6**   Nasal fracture type II. Slanted nose with lateral displacement of the osseous nasal pyramid and fracture of the septum caused by a frontal–lateral impact.

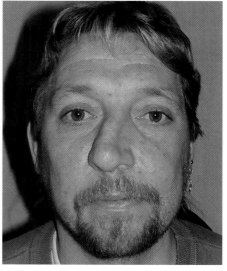

Fig. 13.**7**   Pronounced osseouscartilaginous slanted nose following frontal–lateral trauma. The nasal pyramid is severely deviated and asymmetrically fixed. The consequence of the septum fracture is significant tension formation of the cartilaginous septum towards the right and subluxation of the anterior margin of the septum.

Table 13.**1**   Classification of midfacial fractures

Central midfacial fractures	Lateral midfacial fractures	Centro–lateral midfacial fractures
—Fractures of the nasal pyramid Type I–latera trauma Type II–frontal trauma Type III–fronto–lateral trauma Type IV–caudal–frontal trauma —Fractures of the alveolar process LeFort I LeFort II	—Zygoma complex fracture —Zygoma arch fracture —Orbital fracture Orbital floor Orbital wall	—Naso-orbito-ethmoidal fracture —Le Fort III fracture

marginal depression or an isolated avulsion of the nasal bones from the frontal bone may result. In this case, small step formations form on the nasal dorsum or on the nasion.

Fracture type IV is the result of a trauma striking either in the direction of caudal to cranial or dorsal to the tip of the nose. This causes a compression of the septum cartilage and the surrounding soft-tissue structures. The septum cartilage thus fractures and the osseouscartilaginous connection to the lamina perpendicularis tears and results in a concomitant septum hematoma. The caudal fixation of the septum cartilage and the connection of the cranial septum rim to the cephalic rim of the lower lateral cartilages separates so that a complete or fragmented dislocation of the septum results (Fig. 13.**10**). An indirect sign for this fracture type is a hematoma in the upper

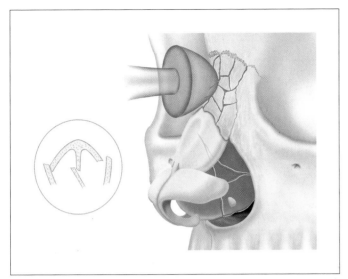

Fig. 13.**8** Nasal fracture type III. Impression of the nasal pyramid with broadening and concurrent septum fracture resulting from a frontal impact.

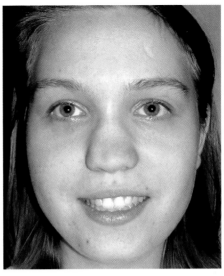

Fig. 13.**9** Saddle nose following frontal trauma. The dissolution of the supporting function of the osseous pyramid and the septum has caused the entire nasal bridge to sink in, resulting in broadening of the nose and deformation of the nose tip. The lateral crus of the lower lateral cartilage are sunk in and the projection of the tip is reduced significantly and at the same time the nostrils clearly appear broadened.

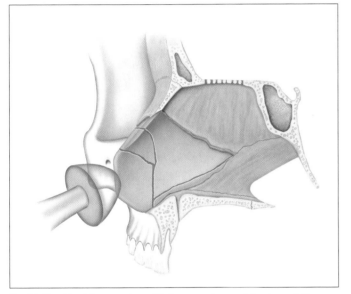

Fig. 13.**10** Nasal fracture type IV. Compression and fracture of the septum resulting from a caudal–cranial impact.

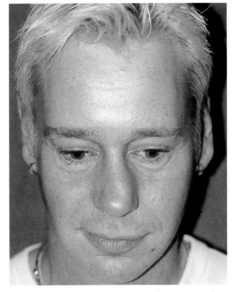

Fig. 13.**11** Substantial septum deviation and cartilaginous slanted nose as a late effect following a septum fracture caused by a caudal–cranial trauma.

lip at the height of the anterior nasal spine. This can be recognized by a cartilaginous saddle formation and rotation of the tip area with a reduction of projection (Fig. 13.**11**).

Naso-orbito-ethmoid Fractures

A classification for the fractures of the naso-orbito-ethmoid complex was suggested by Markovitz et al. (16). Fracture type I consists of a one-sided noncomminuted fracture of the central segment. Two subtypes can be differentiated: a) Avulsion of the medial canthus ligament together with a piece of the lacrimal bone; b) Complete separation of the medial canthus ligament from the medial orbital wall. The consequences are a telecanthus with elapsation of the medial palpebra commisure, narrowing of the palpebral fissure, limpness of the lids, and epiphora. The injuries of type II show one-sided comminutions and dislocations of the medial orbital wall, which, with more severe trauma, can also extend to the orbital roof or floor. The nasomaxillary columns and the maxilla are often affected, but the central segment remains. The clinical signs are similar to those of type I.

In type III, there is such extreme comminution that the central element can no longer be identified and the septum, the nasal bones, and the frontal sinus are affected by the fracture and dislocation. Pronounced flattening and widening of the nasal dorsum and orbital displacement occur (Fig. 13.**12**).

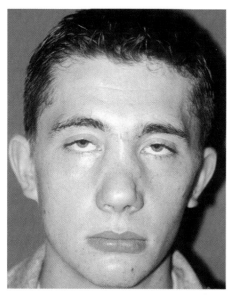

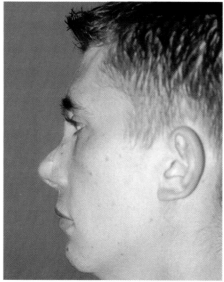

Fig. 13.**12 a, b**   Condition following a naso-orbito-ethmodial fracture. The distinct broadening of the nasal pyramid and the significant flattening of the nasal bridge with cartilaginous and osseous substance deficit are apparent.

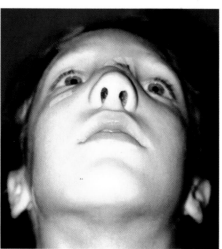

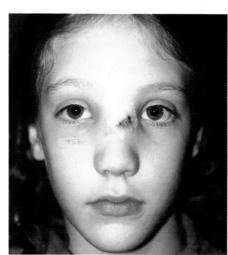

Fig. 13.**13 a, b**   Typical soft-tissue swelling resulting from a subcutaneous hematoma following a blunt trauma to the nose with a nondislocated nasal bone fracture and small skin lacerations on the nasal bridge.

Diagnostics

The clinical examination for nasal trauma with a suspicion of a nasal fracture should be conducted systematically. Because a nasal trauma can also be accompanied by craniofacial and cerebral injuries, the examination must also focus on cranial nerves, the cerebrum, and the eyes. The anamnesis for manifestations of allergic dispositions and chronically infected sinus illnesses is significant.

Inspection and Palpation

The external examination includes the inspection of the soft-tissue injuries, swellings, and deviations, as well as palpation of the nasal skeleton for abnormal movement, crepitation, depressions, a shortening of the nose, and also a possible widening of the nasal base (Fig. 13.**13**). In doing so, in particular, the intercanthal distance should be assessed. If the thumb and forefinger are each placed directly on the fixation point of the medial canthal tendon, the instability of the central fragment can be determined based on the extent of movement. A more sensitive estimation can be made according to the re-

commendations of Paskert and Manson (20) by means of bimanual examination. An instrument inserted in the nose moves the mobile bone fragment against the externally palpating finger. In addition, the "traction test" can be executed by laterally pulling on the external edge of the lower lid. Asymmetries or abnormal movements indicate an avulsion of the medial canthal tendon. The integrity of the nasal framework can be checked through palpation of the nasal dorsum. A lack of resistance indicates a loss of osseous or cartilaginous buttresses in the central element.

Intranasal Diagnostics

Particular attention should be paid to the intranasal examination, for which an endoscope should always be used. It is the most important examination that can ensure a certain determination of the functional and esthetic consequences of the nasal fracture. Verwoerd describes the pathogenesis of septum fractures of three septum zones with thicker cartilage as dorsoposterior, basal, and caudal (32). In contrast, the central section of the septum cartilage is thin. The thick posterior section of the septum cartilage supports the nasal dorsum. Therefore, trauma in the nasal dorsum area can cause caudal–basal to cephalo–dorsal lesions and horizontal fractures of the thin cen-

Table 13.**2** Clinical symptoms of nasal fractures

Extranasal	Intranasal	Concomitant Symptom
—Lacerations, edema, ecchymosis —Decrease of projection —Impression of the nasal dorsum —Widening of the nasal dorsum —Telecanthus —Rounding of medial canthus —Mobility of the central element	—Lacerations of septal mucosa —Septal dislocation —Fracture and commution of bony parts of the septum —Septal hematoma	—Rhinoliquorrhoe —Pneumocephalus —Anosmie —Vertical dystopia —Enophthalmus —Diplopia —Epiphora

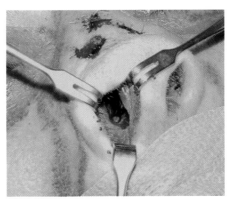

Fig. 13.**14** Mucous membrane avulsion and septum fracture of a naso-orbito-ethmoidal fracture.

tral regions. Fry presents the clear displacement of fractured septum cartilage fragments based on the separation of internal osseous cartilaginous connections (5) (Fig. 13.**14**). Gunter and Rohrich show that the septum has a key function in the optimal care of nasal trauma and of the minimization of secondary deformities (8). All deformities and obstructions can be estimated with a rigid endoscope with a 4-mm optic (0° or 30°). In doing so, one must pay particular attention in the cases of type II and III nasal bone fractures and naso-orbito-ethmoid fractures to the posterior osseous septum sections and to the vomer. A topical local anesthetic with 4 % Pantocain and an additional reduction of the swelling with Naphazolin is necessary in order to carry out a nasal endoscopy on conscious patients. It has been found that the endoscope should first be led along the nasal floor along the lower nasal concha to the posterior end of the septum. In addition to assessing the septum anomalies, the mucous membranes can be investigated for injuries and hematomas. These can occur on one or both sides. The disturbance of circulation to the septum cartilage resulting from the hematoma, which is provided by the perichondrium, can lead to irreversible damage after only three to four days (Fig. 13.**15**). Early recognition of these problems prevents the development of fibroses with ensuing septum displacement, abscess formations, and successive complete necrosis with nasal saddle formations. Pulling back the septum can allow for the recognition of possible injuries to the nasal concha and anything conspicuous, in particular bleeding, in the middle nasal passage.

An epistaxis occurs almost routinely with nasal trauma and is an indication of an injury to the mucous membranes. The intensity of bleeding and the localization of bleeding can indicate the extent of injury. With severe persistent bleeding indicating a capillary rupture, a tamponade must be inserted before the planned repositioning procedure and must be treated accordingly.

An overview shows typical and possible additional and intranasal findings and associated symptoms of nasal traumas (Table 13.**2**).

Imaging Diagnostics

The radiological diagnostics consists of a planar radiograph of the nose laterally (Fig. 13.**16**) and the occipital–mental radiograph (Fig. 13.**17**). These radiograph images show pronounced osseous dislocations or chipping. The images are not absolutely necessary for the diagnosis of an isolated nasal bone

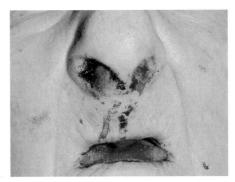

Fig. 13.**15** Pronounced septum hematoma resulting from direct nasal trauma caused by striking the nose tip in a fall.

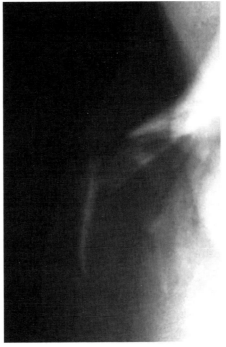

Fig. 13.**16** Radiograph image of a nasal bone fracture following frontal trauma. The nasal bone indicates a dislocation with an impression.

fracture; the diagnosis should be ascertained by the clinical symptoms. Studies by Logan et al. have shown that radiograph examinations are not cost-effective (13) and that a broad misuse of radiological examination techniques exists in the diagnostics for management of nasal trauma (19). In contrast, a

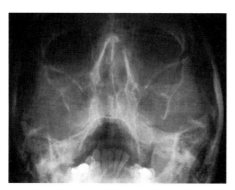

Fig. 13.**17** In the overview of the paranasal sinuses, a fracture of the nasal pyramid is apparent on the left and a fracture in the left orbital floor area is visible.

coronal and axial computed tomography (CT) is necessary for the exact diagnostic of naso-orbito-ethmoid injuries (9, 17). A cross-section of between 1.5 and 2 mm provides an adequate, detailed image. In doing so, particular attention should be paid to the assessment of the central element (Fig. 13.**20**). In the case of an existing fracture, the extent of comminution and the position of the fracture must be taken into consideration in order to determine the exact classification (15). The CT provides information on the integrity of the osseous and cartilaginous septum. In addition, injuries to the sinuses, the nasofrontal duct and the orbits can be analyzed.

Management of Nasal Traumas

Chronological Procedure

In trauma management, the question is always raised as to what the optimal time is for treatment. Only a minority of fractures are treated promptly (within a few hours) following the trauma. At this point in time, the soft-tissue swelling is still minimal and in the case of simple fractures, repositioning can be carried out immediately.

More frequently, injuries are first treated after a longer time interval or after other primary or life-threatening injuries have been treated. With adults, the possibility for primary treatment is limited after a time span of two to three weeks and with children, five to seven days. After that, the improper fixation of fracture fragments must be expected. In the majority of cases, patients come for treatment after a time interval of more than six hours. By then, the palpable fracture findings are masked by the associated edema and an assessment and reliable repositioning procedures are no longer possible. It is recommended that one wait approximately three to five days after the trauma before carrying out any repositioning measures. However, a septum hematoma that occurs in the meantime must on no account be overlooked (23) (Fig. 13.**18**).

Anesthesia

The type of anesthesia required for the treatment of nasal trauma is often discussed. Numerous studies have compared the use of local or general anesthetic for closed repositioning

(3, 6). It has been concluded that in most cases, local anesthetic is sufficiently effective as well as more cost-effective. The choice of anesthetic is also dependent on the seriousness of the nasal trauma and the patient's compliance and pain tolerance. In principal, local anesthetic with or without intravenous sedation can be utilized for central nose bone fractures types I–III. In the case of naso-orbito-ethmoid fractures and in situations in which no adequate repositioning is possible, a general anesthetic should be used. For children and teenagers, a general anesthetic is also recommended, because only in rare cases or with minor dislocation is it possible to successfully manipulate under local anesthetic (3).

Independent of the choice of the anesthesia procedure, the nose should be topically and locally prepared. To do so, following careful cleaning of the main nasal cavity, gauze or cotton soaked with Pantocain and Naphozolin is inserted into the middle and lower nasal passageway and left there for at least 10 minutes. A local anesthetic can be administered by means of an injection of 1% or 2% Xylocain with added epinephrine (1:200 000) intranasally in the nasal dorsum region to block the anterior ethmoidal branches of the trigeminal nerve, and additionally near the maxilla process to block the nasopalatine nerve and the upper dental nerves.

Management of Isolated Central Nose Fractures

A general decision to be made in the treatment of nasal bone fractures is whether open or closed repositioning is to be performed. The closed technique is in principal gentler, but the extent and the overview of the repositioning procedure is more limited. However, in the case of insufficient results following the closed technique, there is always still the possibility of open repositioning either in an early phase or after a longer time interval has passed since the trauma. It must be noted that estimates of the success rate of the closed repositioning technique vary (11, 12, 14, 18, 23, 24, 25, 32). The decisive advantage of open access is the better view of the fractured segments and the possibility of an exact repositioning and fixation. In addition, septum fractures can be precisely analyzed and treated. Studies have shown that theses partially incomplete cartilage fractures lead to an imbalance in the pressure and traction fibers in the external cartilage layers, which then lead to deviations. In addition to the treatment of these recent cartilage injuries, there is the option of removing preexisting bony ridge and spur formations during an open procedure. Clinical reports of good results following open repositioning have been made that support a more generous indication stance on open repositioning (5, 9, 11, 25). However, it is of decisive importance that an exact clinical analysis and assessment based on the force impact corresponding to the stated classification be carried out.

Closed Repositioning Techniques

The treatment, i.e., the repositioning of an osseous fracture should always, if the soft-tissue swelling allows for an appropriate assessment, first be attempted by means of a careful forming the natural nose shape with the fingers. This manipulation is only possible in the case of laterally dis-

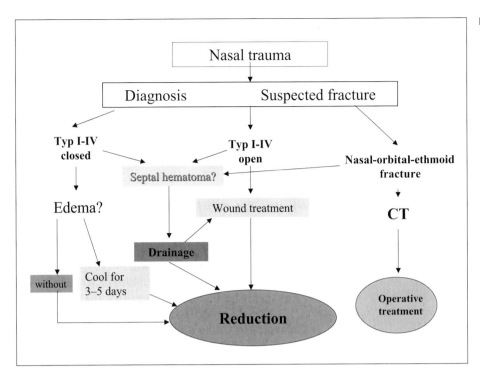

Fig. 13.**18**

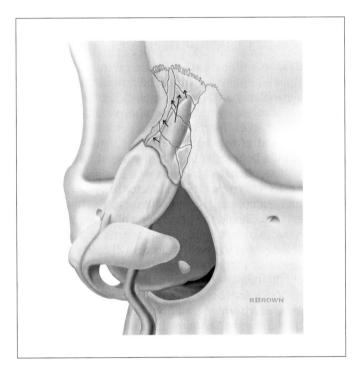

Fig. 13.**19** A powerful repositioning of wedged and depressed fragments can be attained with the solidly built elevator. The rounded outer surface of the tip of the elevator supports the shaping of the repositioned pyramid, while the smooth inner surface prevents the mucosa of the septum from being damaged.

placed fragments. Displaced fragments must be lifted and repositioned. The instruments recommended for this—the Walsham pliers and the Boies elevator—are used for bone repositioning, and the Asch pliers for septum repositioning. The disadvantage of the above-mentioned pliers is the danger of damaging the septum mucous membranes. The elevator as described by Behrbohm and Kaschke has been shown to be a universal elevator that is suited to the repositioning of bone fragments and septum portions as well as to fractures of the midface (Figs. 13.**21**, 13.**19**). It unites the advantages that various sizes of the elevator tip are available with the fact that there is also a round side for the elevation of the bone and a flat side for repositioning the septum. In addition, the design of the handle allows for a subtle movement of bone

fragments, on the one hand, although a powerful elevation of wedged fragments is also possible, on the other (2). The repositioning of the septum should aim to place the fractured septum in the center line of the nasal base. An endoscopic check is essential in order to check the posterior sections. Following this maneuver, stabilization and fixation is required using a splint (e.g., Doyle Splints) for five to six days and additional stabilization with a soft tamponade (e.g., Gelatin, Rhinotamps, etc.). The nasal pyramid should be covered with a dressing of Steri-Strips or bandages. The pressure of the dressing prevents additional hematoma formation. In addition, external splinting by means of a nose cast or a thermoplastic dressing is necessary, which should remain in place for at least one week.

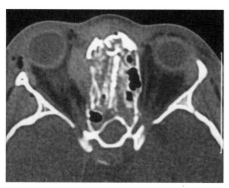

Fig. 13.**20** Axial CT of a naso-orbito-ethmoidal fracture with extensive comminution of the central element.

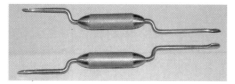

Fig. 13.**21** The elevator enables a specific and controlled repositioning by means of a specially formed tip and a long lever arm.

Septum hematomas must always be relieved. A hemitransfixion incision on the side of the hematoma, careful under-tunneling of the mucous membrane, suction of the hematoma, and the placing of a silicon foil strip for drainage is sufficient. In the case of extensive hematoma findings, the mucous membranes should be compressed using a splint or tamponade positioned on the septum cartilage. Transseptal mattress sutures are also very effective.

Open Repositioning Techniques

Dislocations and injuries of the anterior or posterior septum sections, as seen in central nose bone fractures types II–IV and in naso-orbito-ethmoid fractures, are indications for an acute open septum correction (29). Even when, due to trauma, severe bleeding into the mucosa and small avulsions exist, open reconstruction of the septum should not be avoided in these cases. The high rate of posttraumatic deformities and the associated scarring in the mucosa also make a septum correction at a later point in time more difficult. Access by means of the classical hemitransfixion incision and the under-tunneling of the mucous membranes on both sides of the cartilage has been proved for acute septum corrections. The fragments can thus be replaced with more certainty and bleeding around the nasal base or the posterior sections can be better checked and treated. The danger of new hematoma formation is thereby distinctly reduced. Further recommended measures are mattress sutures with resorbable Vicryl sutures and the placement of Doyle splints for five to six days. None the less, conservative manipulation should principally be preferred in the case of exaggerated cartilage resectioning because of the danger of loss of the support function with saddle nose formations and columella retractions. In the case of mucosa injuries, there is the danger of septum perforation.

The open techniques for repositioning in the acute phase following the trauma are also indicated when repositioning by

means of the closed technique are unsuccessful or if such serious comminution exists that adequate repositioning with sufficient stabilization cannot be carried out. Generally, immediate open treatment is also done in the case of an open tissue wound with simultaneous bone injuries, naso-orbital injuries, or injuries according to LeFort II. All unsatisfactory functional and esthetic later consequences following trauma with or without attempted closed repositioning should principally be remedied by means of rhinoplastic corrections.

The isolated osseous or osseouscartilaginous slanted noses can be corrected in most cases using standardized transcartilaginous or intercartilaginous access. In doing so, it is essential that the incision is made sufficiently wide in the lateral alar of the nostril cartilage extending to the transfixion incision so that broad mobilization of the skin of the nasal dorsum is possible. This is required in order for all fragments to be optimally mobilized and repositioned. Special care must be taken with the elevation of the skin of the nasal dorsum, because submucous layers of the skin can be drawn in and fixated in the fracture gap. While conducting the mobilization maneuver, perforation of the skin or injury to the submucous aponeurotic system can occur as a result of proceeding too abruptly, which in turn can cause acute bleeding and long-term tissue swelling. Therefore, the soft tissue around the fracture gap should be separated very minimally only with direct visual control, and only enough to provide for sufficient fragment mobilization. Overly extensive mobilization reduces the stability that is ensured by the fixation of the soft tissue to the periosteum. The correction of deviations in the late phase requires moving the bony pyramid. In addition, paramedian–oblique as well as complete lateral osteotomies are generally necessary, which are also possible with open transcolumelar access for rhinoplasty.

The method of osteotomy chosen is dependent on the structure of the bony deformity. In the case of an extensively wide nasal base, often in connection with a palpable open roof, a lateral osteotomy must be conducted very wide latero–basally and extending far into the nasion (low-to-high osteotomy) (30). Should the broadening of the nasal base extend to the nasion region, then a paramedian–oblique osteotomy is necessary as well. If there is a distinct concavity in the midsection of the pyramid although the nasal base is of normal width, then lateral osteotomies are necessary in the midsection of the nasal bone (29). This allows for narrow open-roof findings, which often result from frontal traumas, to close anatomically correctly. The most difficult problem arising in the osteotomy of posttraumatic deviations of the nasal pyramid is the exact symmetrical reconstruction. It is often not possible to straighten the pyramid only with a parallel conducted lateral osteotomy. It is often necessary to vary the height of the lateral osteotomy for each side. The osteotomy conducted into the nasion region and the combination with the paramedian-slanted osteotomy must be coordinated based on the findings. A double lateral osteotomy is required in the case of broad concavities of the pyramid in conjunction with a broadening of the nasal base. In doing so, a complete osteotomy of the midsection should always be carried out prior to the osteotomy of the nasal base. This allows one to take advantage of the stability of the base in the maxilla region.

All asymmetries of the cartilage framework can be corrected by means of open transcolumelar access. Traumatically induced deformities of the septum upper rim and its connections to the upper lateral cartilages are easily viewed and can be adequately corrected. The straightening of cartilaginous slanted noses can be made in the case of a traumatically altered and frequently missing or only fragmented septal cartilage by inserting spreader grafts (Fig. 13.**22**). These cartilage strips form a stable connection between the upper lateral cartilages and thus prevent a lateral collapse of the nose as well as the caving in of the nasal dorsum. Through appropriate suture techniques, the paired grafts can be positioned so that a straight alignment of the septum upper rim results and the cartilaginous deviation is counterbalanced. The first choice for a donor region is sufficiently available septal cartilage. However, often septal cartilage is seriously deformed or lacking as a result of the trauma and thus concha cartilage should alternatively be gained. In cases of extensive substance defects of the supporting frame, in particular in the nasal dorsum with saddle formations or also at the tip of the nose with projection loss, the reconstruction can often only be accomplished through the use of rib cartilage. In comparison to ear cartilage, it has the disadvantage of giving a somewhat unnatural firmness to the nasal frame and has a higher resorption than ear cartilage.

Despite intensive repositioning and reconstruction, palpable step formations of the nasal skeleton or around the tip of the nose remain following pronounced combined traumas of the cartilage and bone. This problem can be particularly serious with very thin skin. Cartilage transplants inserted for augmentation of a displaced nasal dorsum can be especially intensively highlighted in the skin, having a negative effect on the overall esthetic impression. A camouflage of the nasal skeleton through autologous facia (M. temporalis) or through nonvital transplants (Tutoplast, AlloDerm) are possible solutions for this. Soft contours and thus harmony of the profile can be achieved once temporary swelling of the soft-tissue structures has subsided. This technique should be considered in particular when major dislocations of the fragments exist and extensive mobilization was necessary during reconstruction. The danger of undesirable fragment mobility is high in these cases and can be reduced by using inserted transplants.

Management of Nasal Traumas in Children

The consequences of nasal trauma in children require differentiated consideration. Although the current extent of the trauma may seem proportionally minor, significant functional and esthetic consequential damage is possible as a result of the trauma. These are caused by the traumatic influences to the growth zones of the nasal septum. Also, intensive manipulation in repositioning following a trauma can influence the integrity of these zones (10, 31). Therefore, the decisions regarding post-trauma treatment should be considered very carefully. Conservative measures should always be preferred, especially because the cartilage is highly flexibility and bone injuries almost always involve greenstick fractures. Dislocations occur very rarely and should be repositioned very carefully using a closed technique and under general anesthetic. Nasal trauma to children almost always results in significant hematoma formation in the nasal dorsum area. The nose should be externally splinted for a sufficiently long period (ca. one week) so that the traumatized cartilage and osseous elements are not dislocated by the hematoma and edema (27). Secondary rhinoplasty that is necessary in children should be postponed until the end of puberty at the earliest, optimally until around age 18 (21).

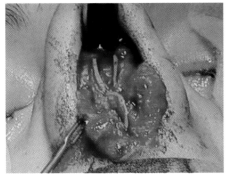

Fig. 13.**22** Stabilization of the partially absent and deviated septum upper margin through the implantation of spreader grafts.

Management of Naso-orbito-ethmoid Fractures

Naso-orbito-ethmoid fractures can be viewed through existing open skin injuries. However, it is usually necessary and recommended to use standardized craniofacial incisions and accesses. The fractures can be widely exposed by means of broad coronal incisions of the scalp with the formation of a galea-periosteum lobe. The supraorbital rim, the supratrochlear column, and the neurovascular column can be carefully identified and treated with care. After removing the column, the nasal bones and the central segment can be completely viewed. A broad subperiosteal separation above the medial orbital wall and the orbital roof is necessary in order to be able to analyze and reposition the fractures of the nasal pyramid (16, 17). The coronal access also provides neurosurgical access to the frontal craniotomy or the repair of an accompanying fracture in the frontal sinus region, in particular repair to the supply of cerebrospinal fluid (CSF) in fractures of the frontal sinus posterior wall (Fig. 13.**23**). Central–lateral midfacial fractures with injuries to the orbital floor are performed by means of a skin incision above the infraorbital rim of the maxilla or transconjunctivally. The caudal section of the central segment can also be viewed and repaired through this access. Direct skin incisions near the glabella or the nasal dorsum are possible, but should be avoided due to visible scarring; a bitemporal incision should be preferred (16).

The exact reconstruction and fixation of the complex of the medial canthal tendon connection for the restoration of the original intercanthal distance is important. Only accurate repair and stabilization can prevent a postoperative telecanthus. Further important aims must be the forming of normal orbital contours and a normal orbital volume, which in turn provides for the restoration of a normal nasal dorsum with normal projection. In addition, all soft-tissue injuries and obstructions of the nose must be treated (33).

The fixation of the fracture fragments can be made with metal wires (cerclage) or more securely and tightly with miniplates and screws (1–1.3 mm). Miniplates are available in various shapes and sizes. In addition, titan nets or plates made of polydioxanon acid (PDS II) are available so that planar comminution and defects can be covered. In the case of multiple injuries to the face, the treatment sequence should always be

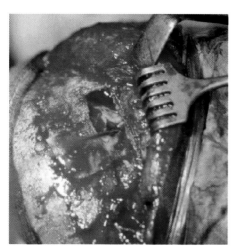

Fig. 13.**23** Exposition and care of a nasal complex fracture above a bicoronal incision. The fracture fissure extends to the posterior wall of the frontal sinus and has led to injury of the dura mater with liquorrhoea.

performed from lateral (i.e., orbital roof or floor) to medial. The fixation of the central element is very dependent upon the type of fracture (9, 33).

Type I Fracture

Type I fractures can be displayed by means of an incision above the medial canthal tendon extending to the lateral eyebrow line. With this opening, the lacrimal sac in the lacrimal cavity is also exposed and the connection of the medial canthal tendon can be checked. A mobile fragment in type I fractures cannot be easily fixated with microplates to the stable osseous processes of the frontal bone and the maxilla. In the case of an isolated separation of the canthal ligament, this can be attached with a secure, nonabsorbable thread to the posterior rim of the lacrimal bone.

Type II Fracture

In type II fractures, it is necessary to fixate the singular fragments with wire cerclage, because the attachment of the medial canthal tendon usually disrupts together with a bone fragment. The area of the trochlea must then be stabilized with a microplate. In addition, transnasal wiring, which begins at the lacrimal cavity and extends across the lamina perpendicularis to the medial upper orbital rim and fixated, has been proved for stabilization. This provides for an optimal adjustment of the intercanthal distance. Care should be taken that the wire does not lie too far ventrally in order to prevent a divergence of the dorsally located fragments. A fracture of the orbital lamina can result in constrictions of the medial rectus muscles and superior oblique muscles, which then causes double vision.

Type III Fracture

Type III of naso-orbito-ethmoid fractures is characterized by osseous comminution and defects and can require primary bone transplantation. This is necessary for the restoration of a central element on which the majority of detached medial canthal tendons can be fixated. The preferred donor region for the bone transplant is the parietal bone of the skull. Transnasal wire cerclages are one possibility for securing the bone transplant in the midline. If at all possible, miniplates and screws

should be the goal in order to increase stability of the nasal pyramid and, finally, to reduce the bone resorption (7).

In many naso-orbito-ethmoid fracture cases a distinct comminution of the bony nose occurs, resulting in a loss of projection and support of the nasal dorsum. In these cases the nasal dorsum and also the stability of the septum should be aspired to by means of primary bone transplants. The insertion of bony transplants is the last step of bony repair and follows the repositioning and fixation of all other fragments of the nose and midface (7).

Management of Soft-Tissue Injuries to the Nose

Open injuries to the nose usually are accompanied by more or less serious contamination of the dermis, which must be eliminated as best as possible before bony repositioning takes place. Brushing out dirt particles with mild soap or saline solution or also iodine-containing solutions is suitable. Intensive rinsing is also often helpful. One should abstain from using hydrogen superoxide because a tissue-toxic exothermal reaction can occur that would compromise the wound healing.

Following the repair of the bony segments, the subtle repair of all lacerations and soft-tissue injuries is carried out. Excisions should only be made to the extent that the wound edges can be precisely adapted. Extensive debridement is not usually necessary because the very good blood circulation of the face generally guarantees good healing and too much debridement produces esthetically unfavorable scarring. If the lesions are highly contaminated and can only be insufficiently cleaned or are contaminated with animal or human saliva, a secondary wound closure should be considered. Primary closure is sufficient for most lesions, even with minor bacterial contamination, because in contrast to the other body regions, infectious inclusion is well tolerated in the facial region due to better blood circulation. The maximum time interval for primary wound closure after an injury to the facial and neck area should be limited to six to eight hours. Beyond that, secondary wound closure should be considered.

The technical implementation of the wound closure is always connected to the precise, tension-free closure of the subcutaneous and epidermal layers. However, generally the loose wound edges must first be undermined, which in turn removes the tension from the skin suture and allows for a better placement of the subcutaneous sutures. Penetrating injuries to the nose are always accompanied by injuries to the mucosa of the main nasal cavity. In order to avoid functionally effective synechia or scar formation in the interior of the nose, a subtle suture of the mucosa is necessary. If the mucosa structures can be adapted free of tension, a quickly absorbable suture material (Vicryl rapid) can be used. If more tension on the suture is expected, then a slowly absorbed, monofile material (PDS II) is used, which guarantees trouble-free healing. An accurate subcutaneous suture reduces the dead space that can form under the skin suture as a result of hematoma and seroma formations. In addition, the tension of the skin suture is reduced and undermined incision edges can be better everted. A precise convergence of the skin edges with minimal tension reduces scarring of the skin. By using monofile, nonabsorbable sutures, bacterial contamination of the skin and introduction of epidermal structures are reduced. Smooth, clean skin lesions can also be adapted well with Steri-Strips or similar microporous bandages. However, the skin must first be carefully cleaned and dried. They are also suited to wound treatment of small children for whom suture removal is difficult.

Contusions are soft-tissue injuries that are always accompanied by hematoma formation. These usually accumulate above the osseous nasal pyramid but can also spread out under the entire nasal dorsum skin. Usually these are spontaneously reabsorbed and only in rare cases does encapsulation occur, requiring expeditious drainage. Abrasions of the upper dermis layer are cleaned with sterile saline, mild soap, or antiseptic solutions and then covered with an antibiotic ointment. Spontaneous healing usually begins quickly.

Long-term Complications Following Nasal Traumas

Potential long-term complications of naso-orbit-ethmoid fractures are telecanthus, obstructions of the tear passage system with the danger of a pussy dacryocystitis, obstructions of the recess and frontal ostium with formation of purulent sinusitis, and chronic headache syndromes. The possibility of rhinoliquorrhea must also be eliminated by means of endoscopic diagnostics and testing of the nasal secretion for β2-transferrin. Further long-term consequences of nontreated type II and III injuries are fixated defective positions and callus formations on the medial orbital wall, the herniation of soft tissue by fracture lines, scarring, and fixations around the orbita, which can lead to cosmetic conspicuities. Corrections at a later date mean that the tissue elasticity is reduced significantly and also that more expansive and sometimes multiple osteotomies are necessary because the callus formation must be overcome. Often a chronic epiphora begins weeks after the trauma, caused by increasing scarring obstruction of the tear passages. A dacryocystorhinostomy, either endoscopically or by means of a medial canthal opening, can establish a drainage path from the lachrymal duct into the nose.

References

1. Becker R, Austermann KH. Frakturen des Gesichtsschädels. In Schwenzer N, Grimm G, *Zahn-Mund-Kiefer-Heilkunde, Band 2, Spezielle Chirurgie*. Stuttgart-New York: Thieme: 1981:464–583.
2. Behrbohm H, Kaschke O. Elevatorium für Frakturen des Os nasale und des Arcus zygomaticus. *Laryngo-Rhino-Otol*. 1998; 77:52–53.
3. Cook JA, McRae DR, Irving RM, Dowie LN. A randomized comparison of manipulation of the fractured nose under local and general anaesthesia. *Clin Otolaryngol*. 1990; 15:343.
4. Donat TL Endress C, Mathog RH. Facial fracture classification according to skeletal support mechanisms. *Arch Otolaryngol Head Neck Surg*. 1998; 124:1306–1314.
5. Fry HJH. Interlocked stresses in human nasal septal cartilage. *Br J Plast Surg*. 1966; 19:276.
6. Green KM. Reduction of nasal fractures under local anaesthetic. *Rhinology*. 2001; 39:43–46.
7. Gruss JS. Nasoethmoid-orbital fractures: classification and the role of primary bone grafting. *Plast Reconstr Surg*. 1985; 75:303–311.
8. Gunter JP, Rohrich RJ. Management of the deviated nose: The importance of septal reconstruction. *Clin Plast Surg*. 1988; 15:43
9. Hoffmann JF. Naso-orbital-ethmoid complex fracture management. *Facial Plast Surg*. 1998; 14:67–81.
10. Holt GR. Biomechanics of nasal septal trauma. *Otolaryngol Clin North Am*. 1999; 32:15–19.
11. Holt GR. Immediate open reduction of nasal septal injuries. *Ear Nose Throat J*. 1978; 57:344–354.
12. Illum P. Legal aspects in nasal fractures. *Rhinology*. 1991; 29:263–266.
13. Logan M, O'Driscoll K, Masterson J. The utility of nasal bone radiographs in nasal trauma. *Clin Radiol*. 1994; 49:192.
14. Marcks R, Pirsig W. Spätergebnisse der Nasenbeinfrakturen bei Erwachsenen. *HNO*. 1977; 25:187–1192.
15. Markowitz BL, Manson P, Sargent L, Van der Kolk C, Yaremchuk M, Galssman D, Crawley W. Management of the medial canthal tendon in nasoethmoid orbital fractures: Importance of the central fragment in classification and treatment. *Plast Reconstr Surg*. 1991; 87:843–853.
16. Markowitz BL, Manson PN. Panfacial fractures: organization of treatment. *Clin Plast Surg*. 1989; 16:105–114.
17. Meleca RJ, Mathog RH. Diagnosis and treatment of naso-orbital fractures. In Mathog RH, Arden RL, Marks SC, eds. *Trauma of the Nose and Paranasal Sinuses*. Stuttgart-New York: Thieme: 1995:65–98.
18. Murray JAM, Maran AGD, MacKenzie IJ, Raab G. Open vs. closed reduction of the fractured nose. *Arch Otolaryngol*. 1984; 110:797–802.
19. Oluwasanmi AF, Pinto AL. Management of nasal trauma—widespread misuse of radiographs. *Clin Perform Qual Health Care*. 2000; 8:83–85
20. Paskert JP, Manson PN. The bimanual examination for assessing instability in naso-orbito-ethmoidal injuries. *Plast Reconstr Surg*. 1989; 83:165–167.
21. Perkins SW, Dayan SH, Sklarew EC, Hamilton M, Bussell GS. The incidence of sports-related facial trauma in children. *Ear Nose Throat J*. 2000; 79:632–638.
22. Pirsig W, Lehmann I. The influence of trauma on the growing septal cartilage. *Rhinology*. 1975; 13:39–46.
23. Renner GJ. Management of nasal fractures. *Otol Clin N Amer*. 1991; 24:195–213.
24. Rohrich RJ, Adams WP. Nasal fracture management: minimizing secondary nasal deformities. *Plast Reconstr Surg*. 2000; 106:266–273.
25. Simmen D. Nasenfrakturen-Indikationen zur offenen Reposition. *Laryngo-Rhino-Otol*. 1998; 77:388–393.
26. Smith D, Mathog RH. Diagnosis and management of acute nasal fracture. In Mathog RH, Arden RL, Marks SC, eds. *Trauma of the Nose and Paranasal Sinuses*. Stuttgart-New York: Thieme: 1995:21–38.
27. Stucker FJ, Bryarly RC, Shockley WW. Management of nasal trauma in children. *Arch Otolaryngol*. 1984; 110:190–192.
28. Tardy ME. Cartilage autograft reconstruction. In Tardy ME, ed. *Rhinoplasty: The art and the science*, Volume 2, Chapter 8. Philadelphia: WB Saunders: 1997:648–723.
29. Tardy ME. Narrowing the nose. In Tardy ME, ed. *Rhinoplasty: The art and the science*, Volume 1, Chapter 5. Philadelphia: W.B. Saunders: 1997:326–373.
30. Tebbetts JB. Osteotomies. In Tebbetts JB. *Primary rhinoplasty: a new approach to the logic and the techniques*. St. Louis: Mosby: 1998:225–260.
31. Verwoerd CDA, Verwoerd HL, Meeuwis CA. Stress and wound healing of the cartilaginous nasal septum. *Acta Otolaryngol*. 1989; 107:441–445.
32. Verwoerd CDA. Present day treatment of nasal fractures: closed versus open reduction. *Facial Plast Surg*. 1992; 8:220.
33. Vora NM, Fedok FG. Management of the central nasal support complex in naso-orbital ethmoid fractures. *Facial Plast Surg*. 2000; 16:181–191.

Postoperative Care and Management

O. Kaschke

Contents

Introduction

Postoperative treatment begins with the application of intranasal packs and splints. Removal of the packs does not mark the end of postoperative care. On the contrary, it is essential to maintain diligent surveillance of intranasal and extranasal wound healing dynamics. In the early postoperative period, the nasal surgeon should support wound healing with specific manipulations and instruct the patient in how to protect the result with proper conduct and self-care.

Endonasal care is particularly important after surgical procedures involving the combined treatment of chronic inflammatory sinus diseases, septal deformities, turbinate hyperplasias, and osseocartilaginous morphological variants. With minimally invasive operative techniques, it is possible to combine functional endoscopic procedures with rhinoplastic procedures, thereby achieving different treatment goals in one operation. This requires a postoperative regimen that is geared toward preventing early and late complications and, if they occur, can ensure the rapid institution of appropriate treatment.

Intraoperative Management

Internal Dressing

Packs

The function of intranasal packs is to provide appropriate tissue compression to approximate the wound surfaces and prevent swelling, bleeding, and hematoma formation. These goals are particularly important when there are large, open wounds in the mucosa, like those resulting from endoscopic sinus surgery or a strip turbinectomy.

Some packing materials for sinus or turbinate wound surfaces are placed temporarily and are generally removed after a period of one to three days. These include silastic-coated foam packs (Rhinotamps, Fig. 14.1), self-expanding polyvinylacetate packs (Merocel, Ivalon, Fig. 14.2), hydrogel-coated packs (Rhino-Force, Fig. 14.3), ointment-impregnated gauze strips (Tampograss, Fig. 14.4), and Telfa gauze. The main selection criterion should be minimal adhesion to the mucosa with a good hemostatic action. Pack removal should be painless and

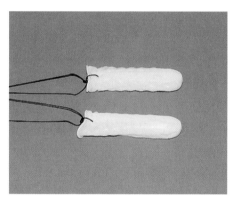

Fig. 14.**1** Silastic-coated foam strips with attached threads (Rhinotamp), used in packing the ethmoid or inferior meatus.

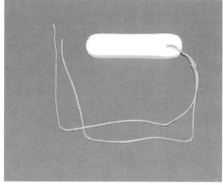

Fig. 14.**2** Polyvinylacetate pack with attached thread (Merocel). The material expands on contact with blood, exerting a compressive effect on the mucosa.

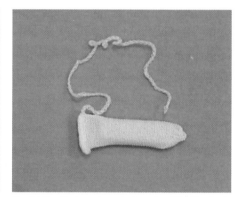

Fig. 14.**3** Hydrogel-coated pack with attached thread (Rhino-Force). This pack can be placed in the ethmoid or inferior meatus. When the pack is moistened, it exudes a gel that promotes platelet aggregation for hemostasis.

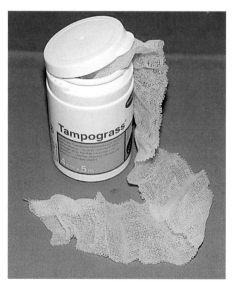

Fig. 14.**4** Paraffin-impregnated gauze for packing the ethmoid and nasal cavity in layers. This material is rarely used nowadays due to the risk of postoperative paraffinoma formation.

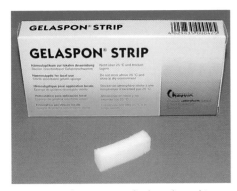

Fig. 14.**5** Gelatin sponge for loosely packing the nasal cavity and ethmoid. The material dissolves in three to five days and can then be suctioned from the nose.

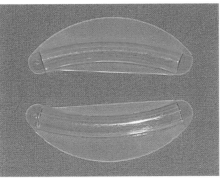

Fig. 14.**6** Doyle intranasal splints. The silastic splints are positioned on the septal mucosa and secured. The small tubes allow for minimal nasal airflow and allow secretions to be suctioned from the nose and nasopharynx.

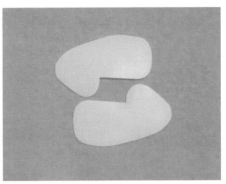

Fig. 14.**7** Reuter splints made of silicone and Teflon.

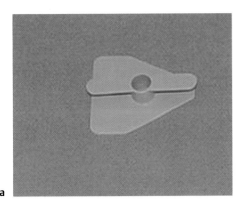

a

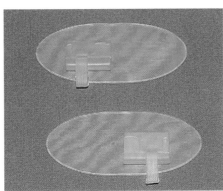

b

Fig. 14.**8 a, b** Stents for maintaining patency of a supraturbinate maxillary sinus window.

should not damage the mucosa. Another option is to use hemostyptic packing materials that liquefy as wound healing progresses and can be removed by means of suction during postoperative care. This eliminates the pack-removal procedure that patients dread. These materials include gelatin sponge (Gelfoam, Gelaspon, Fig. 14.**5**), hyaluronic acid (Merogel), and oxidized cellulose (Tabotamp).

Splints

Internal splints are designed to keep reconstructed portions of the septum from dislodging and prevent hematoma formation about the septum. They are also used to prevent synechia formation between wound surfaces. The most commonly used splints are Doyle nasal airway splints (Fig. 14.**6**) and Reuter silastic or Teflon splints (Fig. 14.**7**). Specially molded stents can be used to maintain the patency of enlarged passages in functional endoscopic sinus surgery (Fig. 14.**8 a, b**).

It is wrong to expect internal packing to salvage a poor postoperative result in the septum, sinus ostia, or external nasal shape. Also, a pack that fits too tightly or is too long will interrupt venous and lymphatic drainage, resulting in unnecessary swelling.

The duration of septal splinting and the danger of submucous hematoma formation can be reduced by placing multiple transseptal mattress sutures (Fig. 14.**9**). We have had good results with doubly armed 4–0 Vicryl sutures on a straight needle.

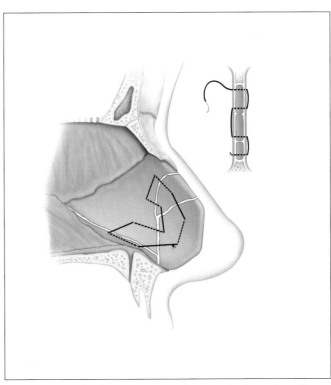

Fig. 14.**9** Principle of mattress suture placement in the septum. The sutures largely prevent the formation of a septal hematoma and give the corrected septum additional stability. They also permit early removal of the septal splints.

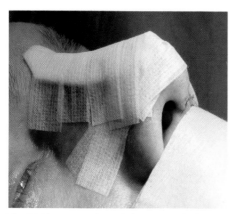

Fig. 14.**10** External nasal dressing with skin-friendly adhesive tapes (Steri-strips). Several overlapping strips are placed across the nasal dorsum, and two longer strips are slung over the nasal tip. A Gelfoam strip has been placed on the nasal dorsum beneath the dressing.

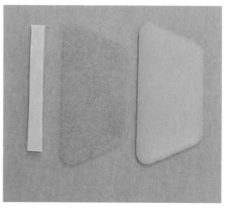

Fig. 14.**11** Denver splint set, consisting of an adhesive strip with Velcro and an aluminum strip, also with Velcro.

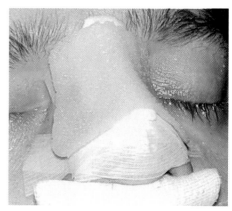

Fig. 14.**12** A thermoplastic splint covers most of the adhesive dressing. The nasal tip and two thirds of the alae are left uncovered.

External Dressing

The function of the external dressing is to secure the mobilized skin on the cartilaginous and bony nasal framework. It should reduce potential spaces that may fill with blood or serum, leading to hematomas and swelling. The external dressing should also protect the mobilized nasal segments from displacement due to external trauma or intranasal swelling.

Like the internal dressing, the external dressing cannot salvage a technically poor result due, for example, to inadequate osteotomies or resections. Before the external dressing is applied, postoperative edema and blood residues should be massaged from the nasal dorsum so that the result can be assessed. The principle of "what you see is what you get" applies.

The external dressing should consist of at least two layers: A skin-friendly adhesive dressing and a firm nasal splint.

The adhesive dressing for the skin consists of several, slightly overlapping adhesive strips that are placed across the nasal dorsum from the root of the nose to the supratip area. They are applied over a Gelfoam strip about 0.5 cm wide that is first placed along the full length of the nasal dorsum. This will facilitate dressing changes. One or two longer adhesive strips are slung over the nasal tip without obstructing the nares (Fig. 14.**10**).

Various materials can be used for the nasal splint. Plaster cast materials are widely used and are easily shaped to fit the individual nose. One disadvantage of casts is that they adhere poorly to the adhesive dressing, and the dressing will tend to loosen as swelling subsides, often requiring additional fixation. Thermoplastics can be trimmed to match the nasal size and can be accurately molded to the postoperative shape. Preshaped thermoplastic splints are supplied with an adhesive surface and adhere well to the adhesive dressing. Malleable aluminum splints are also available. The Denver splint (Fig. 14.**11**) is supplied in three pieces—an adhesive tape to which an aluminum splint is attached with Velcro, padded by a foam strip.

The splint covers the nasal dorsum, the nasal tip, and two thirds of the caudal margin of the alar cartilage (Fig. 14.**12**). A splint that fits too tightly can cause ischemia in the dorsal nasal skin. If pain is reported, therefore, the splint should be changed without delay. Normally the external dressings are removed at one week. The dressing may be extended an additional week, depending on the degree of swelling and the extent of the corrections.

Postoperative Management

First Postoperative Day

Generally the packs are removed from the ethmoid after sinus surgery or from the inferior turbinate after a turbinectomy on the first postoperative day. Pack removal must be done carefully, and spraying pantocaine and naphazoline into the nose will facilitate the procedure.

Slight postoperative bleeding causes blood to collect in the nasal cavity. This blood coagulates and dries, forming blackish crusts. Sinus operations are followed by mucous drainage from the opened sinus, which also dries to form crusts (Fig. 14.**13**). Serous and mucous wound secretions collect on the floor of the nasal cavity and in the sinuses. Patchy fibrin deposits form on surgical mucosal defects, especially on the turbinates, and dry to form crusts (Figs. 14.**14**, 14.**15**).

Early Postoperative Period

Most patients are unfamiliar with the typical changes that occur after their operation. They should be given strict instructions that will help to reduce complications during the postoperative period. These instructions are outlined below:
- The face should be rested for up to eight days after the operation. Excessive facial movements (e.g., prolonged talking, chewing hard foods, vigorous laughter) should be avoided.
- For the first five days after the operation, the patient should sleep with the head and upper body slightly elevated.

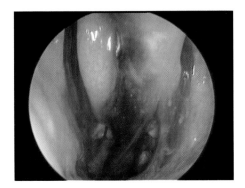

Fig. 14.**13** Endoscopic view of the nasal cavity and excavated ethmoid on the fourth postoperative day. A mucous discharge permeated with clots is draining from the opened sinuses over the back of the inferior turbinates toward the nasopharynx.

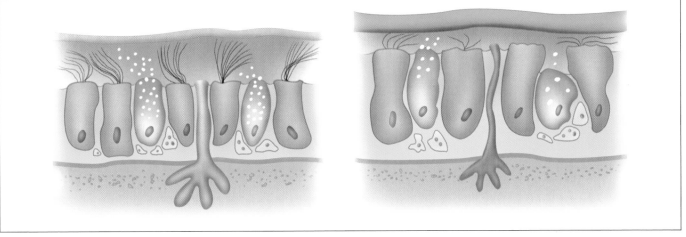

Fig. 14.**14** The respiratory epithelium of the nose and paranasal sinuses is altered by inflammatory disease and by surgery. Epithelial cell formation is altered, and mucociliary clearance is significantly hampered due to ciliary deformity and changes in the periciliary gel and fluid layers.

- Cooling compresses should be regularly applied to the eyes and cheek for the first few days.
- Medications should be taken only as directed. In particular, medications that contain acetylsalicylic acid should be avoided.
- The nose should not be blown, and the mouth should be opened during sneezing.
- Any physical exertion should be avoided for two weeks. Sports and other strenuous physical activities should be avoided for six weeks.
- Glasses should not be worn for at least six weeks after the operation.
- Excessive heat and sun exposure to the nose (including solarium treatment) should be avoided for three months after the operation.
- Smoking and drinking alcoholic beverages should be avoided during the initial weeks after surgery.

The patient should also be informed about necessary measures during postoperative management and the typical changes that may occur. This should include information on follow-up appointments and the schedules for dressing changes and suture removal. Other important points are information on postoperative complaints such as dry mouth, obstructed nasal breathing due to reactive mucosal swelling, transient subfebrile temperatures, and other possible complications. The latter may be classified as typical early postoperative complications or late complications.

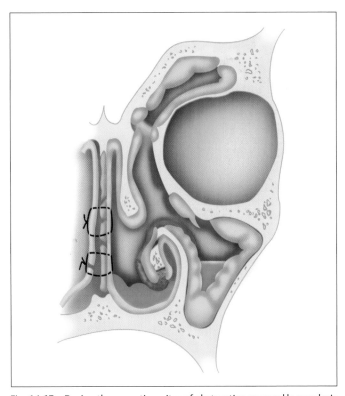

Fig. 14.**15** During the operation, sites of obstructive mucosal hyperplasia are removed and pathogenically active anatomical variants are corrected. If the clearance function of the respiratory epithelium is impaired, the secretions dry out and form crusts. Secretions and clots accumulate in the sinuses. Splints or mattress sutures can reduce the small hematomas and seromas that form under the mobilized layers of the septal mucosa.

Complications in the Early Postoperative Period

The following are external complications that most commonly occur during the early postoperative period.

Extensive edema and swelling can result from traumatizing osteotomies, especially those involving the lateral portions of the nasal pyramid. Vigorous rasping of the nasal bones can evoke similar reactions. The use of narrow chisels 2 or 3 mm wide for micro-osteotomies and the gentle use of rasps and files can significantly reduce the severity of these reactions.

Hematomas usually result from improper dissection outside the standard planes, resulting in excessive tissue traumatization. Unfavorable anesthesia parameters (high ventilatory pressure, high pCO$_2$ values) or poorly regulated circulatory parameters (high blood pressure) during the operation can hamper intraoperative exposure and cause heavy bleeding into the tissues. Hematomas are best treated by intraoperative compression and by applying a sufficiently large external pressure dressing combined with antibiotic coverage. Some hematomas may require incision and drainage. Possible *septal hematomas* are detected by diligent postoperative surveillance. They are treated by drainage and subsequent splinting. Transseptal mattress sutures and the insertion of septal splints (Doyle or Reuter type) will significantly reduce the risk of hematoma formation.

Infections of the skin surface occasionally develop below the external dressing, but most are punctate and resolve quickly in response to local ointment therapy. Subcutaneous abscesses and septal abscesses, on the other hand, are serious complications that result in tissue defects. Abscesses should be drained, and any prosthetic implants must be removed from the affected site.

Another serious complication is *skin necrosis.* It is often due to too much pressure from external and internal dressings, causing circulatory impairment. This problem can be significantly reduced by the use of loose packing materials and suitable external dressings. Skin ischemia can also result from excessive thinning of the dorsal nasal skin or the overtightening of implant fixation sutures. Regular dressing checks will disclose the clinical signs of ischemia or skin necrosis. In this case the dressing should be removed, followed by any revision surgery that may be required.

Common endonasal changes are reactive swelling of the mucosa on the septum and turbinates. Pads of edematous tissue, sometimes of considerable size, can form in the parietal sinus mucosa as a result of obstructed lymphatic drainage. They usually persist for four to six weeks after the operation and also depend on the original sinus pathology. Sites of edematous mucosal swelling are particularly common at the margins of supraturbinate antral windows and in the frontal recess. Often the entire ethmoid region is affected. The reactive swelling can sometimes mimic small polyps. It is common for *infection* to spread on the edematous mucosa, presenting clinically as a putrid nasal discharge.

Headaches are a common side effect of septorhinoplasties combined with endonasal procedures. A frequent endonasal cause is the obstruction of a frontal sinus ostium by reactive mucosal swelling, which usually clears spontaneously within a few days.

Measures During the First Postoperative Week

Secretions and clots should be carefully suctioned from the nasal vestibule for the first few days after the operation. This is easily done with thin suction tips introduced through the breathing tubes of the Doyle splint. Hard blood crusts can be loosened with hydrogen peroxide and then removed with a forceps.

After removal of the Doyle splint or septal splint on the third to fifth postoperative day, the nasal vestibule and floor can be cleaned using a rigid suction probe with fingertip suction control. Great care should be taken to avoid damaging the mucosa by overvigorous probe movements or by aspirating spongy mucosal tissue.

Starting on the fourth postoperative day, wound coatings and crusts may form, obstructing the nasal cavity and sinus ostia. They can be selectively removed with a suction tip, a small hook, or a suitable forceps to improve nasal airflow. These measures should be performed under endoscopic guidance to avoid injury to the regenerating mucosa. The epithelium still has little regenerative capacity before the end of the first postoperative week, however. It is best to avoid instrument manipulations in the excavated ethmoid, frontal recess, or supraturbinate windows at this stage following sinus operations.

Measures After the First Postoperative Week

The external dressing is changed one week after the operation. The tape sling on the nasal tip is divided, and the adhesive strips are carefully lifted from the nasal sidewall to free the dressing. The skin of the nasal dorsum is thoroughly cleaned, and fresh adhesive strips are placed across the nasal dorsum in an overlapping fashion. A firm splint is molded over the adhesive dressing and remains in place for an additional week (Fig. 14.**16**). If there is still much swelling of the dorsal nasal skin after the cast is removed, adhesive strips should be worn on the nose at night for the next two to four weeks. The strips are again placed across the nasal dorsum in an overlapping pattern, using skin-friendly adhesive tape.

Adhesions between opposing, deepithelialized wound surfaces may be encountered in the nose during postoperative care (Fig. 14.**17**). They commonly form between the lateral aspect of the middle turbinates and the lateral nasal wall and also between the septum and the inferior turbinates. The fibrous organization of these fibrin-containing adhesions leads to synechia formation within 10–14 days. These fibrin bridges can be carefully removed with suitable suction instruments under endoscopic guidance, avoiding injury to the regenerating mucosa.

Pharmacological Therapy

Antibiotics (cephalosporins) are administered intraoperatively and for an additional five days after surgery. The intraoperative administration of 250 mg prednisone plus 150 mg on the first and second postoperative days will help to reduce postoperative soft-tissue edema and accompanying ecchymosis.

After intranasal crusts have been selectively removed and secretions aspirated, the epithelial regeneration process can be positively influenced by the application of low-viscosity ointments containing panthenol. Drops of physiological saline solution or, preferably, an isotonic saline spray will reduce the drying of secretions. Adhesions between mucosal surfaces are cleared. Mucolytic agents (e.g., standardized myrtol preparations, Gelomyrtol forte) promote the reactivation of mucociliary clearance.

Late Postoperative Period

The postoperative result after the removal of all dressings is not the final result. When major corrections have been made in the bony and cartilaginous framework of the nose, it is difficult to evaluate the definitive result. Unsatisfactory results and complications relating to faulty surgical techniques may not become apparent until the late postoperative period. Scheduling long-term follow-ups with regular photographic documentation is helpful in monitoring the changes. By critically evaluating the results of the operation, the surgeon can gain experience that is useful in refining his/her operating technique. Endoscopic follow-up is particularly important in the late postoperative period following procedures on the turbinates and paranasal sinuses. Reactive mucosal hyperplasia (Fig. 14.**18**) will regress gradually over a period of several weeks or months.

After the initial six-week follow-up period, additional follow-ups should be scheduled every three months until the end of the first postoperative year. After that, the patient should be present for follow-ups once a year. It is important that the patient be informed about possible late complications.

Late Complications

Late complications result from scar formation due to faulty operating technique, overresection, or from early complications such as infection and hematomas.

The following are typical late complications that may involve the external nose:

Irregularities and deviations of the nasal dorsum. These usually result from excessive surgical trauma with fragmentation of the bony pyramid and subsequent scar traction. Persistent deviations of the pyramid and nasal dorsum can result from inadequate mobilization of the bony structures, insufficient correction of the deviated septum, or existing asymmetries of the upper lateral cartilages. Patients may exhibit bony ridges or persistent bony and cartilaginous humps, especially when the skin is thin (Fig. 14.**19**). Subcutaneous bone grafts may be clearly visible beneath the skin if they were not precisely matched to the recipient defect.

A *paranasal callus* may form as the result of a paranasal hematoma or a bony gap left between fracture fragments. The great majority of these calluses will resolve without treatment.

Pollybeak deformity is a frequent problem after rhinoplasties. A soft-tissue pollybeak is usually based on a lesion of the muscle and connective-tissue layers in the nasal dorsum, with corresponding scar formation. A cartilaginous pollybeak is the result of an inadequate resection of the superior septal margin and a significant loss of tip support. Both deformities are treated by touch-up surgery (Fig. 14.**20**).

Heavy scarring, discontinuities, and asymmetrical resections or sutures in the alar cartilages lead to *nasal tip deformities.* For this reason, the indications for all resections and techniques involving the division of cartilage should be weighed very carefully.

If the mechanisms of nasal tip stability are disregarded and too much tissue is resected, there is a danger of progressive

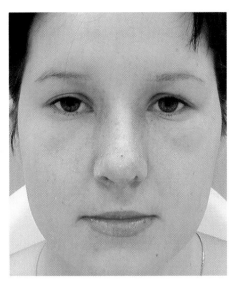

Fig. 14.**16**   The external nasal dressing in this patient has been removed at two weeks postoperatively. The skin is swollen and shows a stippled pattern of inflammation. Hematomas and swelling are still evident about the nose and the upper and lower eyelids.

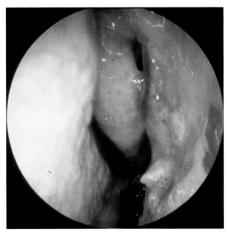

Fig. 14.**17**   Endoscopy approximately 10 days after endonasal sinus surgery shows a distinct fibrin layer on the mucosa of the lateral nasal wall, which creates a nidus for synechiae formation. The fibrin layer should be removed under endoscopic control.

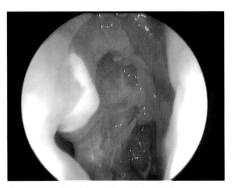

Fig. 14.**18**   View into the ethmoid about two weeks after the operation shows edematous swelling of the parietal mucosa. The supraturbinate maxillary sinus window is visible on the left side of the image, and some fibrin deposit is visible at the top.

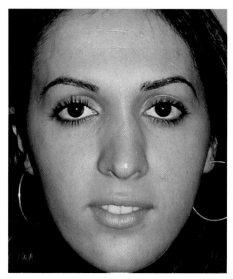

Fig. 14.**19**   Bony deviation of the nose and paranasal callus formation on the left side at 12 months postoperatively. The asymmetry results from an osteotomy that was placed too high. Subsequent scar traction has caused the nasal dorsum to deviate toward the left side.

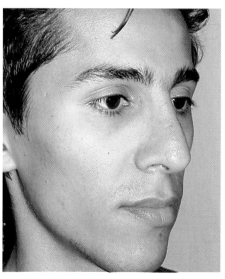

Fig. 14.**20**   Pollybeak deformity caused by inadequate reduction of the superior septal margin. A soft-tissue pollybeak is also present.

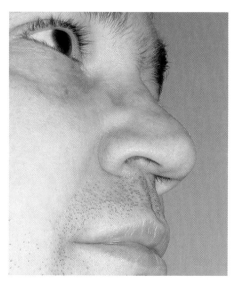

Fig. 14.**21**   Typical appearance of a "hidden columella" prior to operation.

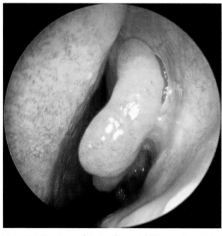

Fig. 14.**22**   Synechia in the middle meatus following ethmoid surgery. The adhesion between the lateral aspect of the middle turbinate and the lateral nasal wall results from organized fibrin deposits as well as inadequate treatment of the middle turbinate.

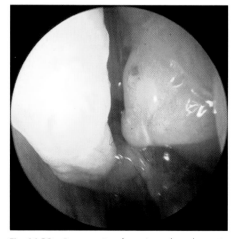

Fig. 14.**23**   Recurrent polyposis and exuberant granulations in the ethmoid two months after surgery.

drooping of the nasal tip. It is normal for nasal tip drooping to occur with aging, however.

The problem of the "hidden columella" represents a severe *columellar retraction*, which can result from excessive resection of the caudal septal margin. Overresection of the caudal and dorsal cartilaginous septal margin and inadequate fixation of the cartilage also lead to dorsal rotation and retraction of the columella (Fig. 14.**21**).

The following are typical endonasal complications:

Scar adhesions between the middle turbinate and lateral nasal wall. These result from the inadequate widening of narrow sites, with opposing wound surfaces. The fibrin bridges that initially form between these wound surfaces become organized through the ingrowth of fibrocytes, which form compact scars. These

scars, in turn, create an obstacle to ventilation and drainage, predisposing to a recurrence of inflammatory sinus pathology. Endoscopic examination shows a corresponding retention of secretions or inflammatory mucosal changes (Fig. 14.**22**).

Scar obliteration of the enlarged sinus ostia. The frontal sinus ostia in particular show a tendency toward restenosis following surgical enlargement. Recurrent frontal headaches are a classic symptom. Persistent mucous secretions in the nose and postnasal drainage are a sign of deficient drainage through the maxillary and sphenoid sinus ostia.

Exuberant *granulations* and *edematous tissue proliferation* ranging to *recurrent polyposis*. These usually result from persistent mucosal infections or may be a manifestation of an eosinophil-dominant mucosal disease (Figs. 14.**23**, 14.**24**).

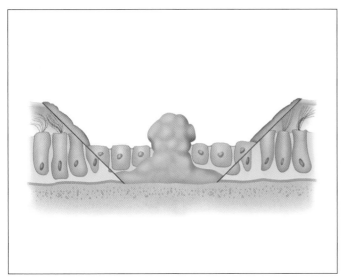

Fig. 14.**24** As a result of small epithelial defects, exuberant granulations can form at sites where wound healing is impaired or where larger exposed bone areas must be overgrown. With a normal progression of wound healing, the epithelial defect will close from the wound margins to form a flat, largely undifferentiated epithelium.

Treatment Strategy During the Late Post-operative Period

Follow-ups should be scheduled at appropriate intervals in the late postoperative period to assess the endonasal status and confirm the regression of postoperative swelling.

The most obvious regression of swelling is noted during the first four weeks after removal of the external dressing. The amount of swelling is variable, depending on the operating technique that was used and the degree of postoperative reactions or complications that have occurred. Aggressive hump removal and multiple osteotomies in the pyramid will cause greater swelling about the nasal bones. An open approach or alar cartilage-splitting approach leads to greater swelling in the nasal tip area. Postoperative swelling will generally subside over a period of 6–12 months, first in the pyramid region, then over the cartilaginous dorsum, and finally in the tip area. A good rule of thumb is that it takes approximately three months for swelling about the nasal pyramid to subside completely. It takes about another three months for swelling to clear over the upper lateral cartilages and 9–12 months over the alar cartilages, depending on the operative technique. These time frames should be kept strictly in mind if follow-ups show that the outcome of the correction is not proceeding as expected and complications are developing. Bony deformities of the pyramid appear relatively early, and so they can be corrected at a relatively early stage. Small asymmetries due to the depression of osteotomized sites or even irregularities in the nasal dorsum can be corrected under local anesthesia.

Asymmetries or pollybeak deformities of the nasal dorsum are often masked by soft-tissue swelling. Generally they are noted only during later follow-ups. Their extent cannot be accurately assessed until all swelling has cleared, however, and a soft-tissue pollybeak will frequently resolve. For this reason, the decision to reoperate should not be made until at least one year after the surgery. On the other hand, cartilaginous pollybeak deformities or asymmetries are clearly detectable by palpation after approximately four to six months, and so these cases can be revised at an earlier time. When patients subjectively appraise the outcome of their surgery, they give particular attention to the nasal tip. The surgeon should keep the timetable for nasal tip healing firmly in mind and should not be pressed into making a premature correction. Overprojection of the tip is usually still present in the early postoperative period, and the tip-defining points cannot yet be recognized because of tip swelling. The supratip break is also obscured because its contours have not yet been defined by postoperative scarring at the upper margin of the alar cartilages. Increasing asymmetries and retraction of the columella may be a sign of developing complications. However, the dynamics of wound healing in the tip area require that any revision surgery on the tip be deferred for at least one year.

Local pharmacological treatment is beneficial in the late postoperative period and is even necessary in many cases. Irrigation of the nose with isotonic saline solution produces a mechanical cleansing effect. The ion concentrations present in various saline solutions also appear to have a supportive effect in boosting ciliary activity, thereby improving mucociliary clearance.

Spraying the nasal mucosa regularly with topical corticosteroids (e.g., Mometason, Fluticason) has a favorable effect on the regression of reactive mucosal swelling. The use of sprays is particularly beneficial for inflammatory mucosal diseases with a high eosinophil content. Third-generation oral antihistamines (e.g., Desloratadin) should be used in patients with an allergic mucosal disease.

References

1. Behrbohm H, Kaschke O, Nachbehandlung nach endoskopischen Nasennebenhöhlen-Operationen. In Behrbohm H, Kaschke O, Nawka T, eds. *Endoskopische Diagnostik und Therapie in der HNO*. Stuttgart: Fischer: 1997:96–102.
2. Daniel RK, Primary rhinoplasty. In Daniel RK, ed. *Rhinoplasty—an atlas of surgical technique*. New York: Springer-Verlag: 1999:279–350.
3. Dorn M, Pirsig W, Verse T, Postoperatives Management nach rhinochirurgischen Eingriffen bei schwerer obstruktiver Schlafapnoe. Eine Pilotstudie. *HNO*. 2001; 49:642–5.
4. Hosemann W, Wigand ME, Gode U, et al., Normal wound healing of the paranasal sinuses: clinical and experimental investigations. *Eur Arch Otorhinolaryngol*. 1991; 248:390–4.
5. Kaschke O, Behrbohm H, *Endoskopische Chirurgie der Nasennebenhöhlen—Die Nachbehandlung*. Arztanleitungen Karl Storz GmbH & Co. Braun Druck 1995.
6. Kuhn FA, Citardi MJ, Advances in postoperative care following functional endoscopic sinus surgery. *Otolaryngol Clin North Am*. 1997; 30:479–90.
7. Leonard DW, Thompson DH, Unusual septoplasty complication: Streptococcus viridans endocarditis. *Ear Nose Throat J*. 1998; 77; 827:830–1.
8. Mang WL, Rhinoplasty. In Mang WL, ed. *Manual of Aesthetic Surgery, Vol. 1*, Berlin: Springer: 2002:3–47.
9. Nolst Trenité GJ, Postoperative care and complications. In Nolst Trenité GJ, ed. *Rhinoplasty—a practical guide to functional and aesthetic surgery of the nose*. The Hague: Kugler Publications: 1998:31–37.
10. Numanoglu A, External cantilever sling in septorhinoplasty: a new technique. *Plast Reconstr Surg*. 1997; 100:250–6
11. Rettinger G, Steininger H, Lipogranulomas as complications of septorhinoplasty. *Arch Otolaryngol Head Neck Surg*. 1997;123:809–14.
12. Stankiewicz JA, Comments about postoperative care after endoscopic sinus surgery. *Arch Otolaryngol Head Neck Surg*. 2002; 128:1207–8
13. Tebbetts JB, Splinting, Dressing and Postoperative Care. In Tebbetts JB, *Primary rhinoplasty: a new approach to the logic and the techniques*. St. Louis: Mosby: 1998:511–526.
14. Thaler ER, Postoperative care after endoscopic sinus surgery. *Arch Otolaryngol Head Neck Surg*. 2002; 128:1204–6.
15. von Szalay L, Bessere Ergebnisse durch frühe Sekundärkorrektur in der Septo-Rhino-Plastik. *HNO*. 1998; 46:611–3.
16. Yavuzer R, Jackson IT, Nasal packing in rhinoplasty and septorhinoplasty: it is wiser to avoid. *Plast Reconstr Surg*. Mar. 1999; 103:1081–2.

of co-ordination
is both valuable and
important to a child's later
development, and this is found,
for instance, in *Finger Rhymes*,
the first book of the six book series.

This series provides an enjoyable introduction to poetry, music and dance for
every young child. Most books of this
type have only a few rhymes for each
age group, whereas each book of this
series is intended for a particular age
group. There is a strong teaching sequence
in the selection of rhymes, from the
first simple ways of winning the child's
interest by toe tapping and palm
tickling jingles, through practice in
numbers, memory and pronunciation,
to combining sound, action and
words. For the first time young
children can learn rhymes
in a sequence that is
related to their age.

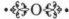

Contents

LEARNING WITH TRADITIONAL RHYMES

Memory Rhymes

by DOROTHY and JOHN TAYLOR

with illustrations by
MARTIN AITCHISON, FRANK HUMPHRIS,
KATHY LAYFIELD & BRIAN PRICE THOMAS
and photographs by JOHN MOYES

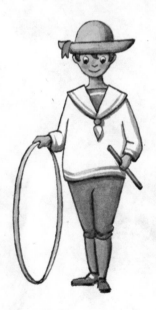

Ladybird Books Ltd Loughborough 1976

Mr East gave a feast

Mr East gave a feast;
Mr North laid the cloth;
Mr West did his best;
Mr South burnt his mouth
With eating a cold potato.

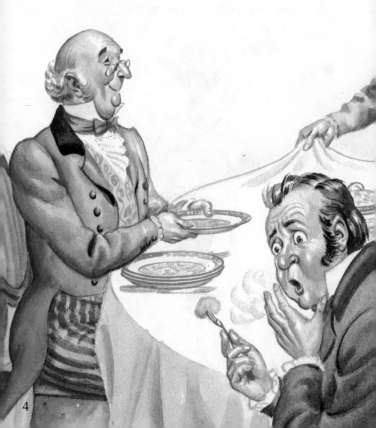

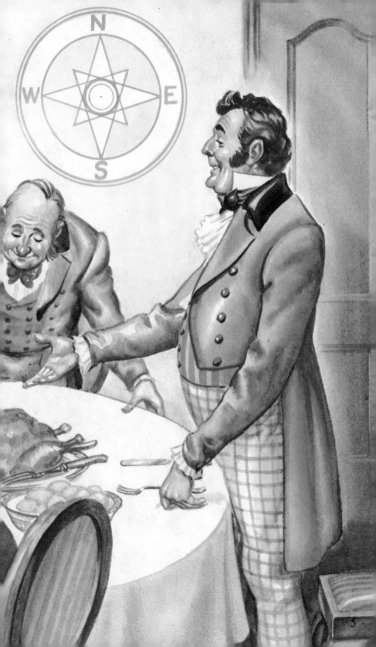

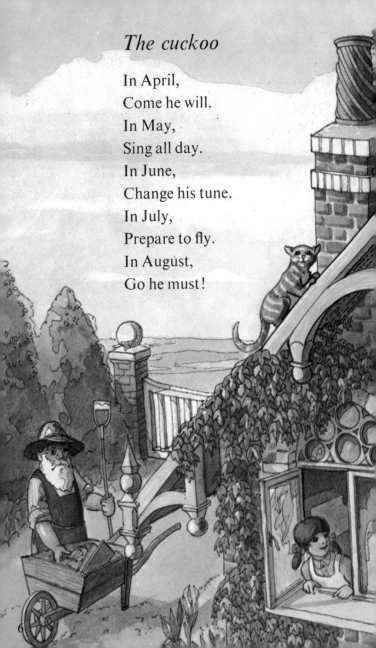

The cuckoo

In April,
Come he will.
In May,
Sing all day.
In June,
Change his tune.
In July,
Prepare to fly.
In August,
Go he must!

6

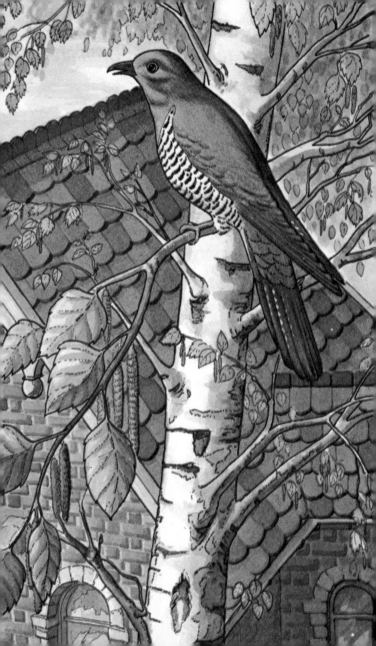

They that wash on Monday

They that wash on Monday
Have all the week to dry;
They that wash on Tuesday
Are not so much awry;
They that wash on Wednesday
Are not so much to blame;
They that wash on Thursday
Wash for very shame;
They that wash on Friday
Wash in sorry need;
They that wash on Saturday
Are lazy folk indeed.

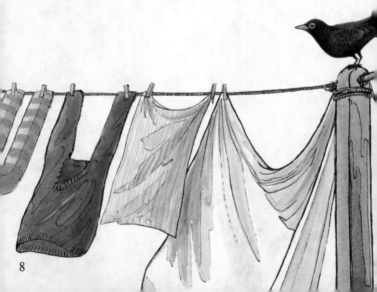

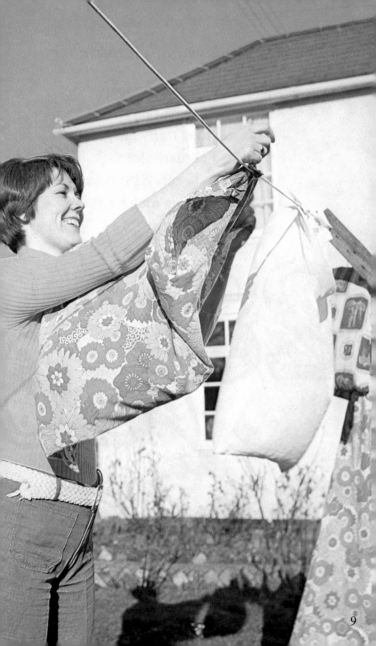

9

Thirty days hath September

Thirty days hath September,
April, June and November;
All the rest have thirty one,
Excepting February alone,
And that has twenty eight days clear
And twenty nine in each leap year.

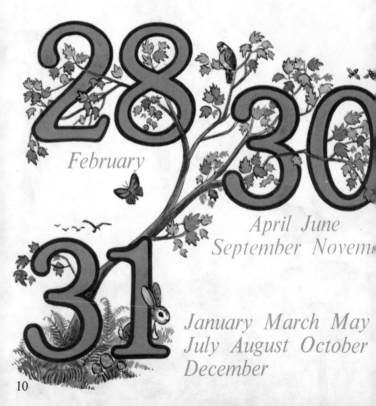

February

28 30

April June
September Novem

31

January March May
July August October
December

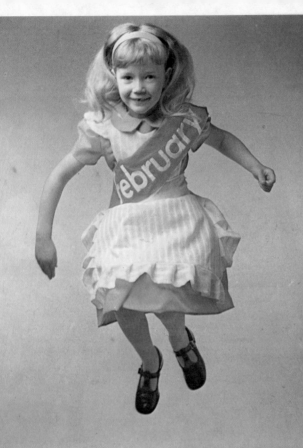

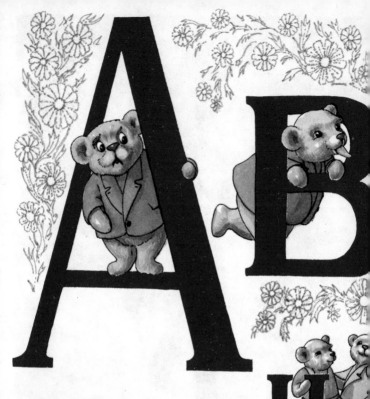

*Great A was alarmed
at B's bad behaviour*

Great A was alarmed at B's bad behaviour,
Because C, D, E, F, denied G a favour,
H had a husband with I, J, K, and L,
M married Mary and taught her scholars how to sp
A, B, C, D, E, F, G, H, I, J, K, L, M, N,
O, P, Q, R, S, T, U, V, W, X, Y, Z.

12

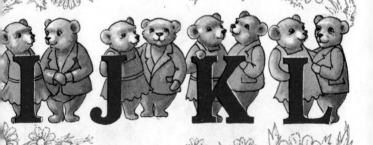

C D E F G

I J K L

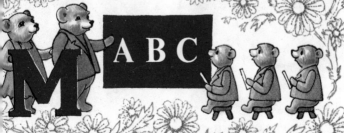

M ABC

13

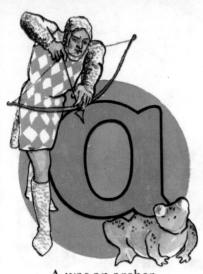
A was an archer,
who shot at a frog;

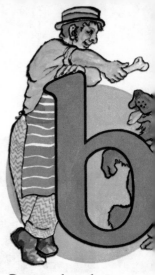
B was a butcher,
and had a great dog.

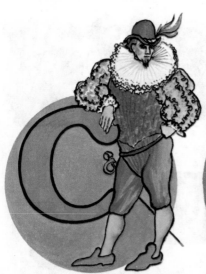
C was a captain,
all covered with lace;

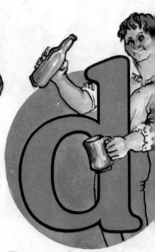
D was a drunkard,
and had a red face.

14

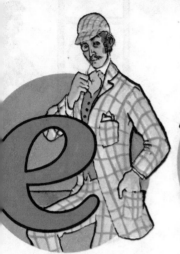

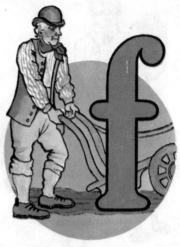

E was an esquire,
with pride on his brow;

F was a farmer
and followed the plough.

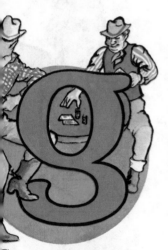

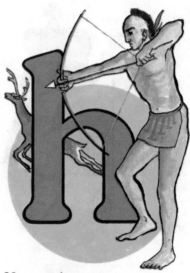

G was a gamester,
who had but ill-luck;

H was a hunter,
and hunted a buck.

15

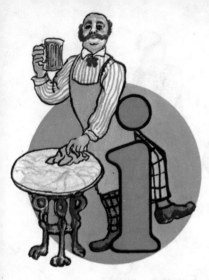

I was an innkeeper,
who loved to carouse;

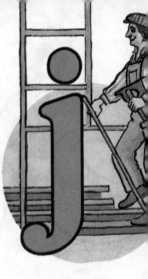

J was a joiner,
and built up a house.

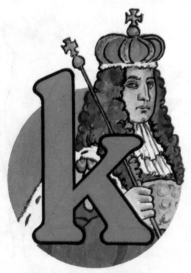

K was King William,
once governed this land;

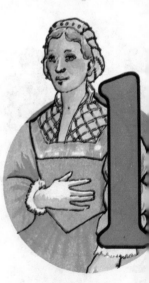

L was a lady,
who had a white hand.

16

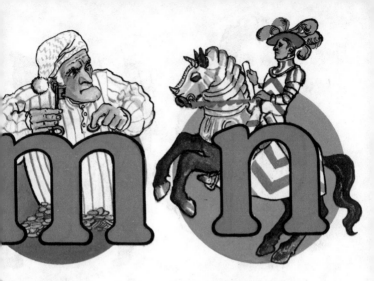

M was a miser,
and hoarded up gold;

N was a nobleman,
gallant and bold.

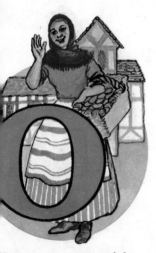

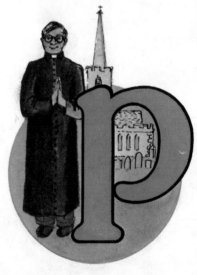

O was an oyster girl,
and went about town;

P was a parson,
and wore a black gown. 17

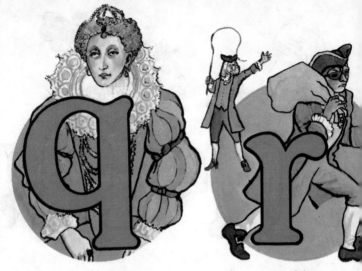

Q was a queen,
who wore a silk slip;

R was a robber,
and wanted a whip.

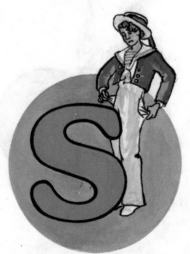

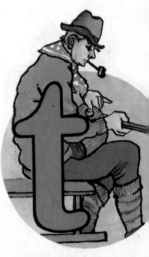

S was a sailor,
and spent all he got;

T was a tinker,
and mended a pot.

18

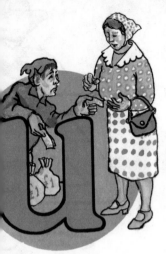

U was a usurer,
miserable elf;

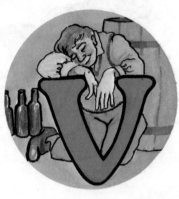

V was a vintner,
who drank all himself.

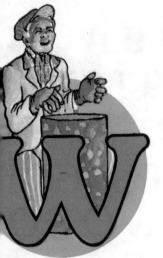

W was a watchman,
and guarded the door;

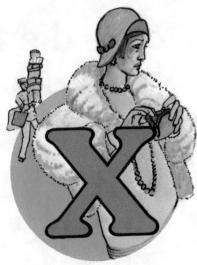

X was expensive,
and so became poor.

19

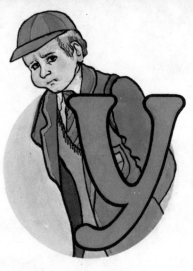

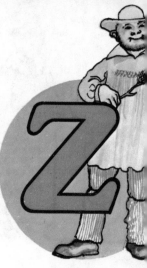

Y was a youth,
that did not love school;

Z was a zany,
a poor harmless fool.

a b c d e f g h i j k
l m n o p q r s t u v
w x y z

A B C D E F G H
I J K L M N O P Q
R S T U V W X Y Z

Sneeze on Monday, sneeze for danger

Sneeze on Monday, sneeze for danger;
Sneeze on Tuesday, kiss a stranger;
Sneeze on Wednesday, get a letter;
Sneeze on Thursday, something better;
Sneeze on Friday, sneeze for sorrow;
Sneeze on Saturday, see your sweetheart tomorrow.

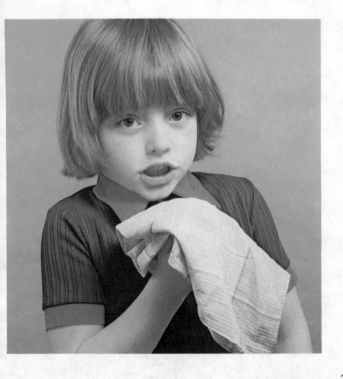

A was an apple pie

A was an Apple pie, B Bit it, C Cut it,
D Dealt it, E Eat it, F Fought for it,
G Got it, H Had it, I Inspected it,
J Joined for it, K Kept it, L Longed for it,
M Mourned for it, N Nodded at it,
O Opened it, P Peeped in it,
Q Quartered it, R Ran for it, S Stole it,
T Took it, U Upset it, V Viewed it,
W Wanted it,
XYZ All wished for a piece in hand.

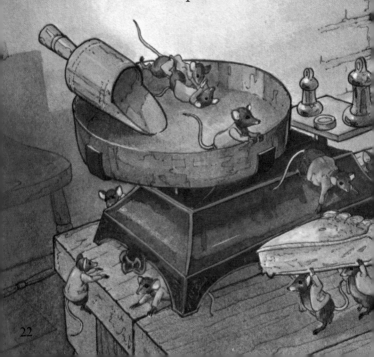

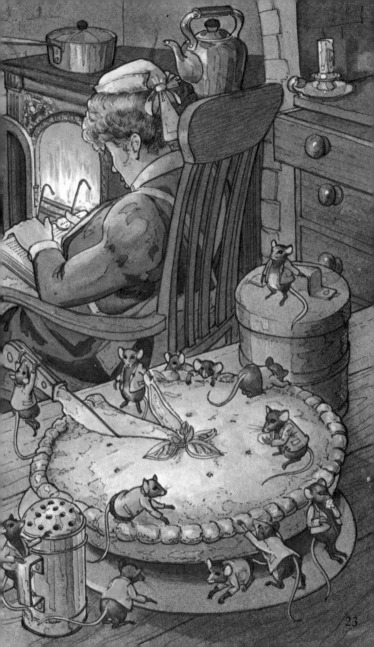

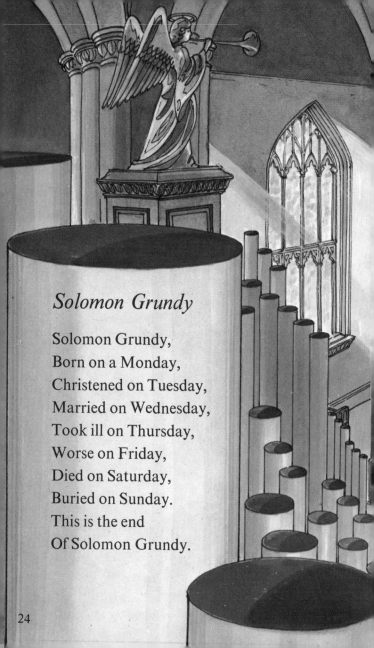

Solomon Grundy

Solomon Grundy,
Born on a Monday,
Christened on Tuesday,
Married on Wednesday,
Took ill on Thursday,
Worse on Friday,
Died on Saturday,
Buried on Sunday.
This is the end
Of Solomon Grundy.

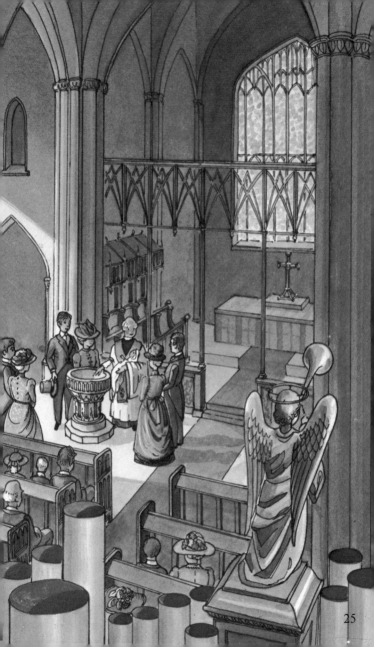

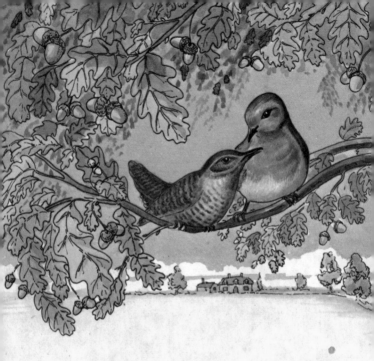

A, B, C, D, E, F, G,
Little Robin Redbreast sitting on a tree;
H, I, J, K, L, M, N,
He made love to little Jenny Wren;
O, P, Q, R, S, T, U,
Dear little Jenny, I want to marry you.
V, W, X, Y, Z,
Poor little Jenny she blushed quite red.

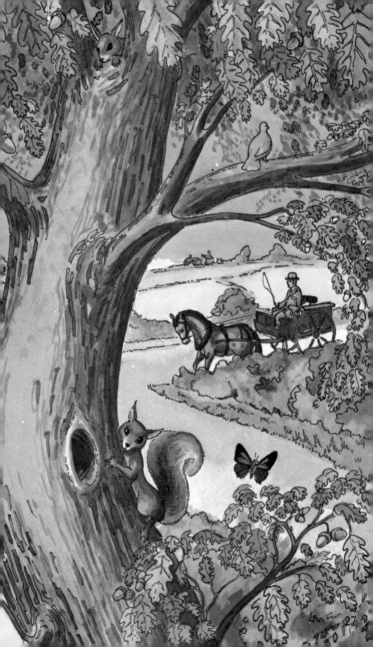

When the wind is in the East

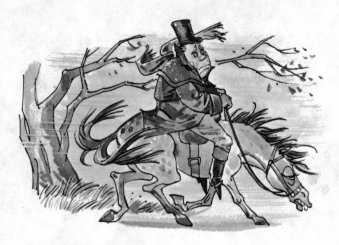

When the wind is in the East
'Tis neither good for man nor beast.

When the wind is in the North
The skilful fisher goes not forth.

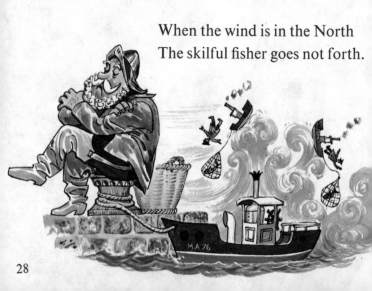

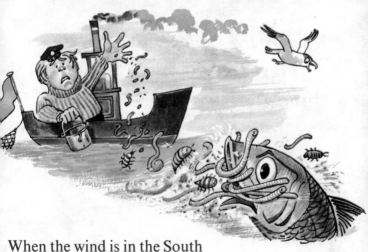

When the wind is in the South
It blows the bait in the fish's mouth.

When the wind is in the West,
Then it is at its very best.

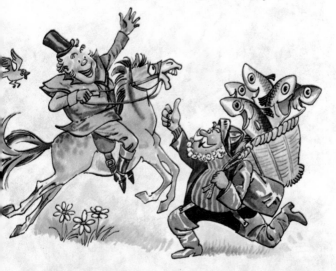

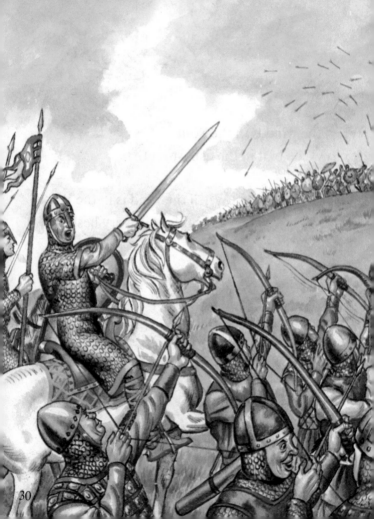

William the Conqueror, ten sixty six

WILLIAM the Conqueror, ten sixty six,
Played on the Saxons oft-cruel tricks.

COLUMBUS sailed the ocean blue,
In fourteen hundred and ninety two.

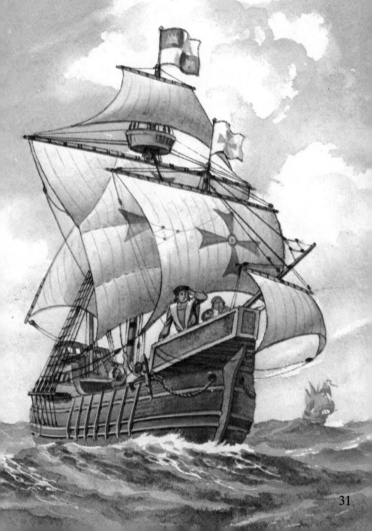

The **SPANISH ARMADA** met its fate,
In fifteen hundred and eighty eight.

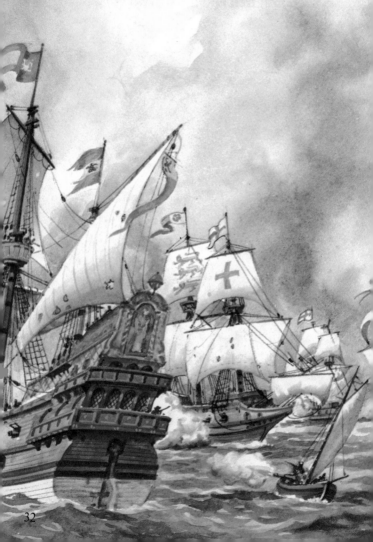

In sixteen hundred and sixty six,
London burnt like rotten sticks.

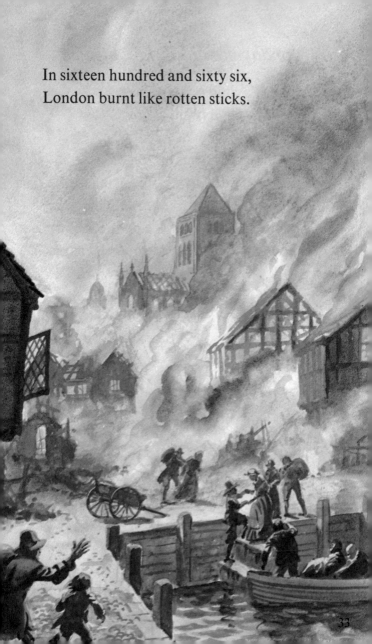

Monday's child is fair of face

Monday's child is fair of face,
Tuesday's child is full of grace,
Wednesday's child is full of woe,
Thursday's child has far to go,
Friday's child is loving and giving,
Saturday's child works hard for a living,
And the child that is born on the Sabbath day
Is bonny and blithe, and good and gay.

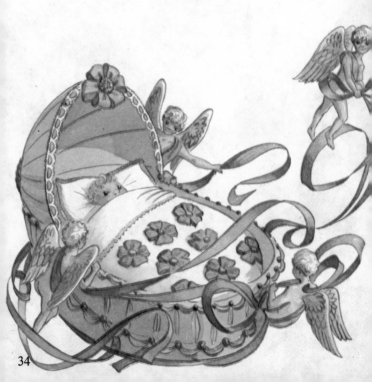

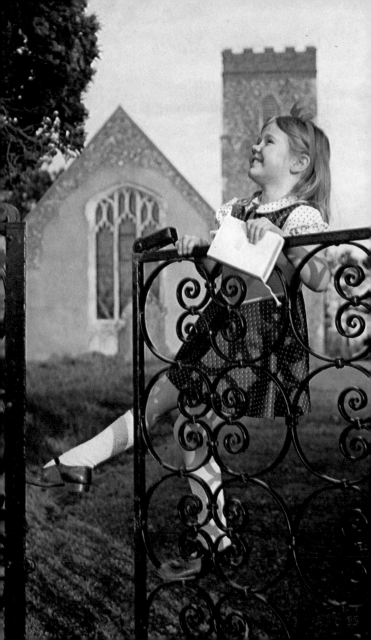

On the first of March

On the first of March
The crows begin to search;
By the first of April
They are sitting still;
By the first of May
They've all flown away,
Coming greedy back again
With October's wind and rain.

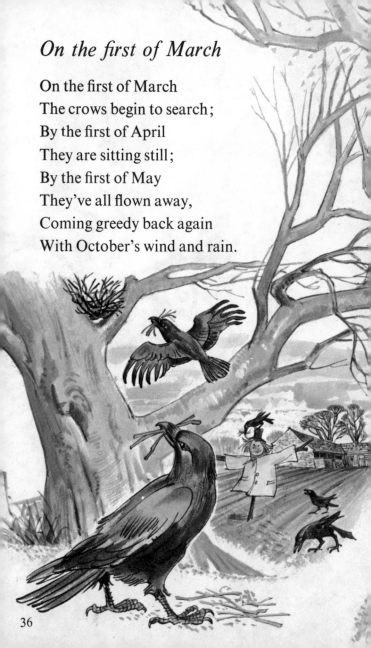

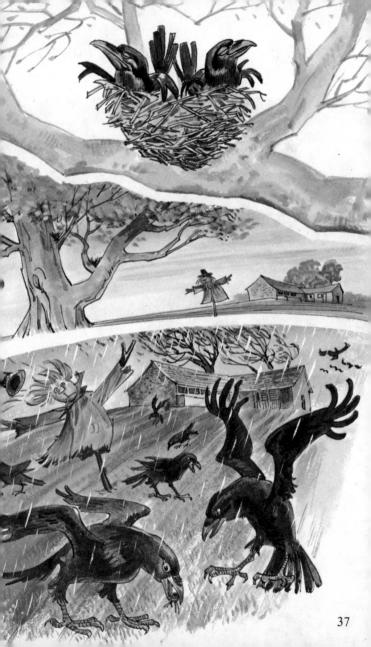

37

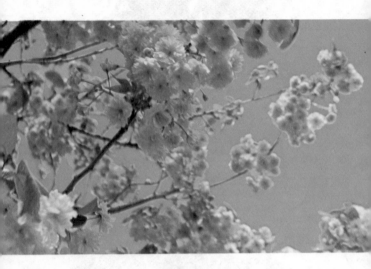

Spring is showery, flowery, bowery;
Summer: hoppy, croppy, poppy;

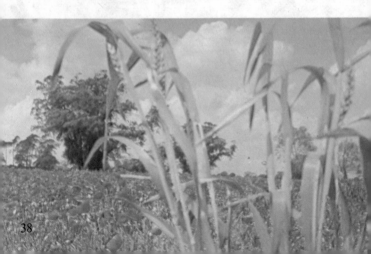

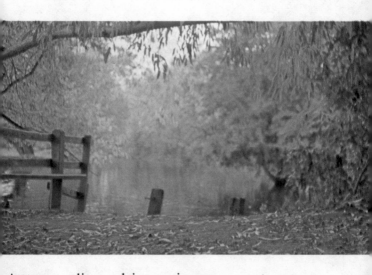

Autumn: slippy, drippy, nippy;
Winter: breezy, sneezy, freezy.

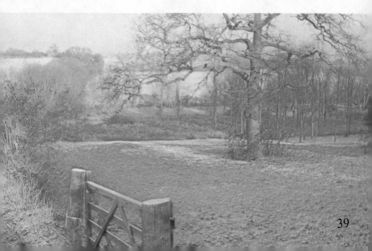

Cut them on Monday,
you cut them for health

Cut them on Monday, you cut them for health;
Cut them on Tuesday, you cut them for wealth;
Cut them on Wednesday, you cut them for news;
Cut them on Thursday, a new pair of shoes;
Cut them on Friday, you cut them for sorrow;
Cut them on Saturday, see your true love tomorrow;
Cut them on Sunday, you cut them for evil,
For all the next week you'll be ruled by the devil.

(To be said whilst cutting toe nails.)

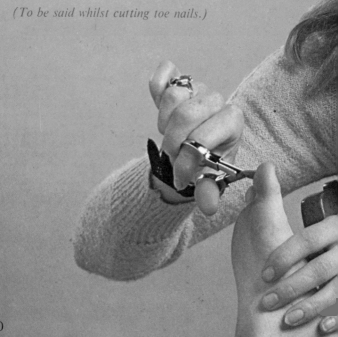

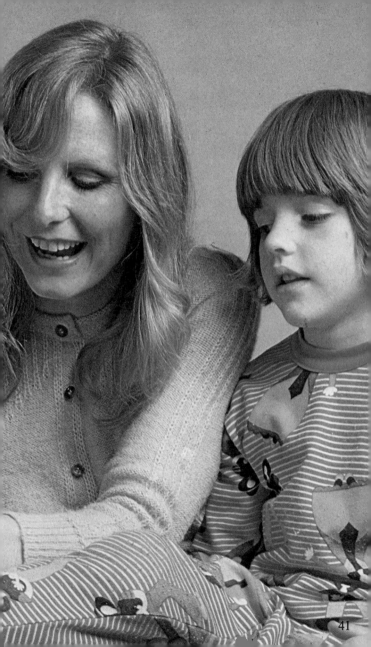

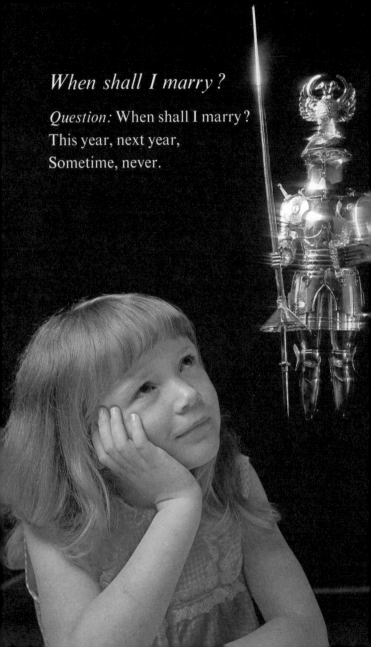

When shall I marry?

Question: When shall I marry?
This year, next year,
Sometime, never.

Question: What is the first letter
of my husband's name?
A, B, C, D, etc.

Question: What is he?
Tinker, tailor, soldier, sailor, rich man, poor man,
 beggar man, thief.

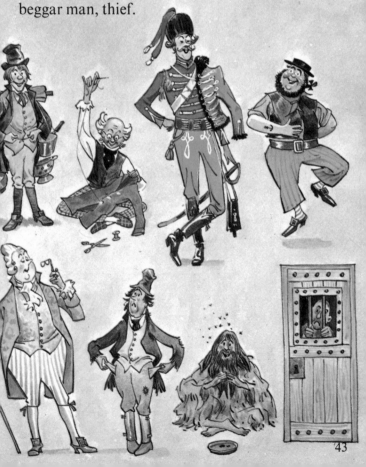

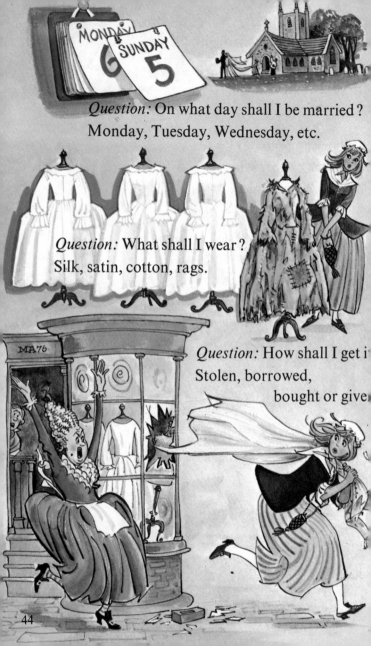

Question: On what day shall I be married?
Monday, Tuesday, Wednesday, etc.

Question: What shall I wear?
Silk, satin, cotton, rags.

Question: How shall I get i
Stolen, borrowed,
        bought or give

44

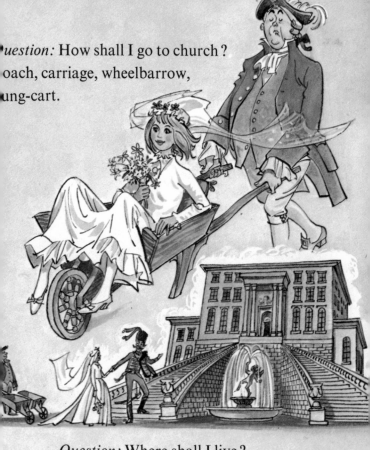

Question: How shall I go to church?
oach, carriage, wheelbarrow,
ung-cart.

Question: Where shall I live?
Big house, little house, pigsty, barn.

Question: How many children
shall I have?
One, two, three, four, etc.

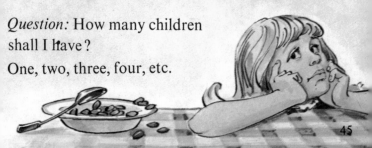

Monday alone

Monday alone,
Tuesday together,
Wednesday we walk
When it's fine weather,
Thursday we kiss,
Friday we cry,

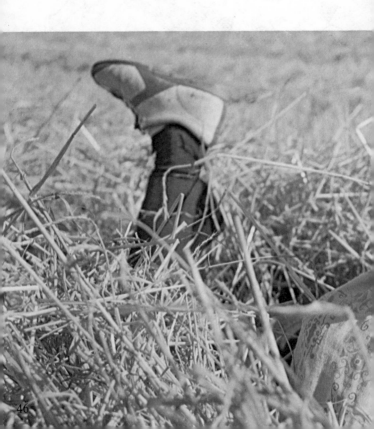

Saturday's hours
Seem almost to fly.
But of all the days in the week
We will call
Sunday the rest day,
The best day of all.

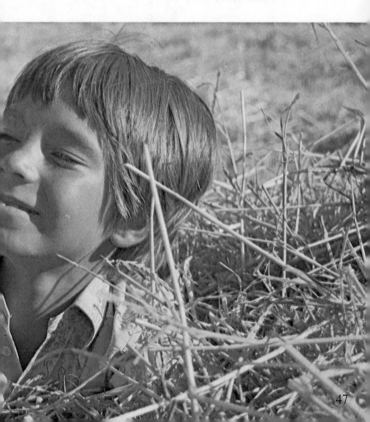

Cut thistles in May

Cut thistles in May,
They grow in a day;
Cut them in June,
That is too soon;
Cut them in July,
Then they will die.

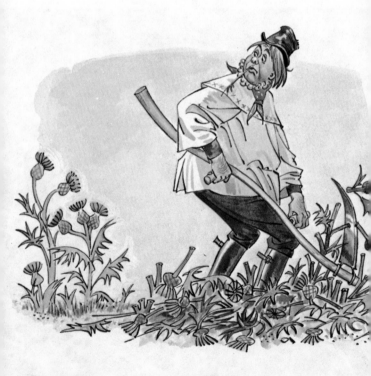

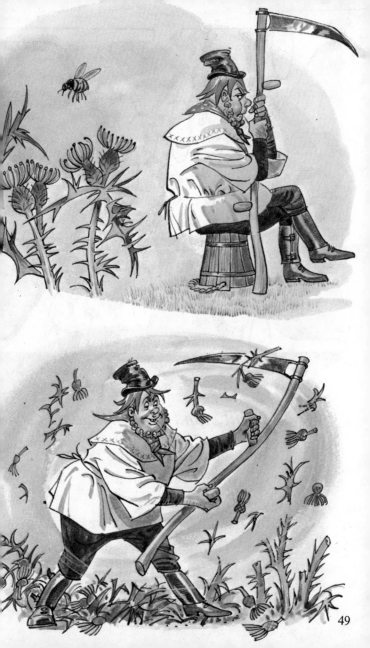

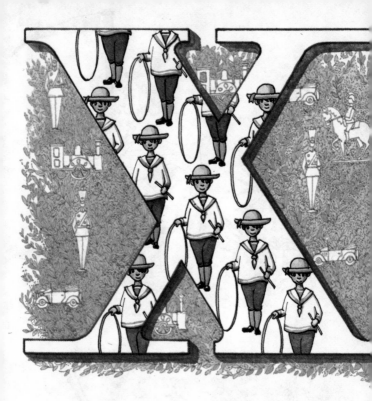

X shall stand for playmates Ten

X shall stand for playmates *Ten*;
V for *Five* stout stalwart men;
I for *One*, as I'm alive;
C for *Hundred*, and D for *Five**;
M for a *Thousand* soldiers true,
And L for *Fifty*, I'll tell you.

*D stands for five *hundred*

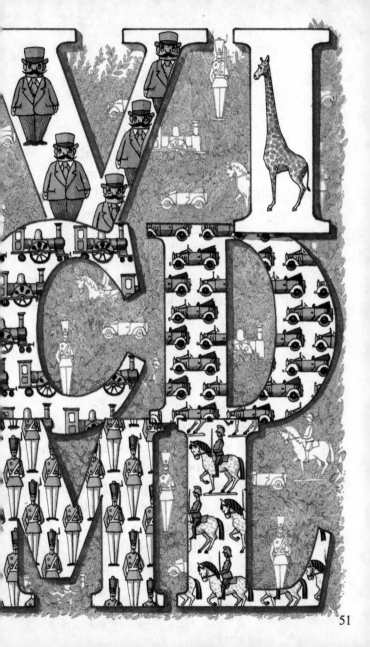

51

·❊O❊·

BOOK ONE
❧ *Finger Rhymes* ❧

A selection of finger
counting, face patting, palm
tickling and toe tapping rhymes to
delight the young child and at the
same time exercise his mind and body.

BOOK TWO
❧ *Number Rhymes* ❧

This book brings together many familiar
and some less well known rhymes which
help with the first steps of arithmetic:
adding, subtracting, multiplying and dividing in their simplest forms.

BOOK THREE
❧ *Memory Rhymes* ❧

A diverse collection of rhymes mainly
concerned with days of the week, months
of the year, points of the compass
and letters of the alphabet. With
these a child learns simple
progressions in an amus-
ing and absorbing
manner.